Advanced Imaging of the Foot and Ankle

Editor

JAN FRITZ

FOOT AND ANKLE CLINICS

www.foot.theclinics.com

Consulting Editor
CESAR DE CESAR NETTO

September 2023 • Volume 28 • Number 3

ELSEVIER

1600 John F. Kennedy Boulevard • Suite 1800 • Philadelphia, Pennsylvania, 19103-2899

http://www.theclinics.com

FOOT AND ANKLE CLINICS Volume 28, Number 3
September 2023 ISSN 1083-7515, ISBN-978-0-443-18187-0

Editor: Megan Ashdown
Developmental Editor: Anita Chamoli

Foot and Ankle Clinics (ISSN 1083-7515) is published quarterly by Elsevier, Inc., 360 Park Avenue South, New York, NY 10010-1710. Months of issue are March, June, September, and December. Periodicals postage paid at New York, NY, and additional mailing offices. Subscription price per year is $362.00 (US individuals), $635.00 (US institutions), $100.00 (US students), $389.00 (Canadian individuals), $762.00 (Canadian institutions), $100.00 (Canadian students), $504.00 (international individuals), $762.00 (international institutions), and $215.00 (international students). To receive student/resident rate, orders must be accompanied by name of affiliated institution, date of term, and the *signature* of program/residency coordinator on institution letterhead. Orders will be billed at individual rate until proof of status is received. Foreign air speed delivery is included in all *Clinics* subscription prices. All prices are subject to change without notice. **POSTMASTER:** Send address changes to *Foot and Ankle Clinics*, Elsevier Health Sciences Division, Subscription Customer Service, 3251 Riverport Lane, Maryland Heights, MO 63043. **Customer Service: 1-800-654-2452 (US and Canada). From outside of the United States and Canada, call 314-447-8871. Fax: 314-447-8029. E-mail: JournalsCustomerService-usa@ elsevier.com (for print support); JournalsOnlineSupport-usa@elsevier.com (for online support).**

Reprints. For copies of 100 or more, of articles in this publication, please contact the Commercial Reprints Department, Elsevier Inc., 360 Park Avenue South, New York, NY 10010-1710. Tel.: 212-633-3874; Fax: 212-633-3820; E-mail: reprints@elsevier.com.

Contributors

CONSULTING EDITOR

CESAR DE CESAR NETTO, MD, PhD
Assistant Professor, Director of the Orthopedic Functional Imaging Research Laboratory (OFIRL), Department of Orthopedics and Rehabilitation, University of Iowa, Carver College of Medicine, Iowa City, Iowa, USA; Division of Orthopedic Foot and Ankle Surgery, Department of Orthopedic Surgery, Duke University, Duke University Medical Center, Durham, North Carolina, USA

EDITOR

JAN FRITZ, MD, PD, RMSK
Associate Professor of Radiology, Chief, Division of Musculoskeletal Radiology, Department of Radiology, NYU Grossman School of Medicine, New York, New York, USA

AUTHORS

SHIVANI AHLAWAT, MD
Associate Professor of Radiology, The Russell H. Morgan Department of Radiology and Radiological Science, The Johns Hopkins Medical Institutions, Baltimore, Maryland, USA

SOHEIL ASHKANI-ESFAHANI, MD
Assistant Professor, Department of Orthopaedic Surgery, Foot and Ankle Research and Innovation Lab (FARIL), Massachusetts General Hospital, Harvard Medical School, Waltham, Massachusetts, USA

NACIME SALOMÃO BARBACHAN MANSUR, MD, PhD
Professor, Department of Orthopedics and Rehabilitation, University of Iowa, Carver College of Medicine, Iowa City, Iowa, USA

BRENNAN BOETTCHER, DO
Senior Associate Consultant, Instructor in Physical Medicine and Rehabilitation, Division of Sports Medicine, Department of Orthopedic Surgery, Rochester, Minnesota, USA

MARCELO BORDALO, MD, PhD
Chief of Radiology, Radiology Department, Aspetar Orthopedic and Sports Medicine Hospital, Doha, Qatar

JAMES J. BUTLER, MB BCh
Orthopaedic Surgery Research Fellow, Foot and Ankle Division, Department of Orthopaedic Surgery, NYU Langone Health, New York, New York, USA

BRUNO CERRETTI CARNEIRO, MD
Department of Musculoskeletal Radiology, Fleury Medicina e Saúde; Department of Diagnostic Imaging, United Health Group Brazil, São Paulo, São Paulo, Brazil

JOHN A. CARRINO, MD, MPH
Attending Radiologist, Department of Radiology, Hospital for Special Surgery, New York, New York, USA

AVNEESH CHHABRA, MD, MBA, FACR
Chief of Musculoskeletal Radiology, Professor of Radiology and Orthopedic Surgery, UT Southwestern Medical Center, Dallas, Texas, USA; Adjunct Faculty, Johns Hopkins University, Baltimore, Maryland, USA; University of Dallas, Richardson, Texas, USA; Walton Centre for Neurosciences, Liverpool, United Kingdom

KEPLER ALENCAR MENDES DE CARVALHO, MD
Department of Orthopedics and Rehabilitation, University of Iowa, Carver College of Medicine, Iowa City, Iowa, USA

CESAR DE CESAR NETTO, MD, PhD
Assistant Professor, Director of the Orthopedic Functional Imaging Research Laboratory (OFIRL), Department of Orthopedics and Rehabilitation, University of Iowa, Carver College of Medicine, Iowa City, Iowa, USA; Division of Orthopedic Foot and Ankle Surgery, Department of Orthopedic Surgery, Duke University, Duke University Medical Center, Durham, North Carolina, USA

MARCOS FELIPPE ED PAULA CORREA, MD
Radiology Department, Hospital Sirio Libanes, São Paulo, Brazil

PATRICK DEBS, MD
The Russell H. Morgan Department of Radiology and Radiological Science, The Johns Hopkins Medical Institutions, Baltimore, Maryland, USA

SCOTT ELLIS, MD
Attending Surgeon, Foot and Ankle Service, Hospital for Special Surgery, New York, New York, USA

LAURA M. FAYAD, MS, MD
The Russell H. Morgan Department of Radiology and Radiological Science, The Johns Hopkins Medical Institutions, Division of Orthopaedic Surgery, Johns Hopkins School of Medicine, Baltimore, Maryland, USA

BENJAMIN FRITZ, MD, PD
Department of Radiology, Balgrist University Hospital, Faculty of Medicine, University of Zurich, Zurich, Switzerland; Department of Orthopaedics and Rehabilitation, University of Iowa, Iowa City, Iowa, USA

JAN FRITZ, MD, PD, RMSK
Associate Professor of Radiology, Chief, Division of Musculoskeletal Radiology, Department of Radiology, NYU Grossman School of Medicine, New York, New York, USA

SAMIR GHANDOUR, MD
Research Fellow, Department of Orthopaedic Surgery, Foot and Ankle Research and Innovation Lab (FARIL), Massachusetts General Hospital, Harvard Medical School, FARIL Center, Waltham, Massachusetts, USA

PRAJWAL GOWDA
Radiology, Orthopedic Surgery, UT Southwestern Medical Center, Dallas, Texas, USA

JÚLIO BRANDÃO GUIMARÃES, MD, PhD
Department of Musculoskeletal Radiology, Fleury Medicina e Saúde, São Paulo, São Paulo, Brazil

JOHN G. KENNEDY, MD, MCh, FFSEM, FRCS (Orth)
Chief of Foot and Ankle Surgery, Foot and Ankle Division, Department of Orthopaedic Surgery, NYU Langone Health, New York, New York, USA

JAEYOUNG KIM, MD
Research Fellow, Foot and Ankle Service, Hospital for Special Surgery, New York, New York, USA

AJIT KOHLI, DO
Radiology, Orthopedic Surgery, UT Southwestern Medical Center, Dallas, Texas, USA

RYAN C. KRUSE, MD
Assistant Professor, Department of Orthopedics and Rehabilitation, University of Iowa Sports Medicine, Iowa City, Iowa, USA

JOHN Y. KWON, MD
Associate Professor, Department of Orthopaedic Surgery, Foot and Ankle Research and Innovation Lab (FARIL), Massachusetts General Hospital, Harvard Medical School, FARIL Center, Waltham, Massachusetts, USA

WILLIAM B. MORRISON, MD, FACR
Professor of Radiology, Director, Division of Musculoskeletal Imaging and Intervention, Department of Radiology, Thomas Jefferson University Hospital, Philadelphia, Pennsylvania, USA

ALÍPIO G. ORMOND FILHO, MD
Department of Musculoskeletal Radiology, Fleury Medicina e Saúde, São Paulo, São Paulo, Brazil

CHRISTIAN PLAASS, MD
Senior Physician, Department for Foot and Ankle Surgery, DIAKOVERE Annastift, Orthopedic Clinic of the Hannover Medical School, Hannover, Germany

ALI RASHIDI, MD
Assistant Specialist, Department of Radiology, Molecular Imaging Program at Stanford, Stanford University, School of Medicine, Stanford, California, USA

ALENA RICHTER, MD
Department of Foot and Ankle Surgery, DIAKOVERE Annastift, Orthopedic Clinic of the Hannover Medical School, Hannover, Germany

CHRISTINA STUKENBORG-COLSMAN, MD
Chief Physician, Department of Foot and Ankle Surgery, DIAKOVERE Annastift, Orthopedic Clinic of the Hannover Medical School, Hannover, Germany

TAYLOR WINGO, MD
Orthopaedic Surgery Resident, Foot and Ankle Division, Department of Orthopaedic Surgery, NYU Langone Health, New York, New York, USA

EDUARDO YAMASHIRO, MD
Consultant Radiologist, Radiology Department, Aspetar Orthopedic and Sports Medicine Hospital, Doha, Qatar

ISLAM ZAKI, MBBCh
Radiology Resident, Department of Radiology, Benha University Hospital, El-Shaheed Farid Nada, Qism Banha, Al Qalyubia Governorate, Banha, Egypt

Editorial Advisory Board

Contents

Total ankle arthroplasty (TAA) is an effective alternative for treating patients with end-stage ankle degeneration, improving mobility, and providing pain relief. Implant survivorship is constantly improving; however, complications occur. Many causes of pain and dysfunction after total ankle arthroplasty can be diagnosed accurately with clinical examination, laboratory, radiography, and computer tomography. However, when there are no or inconclusive imaging findings, magnetic resonance imaging (MRI) is highly accurate in identifying and characterizing bone resorption, osteolysis, infection, osseous stress reactions, nondisplaced fractures, polyethylene damage, nerve injuries and neuropathies, as well as tendon and ligament tears. Multiple vendors offer effective, clinically available MRI techniques for metal artifact reduction MRI of total ankle arthroplasty. This article reviews the MRI appearances of common TAA implant systems, clinically available techniques and protocols for metal artifact reduction MRI of TAA implants, and the MRI appearances of a broad spectrum of TAA-related complications.

Use of SPECT/CT (Single Photon Emission Computed Tomography/Computed Tomography) is increasing providing additional information in patients with inconclusive clinical examination and unremarkable imaging findings presenting with chronic pain after total ankle arthroplasty. To differentiate the cause of pain after total ankle arthroplasty can be challenging. SPECT/CT combines structural and metabolic imaging as a hybrid tool leading to higher specificity and overall diagnostic accuracy presumably in cases of gutter impingement, prosthetic loosening, and osteoarthritis of adjacent joints. Moreover, SPECT/CT can complement diagnostic work up in periprosthetic joint infections. Basal tracer enhancement has to be considered for the interpretation of imaging findings.

Weight-bearing computed tomography has multiple advantages in evaluating the hindfoot and ankle. It can assess hindfoot and ankle alignment, pathology in ankle arthritis, and complications related to total ankle replacements. It is an essential tool in ankle osteoarthritis diagnostic, pre-operative planning, and total ankle replacement outcomes. It allows for better accuracy and reproducibility of alignment and implant size. In addition, it has the potential to more assertively detect complications related to weight bearing.

Benjamin Fritz, Cesar de Cesar Netto, and Jan Fritz

MRI is a valuable tool for diagnosing a broad spectrum of acute and chronic ankle disorders, including ligament tears, tendinopathy, and osteochondral lesions. Traditional two-dimensional (2D) MRI provides a high image signal and contrast of anatomic structures for accurately characterizing articular cartilage, bone marrow, synovium, ligaments, tendons, and nerves. However, 2D MRI limitations are thick slices and fixed slice orientations. In clinical practice, 2D MRI is limited to 2 to 3 mm slice thickness, which can cause blurred contours of oblique structures due to volume averaging effects within the image slice. In addition, image plane orientations are fixated and cannot be changed after the scan, resulting in 2D MRI lacking multiplanar and multiaxial reformation abilities for individualized image plane orientations along oblique and curved anatomic structures, such as ankle ligaments and tendons. In contrast, three-dimensional (3D) MRI is a newer, clinically available MRI technique capable of acquiring high-resolution ankle MRI data sets with isotropic voxel size. The inherently high spatial resolution of 3D MRI permits up to five times thinner (0.5 mm) image slices. In addition, 3D MRI can be acquired image voxel with the same edge length in all three space dimensions (isotropism), permitting unrestricted multiplanar and multiaxial image reformation and postprocessing after the MRI scan. Clinical 3D MRI of the ankle with 0.5 to 0.7 mm isotropic voxel size resolves the smallest anatomic ankle structures and abnormalities of ligament and tendon fibers, osteochondral lesions, and nerves. After acquiring the images, operators can align image planes individually along any anatomic structure of interest, such as ligaments and tendons segments. In addition, curved multiplanar image reformations can unfold the entire course of multiaxially curved structures, such as perimalleolar tendons, into one image plane. We recommend adding 3D MRI pulse sequences to traditional 2D MRI protocols to visualize small and curved ankle structures to better advantage. This article provides an overview of the clinical application of 3D MRI of the ankle, compares diagnostic performances of 2D and 3D MRI for diagnosing ankle abnormalities, and illustrates clinical 3D ankle MRI applications.

Prajwal Gowda, Ajit Kohli, and Avneesh Chhabra

This article is meant to serve as a reference for radiologists, orthopedic surgeons, and other physicians to enhance their understanding of progressive collapsing foot deformity, also known as adult acquired flat foot deformity. Pathophysiology, imaging findings, especially on MRI and 3-dimensional MRI are discussed with relevant illustrations so that the readers can apply these principles in their practice for better patient managements.

FOOT AND ANKLE CLINICS

RELATED SERIES

Orthopedic Clinics
Clinics in Sports Medicine
Physical Medicine and Rehabilitation Clinics

THE CLINICS ARE NOW AVAILABLE ONLINE!
Access your subscription at:
www.theclinics.com

Preface

Advanced Foot and Ankle Imaging: Breaching New Frontiers for More Accurate Diagnosis and Post-Operative Care

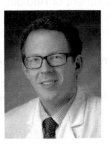

Jan Fritz, MD, PD, RMSK
Editor

Imaging is a critical component in diagnosing ankle conditions and postoperative care. While radiography remains the bedrock of first-line imaging, MRI, computed tomography, and ultrasonography permit the noninvasive diagnosis of a broad spectrum of injuries, conditions, and abnormalities of bones, joints, ligaments, muscle-tendon units, nerves, and vessels.

Exciting innovations and developments have substantially improved the spatial resolution of cross-sectional imaging, contributing to improved abilities to visualize the smallest anatomic structures in the foot and ankle for improved preoperative diagnoses.

2D and 3D MRI is now clinically available by multiple vendors. Artificial intelligence and deep learning have markedly shortened the acquisition time of 2D MRI, whereas 3D MRI provides unprecedented spatial resolution and postprocessing capabilities for visualizing obliquely oriented ligaments and unfolding multidirectional tendon courses into single-image planes. High-resolution 3D MR neurography techniques and many imaging centers are now broadly available.

Similarly, the diagnostic capabilities of ultrasonography have undergone tremendous advancements in image contrast, resolution of small anatomic detail, and speed of real-time imaging. In addition, the base of proficient radiologists, surgeons, podiatrists, sports imaging physicians, and other practitioners has markedly broadened, resulting in a more ubiquitous availability of foot and ankle ultrasonography.

Computed tomography has seen tremendous developments, including the broadening availability of cone beam scanners facilitating weight-bearing and positional

Foot Ankle Clin N Am 28 (2023) xv–xvi
https://doi.org/10.1016/j.fcl.2023.05.013
1083-7515/23/© 2023 Published by Elsevier Inc.

cross-sectional and 3D computed tomography visualization of many foot and ankle conditions before and after surgery.

Last, ultrasonography is crucial for a broad spectrum of minimally-invasive injection procedures, facilitating highly accurate delivery of injectants for pain relief, inflammation control, and tissue regeneration.

I am grateful to each author team for their expert contributions, enormous attention to detail, and superb illustrations.

I thank Dr Netto for entrusting me with the guest editor role in this issue.

Jan Fritz, MD, PD, RMSK
New York University School of Medicine
Department of Radiology
Division of Musculoskeletal Radiology
NYU Grossman School of Medicine
660 1st Avenue, 3rd Floor, Room 313
New York, NY 10016, USA

E-mail address:
jan.fritz@nyulangone.org

Magnetic Resonance Imaging of Total Ankle Arthroplasty

State-of-The-Art Assessment of Implant-Related Pain and Dysfunction

Jan Fritz, MD, PD, RMSK[c],*, Ali Rashidi, MD[a],
Cesar de Cesar Netto, MD, PhD[b]

KEYWORDS

- Ankle arthroplasty • Complications • Metal artifact reduction (MARS)
- Magnetic resonance imaging (MRI)

KEY POINTS

- Metal artifact reduction MRI is useful for evaluating pain and dysfunction after TAA due to its high accuracy in detecting and characterizing pain generators and a broad spectrum of complications.
- Multiple vendors offer effective, clinically available MRI techniques for metal artifact reduction MRI evaluation of pain and dysfunction after total ankle arthroplasty.
- Metal artifact reduction MRI can contribute to timely diagnoses of TAA-related complications and aid management decisions, surgical planning, and prognosis.
- We use metal artifact reduction MRI as a problem-solving tool in symptomatic patients with negative radiographs and to further characterize radiographic findings.

INTRODUCTION

Osteoarthritis and inflammatory arthritis of the ankle are common, chronic, progressive, and often disabling conditions that can substantially impact the quality of life. Post-traumatic arthrosis is most common in the ankle joint, followed by rheumatoid arthritis, other inflammatory conditions, and infection.[1,2] Traditionally, treatment

[a] Division of Musculoskeletal Radiology, Department of Radiology, NYU Grossman School of Medicine, 660 1st Ave, 3rd Floor, Rm 313, New York, NY 10016, USA; [b] Department of Radiology, Molecular Imaging Program at StanDepartment of Radiology, Molecular Imaging Program at Stanford, Stanford University School of Medicine, Stanford, CA, USA; [c] Department of Orthopedic Surgery, Division of Foot and Ankle Surgery, Duke University, Durham, NC, USA
* Corresponding author.
E-mail address: jan.fritz@nyulangone.org

Foot Ankle Clin N Am 28 (2023) 463–492
https://doi.org/10.1016/j.fcl.2023.05.012
1083-7515/23/© 2023 Elsevier Inc. All rights reserved.

foot.theclinics.com

options include surgical joint debridement, osteotomy, and distraction arthroplasty, whereas arthrodesis has been the preferred choice recently.[3]

Total ankle arthroplasty (TAA) was introduced in the early 1970s[4,5] as an effective alternative for arthrodesis in patients with end-stage ankle joint arthrosis and arthritis, with advantages including the restoration of mobility and anatomy. Over the last decade, TAA has been increasingly used to manage patients with end-stage osteoarthritis, producing encouraging outcomes in pain relief and improving function, gait, and quality of life.[1,4–8] However, TAA is associated with higher complication risks and implant failure than hip and knee arthroplasty.[9] Therefore, effective surveillance with imaging modalities that can detect failure early and identify complications accurately is important for optimal management and appropriate timing of revision surgery.[5,10,11]

Radiography, computed tomography (CT), single-photon-emission CT (SPECT), and magnetic resonance imaging (MRI) have different strengths and limitations for the surveillance of well-functioning TAA implants and the evaluation of painful and dysfunctional TAA.[12–17]

Like hip and knee arthroplasty implants,[13–15] MRI uniquely characterizes intact TAA implants and diagnoses TAA-related periprosthetic abnormalities.[16–18] However, when applying conventional MRI techniques, TAA implant-induced metal artifacts substantially degrade images and may render non-diagnostic interpretations of periprosthetic bone and soft tissues. Metal artifact reduction MRI represents a growing, now widely available group of dedicated MRI techniques with unprecedented capabilities to reduce image-degrading effects of arthroplasty implants [16,17,19–21] and optimize MRI for evaluating bone and soft tissues around TAA implants.

This article reviews the MRI appearances of common TAA implant systems, clinically available techniques and protocols for successful metal artifact reduction MRI of TAA implants, and the MRI appearances of a broad spectrum of TAA-related complications.

TOTAL ANKLE ARTHROPLASTY SYSTEMS

Since the introduction of TAA in the early 1970s, different types of implants have been designed. The first-generation TAA implant systems were cemented, requiring a substantial osseous resection.[22] Although they were considered stable implants, their highly constraint design was associated with unacceptably high rates of osteolysis and loosening.

Second-generation TAA implant systems required less osseous resection featured a semi-constrained design with an increased range of ankle motion, allowed for cementless implantation, and featured a two-component design. While the rates of implant loosening were lower, polyethylene wear compromised component stability and contributed to high failure rates due to implant dislocation.

The third generation of TAA implants, currently widely used in the United States, feature semi-constrained designs with 2 or 3 implant components, typically including metallic tibial and talar components with an interposed ultra-high molecular weight polyethylene insert. The designs minimize osseous resection and allow multiplanar ankle motion. However, postoperative pain and dysfunction occur.[22–25]

In 2022, approximately 14 TAA implant systems have been approved by the United States Food and Drug Administration (FDA),[23] most of which feature cobalt-chromium and titanium alloys, porous interface surfaces, and highly cross-linked polyethylene components.[26] Many TAA systems have characteristic component designs and unique features (**Table 1**. Total Ankle Arthroplasty Systems), which allow for imaging

Table 1
Total ankle arthroplasty systems

Implant (Manufacturer)	Components	Constraint	Bearing	Surgical Approach	Characteristic Imaging Features
Scandinavian Total Ankle Replacement (STAR) (Waldemar Link, Hamburg, Germany)	Three	Semiconstrained	Mobile	Anterior	Two characteristic 6.5 mm parallel anteroposterior bars mounted on the tibial component and a fin-like edge on the talar component
Salto Talaris Anatomic Ankle (Tornier, Saint Ismier, France)	Two	Semiconstrained	Fixed	Anterior	Talar component with a curved groove in the sagittal plane of the talar component and the tibial component, which is fixed to the tibial bone
INBONE I Total Ankle System (Wright Medical Technologies, Arlington, TN)	Two	Semiconstrained	Fixed	Anterior	Tall modular talar component stem
INBONE II Total Ankle System (Wright Medical Technologies, Arlington, TN)	Two	Nonconstrained	Fixed	Anterior	Tall modular talar component stem
INFINITY Total Ankle System (Wright Medical Technology, Arlington, TN)	Three	Semiconstrained	Fixed	Anterior	Three press-fit tibial component pegs and two talar component pegs
Trabecular Metal Total Ankle (Zimmer Biomet, Warsaw, IN)	Two	Semiconstrained	Fixed	Lateral	Two mediolateral bars of the tibial and talar components

identification, such as with radiography and MRI. We will briefly discuss the salient features and surgical approaches of the most widely used 3rd generation TAA implant systems.

SCANDINAVIAN TOTAL ANKLE REPLACEMENT

The STAR *(Waldemar Link, Hamburg, Germany)* TAA implant system was introduced in 1978[25–27] and has undergone multiple design iterations. The most recent version features a cementless, mobile-bearing, three-component design[28] (**Fig. 1**). The system is implanted through an anterior approach. Characteristic MRI-visible features are two 6.5 mm parallel anteroposterior bars mounted on the tibial component, which anchor into the tibial osteotomy surface. The talar component has a fin-like keel that anchors into the talar bone and a crest along the articular surface that accommodates the polyethylene meniscus and stabilizes the anteroposterior motion.[29]

SALTO TALARIS ANATOMIC ANKLE

The Salto Talaris *(Tornier, Saint Ismier, France)* TAA system features a fixed-bearing, semi-constrained design, representing a modified version of an earlier European version[26] (**Fig. 2**). The tibial and talar components are cobalt-chromium alloys with interposed polyethylene insert.[22,23,25] The implantation is performed through an anterior approach.[30] A feature is a talar component with 2 different radii. The medial radius is smaller than the lateral radius, mimicking the ankle's normal anatomy and providing equal force to collateral ligaments. A curved groove facilitates ankle rotation in the sagittal plane of the talar component. The polyethylene component is bonded to the tibial component.[26] The dominant MR-visible feature is a single raised central tibial component bar.

INBONE TOTAL ANKLE SYSTEM

The INBONE *(Wright Medical Technologies, Arlington, TN)* TAA system is a two-component fixed-bearing system that was FDA-approved in 2005 (INBONE I, semi-constrained design) and 2010 (INBONE II, non-constrained design).[22,25,26] The implantation is performed through an anterior approach. The dominant characteristic feature is a tall modular talar component stem (**Fig. 3**).

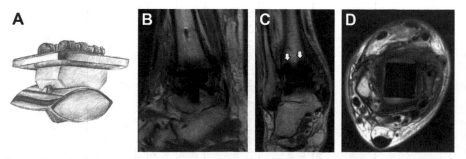

Fig. 1. Scandinavian Total Ankle Replacement (STAR). (*A*) Illustration of the STAR implant system. Sagittal (*B*), coronal (*C*), and axial (*D*) intermediate-weighted SEMAC MRI of the STAR implant system. The STAR implant system features two characteristic parallel anteroposterior bars mounted on the tibial component (*arrows* in *C*) and a fin-like keel on the talar component (visible in *B*).

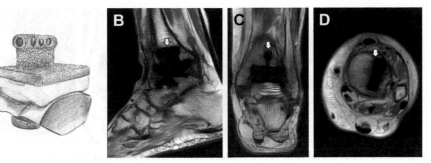

Fig. 2. Salto Talaris Total Ankle Replacement (*A*). A: Illustration of the Salto Talaris implant system. Sagittal (*B*), coronal (*C*), and axial (*D*) intermediate-weighted SEMAC MRI of the Salto Talaris implant system. The Salto Talaris implant system features a single elevated bar mounted on the tibial component (*arrows*).

TRABECULAR METAL TOTAL ANKLE (ZIMMER)

The Trabecular Metal (*Zimmer Biomet, Warsaw, IN*) TAA system is a third-generation, semi-constrained, two-component, fixed-bearing design. Implantation requires a transfibular approach with fibular shaft osteotomy, anterior tibiotalar and talofibular ligaments division, and final fibular plate and screw fixation.[31] Characteristic MRI-visible features are two mediolateral bars of the tibial and talar components (**Fig. 4**).

IMAGING MODALITIES

Radiographs are the first-line imaging modality for the postoperative evaluation of implant component position, alignment, bone-implant interfaces, and periprosthetic bone.[32] Anteroposterior and lateral radiographs in maximal dorsiflexion and maximal plantar flexion can be used to evaluate the postoperative range of motion and alignment of implants.[32,33] TAA implants typically do not cause degrading metal artifacts on radiography. However, the reliability of different measurements for evaluating prosthesis position and detecting TAA complications on postoperative radiographs may vary.[34]

Computed tomography (CT) is more accurate than radiography for detecting early bone resorption and osteolysis at the bone-implant interfaces, characterizing implant

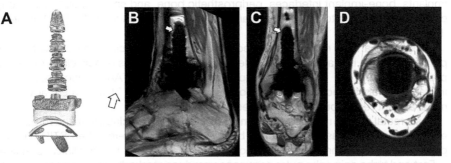

Fig. 3. INBONE II Total Ankle Ankle Replacement. (*A*) Illustration of the INBONE implant system. Sagittal (*B*), coronal (*C*), and axial (*D*) intermediate-weighted SEMAC MRI of the INBONE implant system. The INBONE implant system features a tall modular talar component stem (*arrows*).

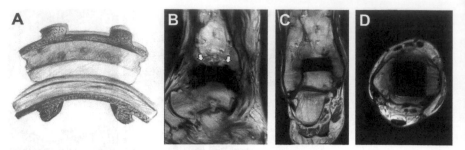

Fig. 4. Trabecular Metal Total Ankle Replacement. (*A*) Illustration of the trabecular metal total ankle system. Sagittal (*B*), coronal (*C*), and axial (*D*) intermediate-weighted SEMAC MRI of the implant system. The implant system features anterior and posterior tibial (*arrows*) and talar component cross bars.

position, and diagnosing subtle fractures.[22,32,35] Dedicated techniques can reduce implant-induced streak artifacts, including dual energy-based monoenergetic extrapolation and iterative metal artifact reduction reconstructions.[36,37] However, substantial metal artifacts frequently remain on smooth kernel soft-tissue window images, which is critical to evaluate the synovium, fluid, tendons, ligaments, and nerves.

Single-photon-emission CT (SPECT) can help visualize increased bone activity at the bone-implant interface associated with pain and periprosthetic infection.[38] However, due to the bone remodeling following the joint replacement, radiotracer activity at the bone-implant interfaces carries low specificity.[38] Adding CT to the SPECT (SPECT-CT) can increase the specificity.[39]

Cone-beam CT is a more recently introduced three-dimensional technique that displays bones and soft tissues at a low radiation dose and has been utilized successfully for weight-bearing assessments.[40,41] However, metal artifacts and low soft tissue contrast remain limitations.

Both radiography and CT result in image acquisition-related radiation exposure and have inherently low contrast resolution to detect bone marrow and periprosthetic soft tissue abnormalities.

METAL ARTIFACT REDUCTION MAGNETIC RESONANCE IMAGING

Metal artifact reduction MRI represents a group of techniques that reduce metallic orthopedic implant-related artifacts and improve the visualization of TAA arthroplasty implants, bone-implant interfaces, periprosthetic bone, and soft tissues.[42] The group can be categorized into basic and advanced metal artifact reduction MRI techniques[43] (**Fig. 5**) (**Table 2**).

Basic metal artifact reduction MRI techniques provide sufficient image quality in the periphery of TAA implants. However, degrading metal artifacts remain close to the implants, rendering the MR images inadequate to evaluate TAA components, bone-implant interfaces, and closeby periprosthetic soft tissues.[44] This is where advanced metal artifact reduction MRI techniques are most valuable.

Basic metal artifact reduction sequence MRI techniques include fast and turbo spin-echo pulse sequences, high receiver bandwidth, bandwidth-matched STIR fat suppression, and the thinnest possible slice thickness, usually 3 mm in clinical practice.

Fast and turbo spin echo pulse sequences produce markedly smaller metal artifacts than gradient-echo pulse sequences.[20] Contrary to previous assumptions, the isolated increase of the echo train length of fast and turbo spin-echo pulse sequences does not reduce metal artifacts but may result in substantial blurring.[45]

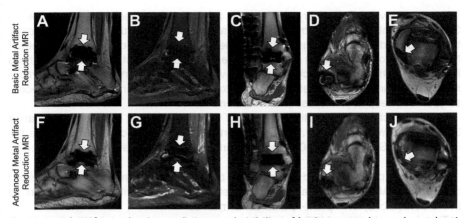

Fig. 5. Metal artifact reduction and structural visibility of basic versus advanced metal artifact reduction MRI. (*A-E*): Sagittal (*A* and *B*), coronal (*C*), and axial (*D* and *E*) basic proton density-weighted (*A, C, D,* and *E*) and STIR (*B*) metal artifact reduction MRI using high receiver bandwidth turbo spin echo MRI pulse sequences. F-G: Sagittal (*F* and *G*), coronal (*H*), and axial (*I* and *J*) advanced proton density-weighted (F, H, I, and J) and STIR (*B*) metal artifact reduction MRI using SEMAC turbo spin echo MRI pulse sequences. Advanced metal artifact reduction results in near complete elimination of metal artifacts, affording better visibility of (*arrows* in F, G, and H), peroneal tendons adjacent to a fibular plate (*arrow* in *I*), and long flexor tendons (*arrow* in *J*).

A high receiver or readout bandwidth of approximately 500 Hz per pixel will reduce in-plane signal displacement and image distortions.[42,46] Increasing the matrix size will result in higher spatial resolution but may not reduce the degree of metallic artifacts.

The bandwidth of the slice-encoding gradient can be increased by reducing slice thickness. However, thin slice thickness is practically limited by the associated loss of MRI signal.[47] In our experience, 3 mm is the practical lower limit of slice thickness for MRI of TAA implants.

Table 2
Summary of basic metal artifact reduction techniques and mechanisms for reducing metallic artifacts on MR images

Metal Artifact Reduction MRI Techniques	Mechanism Resulting in Reduced Metal Artifacts on MRI
Use of fast and turbo spin echo pulse sequences instead of gradient echo pulse sequences	Decreases spin dephasing due to radiofrequency-induced refocusing, as opposed to gradient inversion-induced spin refocusing with gradient echo pulse sequences
Higher receiver bandwidth at 500 Hz/pixel	Reduces signal displacement in the in-plane direction
Thin slice thickness of 3 mm	Reduces through-plane displacement secondary to steepening of the slice encoding gradient
STIR fat suppression with the matching of excitation and read-put bandwidths	STIR fat suppression technique is the most robust because it depends on T1 relaxation constants, which are inert to implant-related effects.
Lower field strength magnet	Minimization of the field-induced inhomogeneity

Short tau inversion recovery (STIR) is the fat suppression technique of choice, as STIR is inherently unaffected by metallic implants. STIR may require matching the excitation and readout bandwidths for homogeneous fat suppression.[48] For postcontrast MRI, subtraction of matching non-fat-suppressed pre-and postcontrast T1-weighted MR images is the method of choice.[49] However, contrast-enhanced MRI with intravenous gadolinium contrast rarely adds value to TAA evaluation and is usually unnecessary, unless neoplastic disease is the concern.[50]

Metal artifact reduction MRI at 0.55 - 1.5 T will result in fewer metal artifacts than at 3.0 T[51,52]; however, with advanced metal artifact reduction techniques, such as the Compressed Sensing SEMAC pulse sequence, similar results may be achieved at 3.0 T.[15,53,54]

A recently published study comparing optimized 1.5T and 3.0T Compressed Sensing SEMAC MRI in total ankle arthroplasty implants demontrasted no differences in the detectability of implant-related abnormalities [120]

The view angle tilting (VAT) technique can result in smaller metal artifacts at lower receiver bandwidth of around 150 Hz/pixel. However, the metal artifact-reducing effects of VAT at high-receiver bandwidth of 500 to 600 Hz per pixel are minimal but can result in substantial blurring.[55]

SEMAC TSE and MAVRIC FSE are advanced metal artifact reduction MRI techniques that substantially reduce metal artifacts in the slice direction.[56,57] Additional phase and frequency encoding steps are employed to sample through-plane displaced signals, which are then used to form final composite MR images with minimal residual TAA implant-induced metallic artifacts (**Fig. 6**). SEMAC TSE and MAVRIC FSE have typically combined with the basic metal artifact reduction MRI techniques. Higher numbers of phase and frequency encoding steps result in more metal artifact reduction at the expense of longer acquisition times.[45] Compressed sensing-based undersampling can reduce the acquisition times of SEMAC TSE by 60% to 70%.[16,58–60] In addition, artificial intelligence and deep learning image reconstruction promise additional meaningful image acceleration.[61–64]

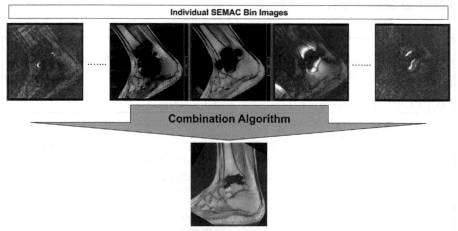

Fig. 6. SEMAC metal artifact reduction MRI technique. Individually phase-encoded SEMAC bin images collect MR signal displaced by effects of the ankle arthroplasty implants into the parent slice (central image in the top row). A mathematical combination algorithm creates the final SEMAC composite image MR images with near-completely eliminated metal artifacts (bottom image).

Table 3 shows our institutional metal artifact reduction MRI protocol for total ankle arthroplasty at 1.5 T field strength.

NORMAL MAGNETIC RESONANCE IMAGING FINDINGS OF TOTAL ANKLE ARTHROPLASTY

Postoperative MRI findings following a TAA vary according to the postoperative interval at the time of imaging, surgical approach, and type of implant. In the immediate and perioperative phases, soft tissue edema and synovitis are considered normal MRI findings that can persist for months. The healed pseudocapsule is expected to be seen as a hypointense thin continuous rim on all pulse sequences. A thin synovial lining without debris and a small volume of joint fluid are common and possible persistent normal MRI findings in postoperative settings. Except for the bone reaming, which can result in adjacent marrow edema signal for more than 12 months following the surgery,[65] in patients with no underlying infiltrative disease, the periprosthetic cancellous bone should have a similar signal intensity to native bone. Although the most desirable outcome of implantation is direct ingrowth with MRI demonstrating solid, uninterrupted contact at the osseous bone-implant interface, a < 2 mm intermediate to high signal intensity fibrous pseudomembrane layer at the bone-implant interface may be considered a finding indicating solid implant fixation.[66]

MAGNETIC RESONANCE IMAGING OF TOTAL ANKLE ARTHROPLASTY COMPLICATIONS

The triple-component design of the ankle prosthesis reduced the incidence of prosthesis loosening and wear.[67] However, inevitable repetitive axial loading and shear forces on the ankle joint predispose ankle prostheses interfere with implant longevity.[68] The reported incidences of TAA complications vary.[1,10,69,70] A meta-analysis comparing the outcomes of TAA and ankle arthrodesis found a 19.7% complication rate in 2239 ankle arthroplasties,[71] whereas another study found a 23% complication rate in 217 TAA.[72]

Intraoperative and postoperative complications can be categorized based on the timing of the diagnosis and the interval since surgery (**Box 1**).[69,73] TAA complications can also be categorized into low-grade, intermediate-grade, and high-grade.[32] The most frequent complications are aseptic loosening, wound complications, fractures, and deep infections.[71] Radiography, CT, and MRI have varying strengths and weaknesses in evaluating postoperative complications (**Table 4**).

OSSEOINTEGRATION AND ASPECTIC LOOSENING

Loosening, describing the partial or complete loss of implant fixation from the host bone, represents the most frequent complication of TAA.[23,69,71] The term aseptic loosening indicates a negative infection work-up.[19] Inadequate bone ingrowth, insufficient prosthesis cementing, higher forces at the bone-prosthesis interface, and malalignment can contribute to loosening.[32,69,74] In addition, bone resorption as a physiologic periprosthetic response to asymmetrical mechanical overload is a common cause of loosening as a late complication.[32] Body weight, activity level, age, and genetics are also linked to developing aseptic loosening.[75]

On radiographs and CT images, linear periprosthetic lucency greater than 2 mm width suggests loosening,[19,23,66,68,74] whereas CT is thought to be more accurate.[76,77] On MRI, a sharply demarcated bone-implant interface with host bone directly contacting the implant surface equates to complete osseous integration (**Fig. 7**).[16] A 1 to 2 mm

Table 3
Metal artifact reduction protocols for MRI of ankle arthroplasty implants at 1.5 T

Parameters	Sagittal		Coronal			Axial		
Type	CS-SEMAC	CS-SEMAC	CS-SEMAC	CS-SEMAC	High-Bandwidth	CS-SEMAC	High-Bandwidth	CS-SEMAC
Weighting	Proton density	STIR	Proton density	STIR	Proton density	Proton density	STIR	STIR
Repetition time/echo time (ms)	3800/28	3500/7.5	3800/28	3700/7.5	3800/31	3800/31	4540/4.6	4620/7.5
Receiver bandwidth (Hertz/pixel)	601	601	601	601	587	601	592	601
Number of slices/Flip angle (degree)	32/135	22/150	34/135	24/150	41/135	41/135	30/140	30/140
Field-of-view (mm²)	170 × 170	190 × 190	170 × 118	190 × 137	170 × 118	170 × 118	180 × 118	180 × 118
Matrix	320 × 240	256 × 204	320 × 240	256 × 204	320 × 240	320 × 240	256 × 204	256 × 204
Slice thickness/gap (mm)	3/0	4/0	3/0	4/0	3/0	3/0	4/0	4/0
Number of excitations/concatenations	1/1	1/2	1/1	1/2	3/2	1/1	2/2	1/2
Turbo factor/acceleration factor	11/8	17/8	11/8	19/8	19/1	11/8	16/1	19/8
SEMAC steps	19	19	19	16	-	19	-	19
View-angle tilting	100%	100%	100%	100%	100%	100%	100%	100%
Acquisition time	4:35	4:56	4:39	4:35	5:06	4:39	5:02	5:16

Abbreviations: CS-SEMAC, compressed sensing slice-encoding for metal artifact correction; STIR, short tau inversion recovery.

Box 1
Classification of total ankle arthroplasty complications based on time of finding

Intraoperative Complications

Intraoperative fracture

Accidental osteotomy of the lateral malleolus

Tibial nerve injury

Postoperative Complications

Aseptic/mechanical loosening

Geographic/ballooning osteolysis

Postoperative early fracture (<4 months)

Postoperative late fracture (>4 months)

Component mispositioning

Wound-healing problems

Superficial and deep/periprosthetic infection

Polyethylene fracture/dislocation

Edge loading

Gutter impingement

Residual pain

Stiffness

Soft-tissue injuries (nerve/tendon)

Subsidence

Thromboembolism

Chronic regional pain syndrome

Superficial and deep peroneal dysesthesias

Table 4
Relative strengths and weaknesses of radiography, computed tomography, and magnetic resonance imaging for diagnosing total ankle arthroplasty complications

Complication	Radiography	Ultrasonography	CT	MRI
Aseptic/mechanical loosening	+	-	++	+++
Geographic/ballooning osteolysis	+	-	++	+++
Infection	+	+	+	+++
Periprosthetic osseous stress reaction	-	-	-	+++
Periprosthetic fracture	+	-	++	+++
Immature heterotopic ossification	+	+	++	+++
Mature heterotopic ossification	+	+	+++	++
Polyethylene fracture or displacement	+	-	++	++
Nerve injury and neuropathy	-	++	-	+++
Tendon and ligament injury	+	++	+	+++

Abbreviations: CT, computed tomography; MRI, magnetic resonance imaging.

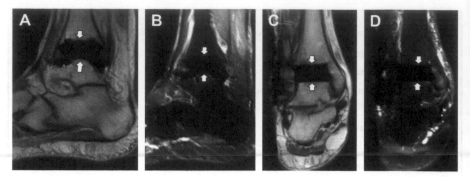

Fig. 7. MRI appearance of intact bone-implant interfaces. Sagittal (*A* and *B*) and coronal (*C* and *D*) intermediate-weighted (*A* and *C*) and STIR (*B* and *D*) SEMAC MR images demonstrate sharply demarcated bone-implant interfaces (*arrows*) with cancellous bone directly contacting the implant surfaces, indicating successful and complete osseointegration.

thick layer of intermediate signal intensity on proton density-weighted and STIR MR images interposed between the implant surface and periprosthetic bone suggests fibrous membrane formation, which may be considered meta-stable and followed. Abnormal signal intensity measuring greater than 2 mm width is considered absent osseointegration or bone resorption if osseointegration occurred previously (**Fig. 8**). In most cases, bone resorption occurs locally or regionally involving parts rather than complete bone-implant interfaces but may eventually progress to involve the entire bone-implant interface. The imaging diagnosis of implant loosening, synonymous with complete loss of implant fixation, requires bone resorption along the entire bone-implant interface and signs of implant subsidence, rotation, shift, or frank displacement to be certain.[14,19]

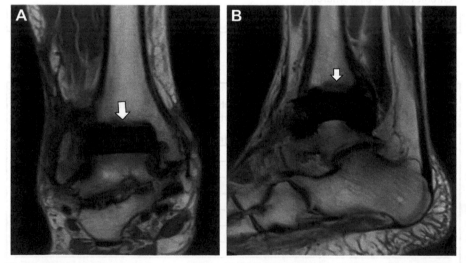

Fig. 8. MRI appearance of bone resorption at the bone-implant interfaces. Coronal (*A*) and sagittal (*B*) intermediate-weighted SEMAC MR images demonstrate regional bone resorption along the tibial bone-implant interface (*arrows*) with a sclerotic line and interposition of fluid-like signal. The talar bone-implant interface is intact, indicated by bone directly contacting the implant surfaces.

OSTEOLYSIS

Geographic or "ballooning" osteolysis describes "osteolytic cavities" or "cavitation" adjacent bone-implant interfaces. Osteolyses are associated with regional loss of implant fixation and bone weakening and hence, are considered a risk factor for prosthesis failure.[78] Fretted implant particles and wear debris from articulating bearing and non-articulating implant interfaces contribute to lymphocyte and macrophage activation, cytokine production, osteoclasts activation, and subsequent bone destruction and osteolysis.[79] Exacerbating factors include an exaggerated host immune response to the where particles, high metal bone interface loading pressure, inaccurate implant positioning resulting in excessive shear stress, and wear of the hydroxyapatite coating of the implant components.[78,80] The detection accuracy of osteolysis is higher with CT than radiography; however, MRI is most accurate for detecting periprosthetic osteolyses.[14,19,81,82]

On MRI, periprosthetic osteolyses usually appear as well-marginated cavities in the host bone. In the early phase, surrounding bone marrow edema may be present (**Fig. 9**), whereas in the later stages, no surrounding bone marrow edema is typically present.[16] The surrounding bone marrow edema may be part of the osteoclast activity or indicate an associated localized stress reaction. Osteolysis may be filled with simple joint fluid or demonstrate internal complexity with mixed fluid and debris components. Polyethylene-based debris conglomerates within osteolyses often demonstrate similar signal intensities and texture to muscle tissue on proton density-weighted nonfat suppressed MR images. Metallic debris is typically dark on all pulse sequences and may show blooming artifacts.

INFECTION

Postoperative infections include superficial wound infections and deep periprosthetic infections. Superficial wound infections result in delayed wound healing, whereas deep periprosthetic infections extend to the joint capsule, implant surfaces, and

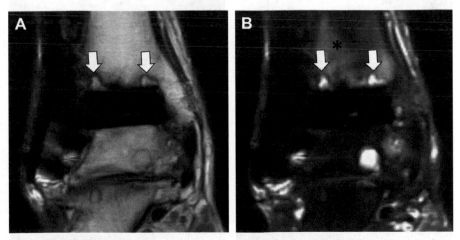

Fig. 9. MRI appearance of geographic/ballooning osteolysis at the bone-implant interfaces. Coronal intermediate-weighted (A) and STIR (B) SEMAC MR images demonstrate cystic osteolysis lesions (arrows) at the tibial bone-implant interface. The talar bone-implant interface is intact, indicated by bone directly contacting the implant surfaces. The asterisk indicates surrounding bone marrow edema in the distal tibia, suggesting increased stress.

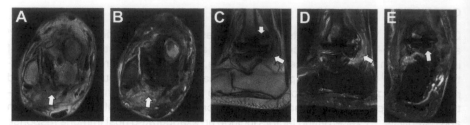

Fig. 10. MRI appearance of periprosthetic joint infection after total ankle arthroplasty. Axial (*A* and *B*), sagittal (*C* and *D*), and coronal (*E*) intermediate-weighted (*A* and *C*) and STIR (*B, D,* and *E*) SEMAC MR images demonstrate infectious talocrural synovitis (*arrows* in *A–D*), characterized by pseudo-capsular edema, thickening, and layering, as well as prominent diffuse pericapsular edema. The coronal images demonstrate near complete bone resorption along the talar bone-implant interface (*arrow* in *E*), indicating loss of fixation.

periprosthetic bone. The rate of postoperative wound complication reports ranges between 1.1% and 16.9%.[83–85] A systematic review and meta-analysis of 7942 TAA found 2.4% superficial and 1.1% deep infections.[1] Predisposing factors of deep infections after TAA include previous ankle surgery, prolonged surgical time during TAA, preexisting diabetes mellitus, and impaired wound healing beyond 14 days following surgery.[86] Serological tests, including erythrocyte sedimentation rate, C-reactive protein, and white blood cell count, have low specificity but high sensitivity for diagnosing

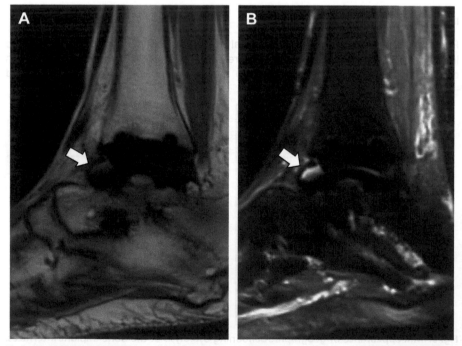

Fig. 11. MRI appearance of normal joint fluid after ankle arthroplasty. Sagittal intermediate-weighted (*A*) and STIR (*B*) SEMAC MR images demonstrate normal synovial fluid volume and simple fluid texture (*arrows*) after ankle arthroplasty. Note the normal thin hypointense appearance of the joint capsule.

periprosthetic joint infection.[14] The inability to reliably differentiate infection from other complications, such as aseptic loosening, limits the utility of radiographs in diagnosing periprosthetic joint infections.

Traditional bone scan scintigraphy may help to differentiate periprosthetic infection from loosening in a small subset of cases. Late focal radiotracer activity favors loosening, whereas intense and diffuse early and late periprosthetic radiotracer activity may indicate infection. However, persistent radiotracer activity along bone-implant interfaces and noninfectious synovitis interfere with bone scan accuracy.[87]

Single-photon emission computed tomography (SPECT) with computed tomography (SPECT-CT) holds promise for improved accuracy over traditional bone scans in diagnosing periprosthetic infection.[88]

The MRI appearance of septic arthritis in the setting of periprosthetic joint infection is similar to the MRI appearance in hip, knee, and shoulder arthroplasties.[13–16,43,89] On MRI, the combination of complex synovial fluid, edematous synovial thickening, and periprosthetic soft tissue edema suggests periprosthetic infection (**Fig. 10**).[16] Regional bulky lymphadenopathy is an uncommon finding in periprosthetic TAA infections. In addition, MRI can directly visualize sinus tract connections between skin and implant surfaces as a major criterion for periprosthetic joint infection. Periprosthetic joint infections may include osteomyelitis, which has the typical MRI appearance of altered marrow fat, including ill-defined T1 and proton density signal hypointensity and edema-like STIR signal hypointensity.[90] Periprosthetic bone marrow edema carries a low accuracy for diagnosing periprosthetic joint infections, as edema related to osteotomy and implantation can persist for many months to years.[65]

Synovial aspiration and tissue sampling facilitate cell count, synovial analysis, culture, and sensitivity testing.[14,91]

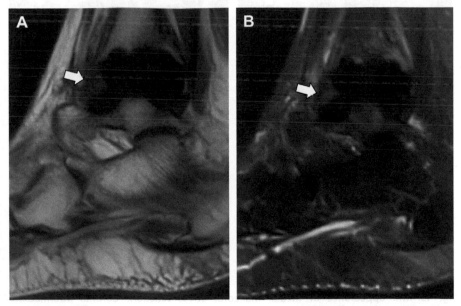

Fig. 12. MRI appearance of arthrofibrosis in a patient with ankle stiffness after ankle arthroplasty. Sagittal intermediate-weighted (A) and STIR (B) SEMAC MR images demonstrate prominent scarring of the anterior capsule and fibrous material filling the joint recess (arrows) without synovial fluid signal.

PSEUDOCAPSULE

MRI is the most accurate technique for visualizing the pseudocapsule and characterizing the synovial fluid. A small amount of simple synovial fluid is a normal finding after ankle arthroplasty (**Fig. 11**). In the setting of stiffness after TAA, arthrofibrosis is characterized by diffuse pseudocapsule thickening and replacement of the typically present joint fluid by fibrous tissue (**Fig. 12**).

PERIPROSTHETIC OSSEOUS STRESS REACTION AND FRACTURE

Intraoperative and postoperative periprosthetic fractures are TAA's most common intraoperative complication, occurring in up to 10% of TAA cases[10,43,92] and contributing to up to 3.2% of revisions.[93] Intraoperative fractures may occur in osseous fragility secondary to osteoporosis, infiltrative marrow diseases, and disuse osteopenia.[94,95] Postoperative fractures may be associated with implant failure in up to 50%.[32,96] Postoperative fractures can be categorized into traumatic and stress-induced

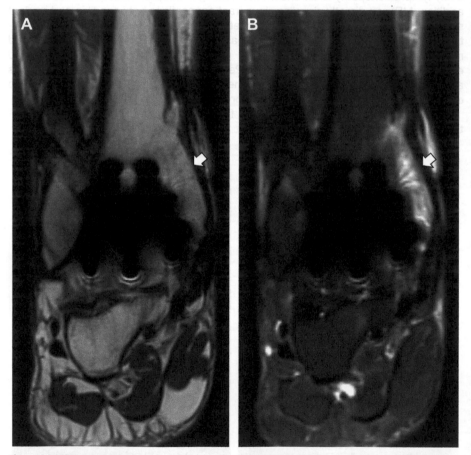

Fig. 13. MRI appearance of medial malleolus stress reaction. Coronal intermediate-weighted (A) and STIR (B) SEMAC MR images demonstrate localized bone marrow edema of the medial malleolus (arrows), indicating a local stress reaction. The bone-implant interfaces of the talar and tibial components are intact without findings to suggest bone resorption or osteolysis. A healed medial metaphyseal cortical tibia fracture is partially seen.

fractures.[94] Sizable bone resection, oversized implants, and mispositioned components increase the risk of postoperative fracture.[10]

The medial malleolus is the most prevalent site of osseous stress reactions and fractures (**Fig. 13**). Restoration of sagittal and coronal plane alignment,[17] higher mechanical loading on the medial malleolus due to varus positioning of the prosthesis, patient
noncompliance with postoperative weight-bearing instructions, talar medialization,
and excessive bone resection of the distal tibia contribute to osseous stress reactions
and stress fractures of the medial malleolus.[23,94,95]

Radiographs and CT scans accurately diagnose periprosthetic fractures with
distinct fracture lines and displacement.[97] However, nondisplaced fractures without
distinct fracture lines and osseous stress reactions without fracture lines, sclerosis,
osseous remodeling, or mineralized periosteal reaction are occult on radiographs
and CT.[98]

MRI is the most accurate imaging test for detecting and characterizing the spectrum
ranging from osseous stress reactions to nondisplaced fractures. MRI is particularly
valuable for diagnosing incomplete and nondisplaced fractures and osseous stress reactions before osseous remodeling and mineralized periosteal reactions occur and
become visible on radiographs and CT.

Typical MRI appearances of osseous stress reactions include regional STIR signal
hyperintensity of cancellous bone,[14] indicating bone marrow edema, optional cortical
and periosteal edema, and absent fracture lines and cortical deformity (**Fig. 14**). MRI
appearances of nondisplaced fractures feature distinct fracture lines on proton
density-weighted, T1-weighted, and STIR MR images through the cortex, cancellous

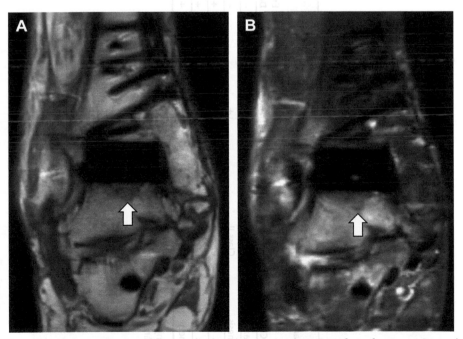

Fig. 14. MRI appearance of a nondisplaced bone-implant interface fracture. Coronal
intermediate-weighted (*A*) and STIR (*B*) SEMAC MR images demonstrate a nondisplaced
fracture line (*arrow*) subjacent to the talar bone-implant interface and surrounding bone
marrow edema of the talus.

Table 5
Seddon and Sunderland nerve injury classification with structural correlation

Seddon Classification	Sunderland Classification	Axonal Disruption	Endoneurium Disruption	Perineurium Disruption	Epineurium Disruption	Wallerian Degeneration
Neurapraxia	Class I	-[a]	-	-	-	-
Axonotmesis	Class II	+	-	-	-	+
	Class III	+	+	-	-	+
	Class IV	+	+	+	-	+
Neurotmesis	Class V[b]	+	+	+	+	+

[a] Axonal injury without disruption.
[b] Nerve transection.

bone, or both. Nondisplaced subcortical fractures typically parallel the cortex. Similar fractures may occur at the bone-implant interface.

HETEROTOPIC OSSIFICATION

Heterotopic ossification describes the presence of bone in soft tissues.[10,99] Heterotopic ossification is thought to occur as a response to local tissue trauma and undergoes different stages, starting with localized tissue inflammation, which may present clinically similar to infection. Soft tissue conglomerates do not demonstrate mineralization in the immature stage on radiographs and CT. In the mature stage, heterotopic ossification demonstrates cortex and cancellous bone matrix, similar to normal bone. Heterotopic bone formation poses challenges in the immature stage. Radiographic or CT follow-up helps to document progressive mineralization and maturing bone formation and confirm a working diagnosis.

Heterotopic ossification after TAA can cause pain and restricted joint mobility.[10,100] The reported incidence of heterotopic ossification after TAA ranges between 3.8% and 91%.[100,101] The wide range is likely due to different sizes, whereas large mechanically more meaningful clusters of heterotopic ossification are less common than smaller clusters. Risk factors may include male gender, use of undersized prosthesis, periosteal irritation, prolonged operation time, osseous debris, ankylosing spondylitis, infection, and previous history of heterotopic ossification in the operative bed or elsewhere.[10,99,102]

Modifications of Brooker's heterotopic ossification classification system after hip arthroplasty has been proposed for TAA[99,103,104] considering location, joint involvement, and osseous bridging.

Radiography is accurate for detecting larger mature areas of heterotopic ossification; however, immature heterotopic ossification and smaller areas of heterotopic ossification may go undetected. CT is most accurate for detecting mature heterotopic ossification of any size. CT is also more accurate than radiographs for diagnosing and localizing osseous bridging due to its cross-sectional nature and lack of projection superposition of structures.

Neither radiography nor CT may accurately depict immature heterotopic ossification because of the lack of mineralization.[105] MRI is most sensitive for visualizing immature heterotopic ossification; however, the MRI appearances are not specific, overlapping with localized soft tissue inflammation, soft tissue infection, and hematomas at various stages. On MRI, mature heterotopic ossification presents with all

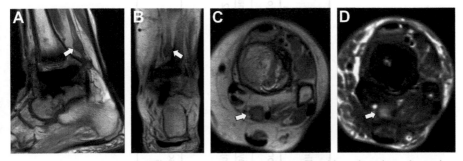

Fig. 15. MRI appearance of a tibial nerve transection after total ankle arthroplasty through an anterior implantation approach. Sagittal (A), coronal (B), and axial (C) intermediate-weighted and axial STIR (D) SEMAC MR images demonstrate a transected tibial nerve (arrows) with end-bulb neuroma.

Table 6
MRI findings in nerve injuries

	Neurapraxia	Axonotmesis	Neurotmesis
Nerve Conduction Study	Slowing or focal conduction block	Initial conduction block followed by recovery	Persistent conduction block
Electromyography	No or minimal denervation	Denervation occurs after 2–3 wk	Persistent denervation.
MRI of Injured Nerve	Abnormal T2 signal hyperintensity	Nerve enlargement and abnormal T2 signal hyperintensity distal to injury followed by normalization with nerve regeneration.	Nerve discontinuity with abnormal T2 signal hyperintensity distal to injury followed by delayed normalization.
MRI Muscle Denervation Effects	None	Muscle edema pattern, followed by normalization with nerve regeneration.	Muscle edema pattern, followed by progressive atrophy and fatty infiltration.

features and signatures of healthy bone, including cortex, cancellous matrix, and fatty marrow. However, because of the similarity with surrounding fatty tissues, mature heterotopic ossification may blend with the surrounding tissues, requiring careful imaging review for detection.[14]

POLYETHYLENE FRACTURE AND DISPLACEMENT

Ultra-high molecular weight polyethylene TAA components facilitate improved ankle motion and lower bone-implant interface loading. Polyethylene fractures and dislocation are rare.[10,23,106] Abnormal tibiotalar alignment and metallic markers displacement may indicate polyethylene fracture or dislocation on radiographs,[10] whereas CT is more accurate for differentiating dislocation and fracture.[10,23] MRI can directly visualize polyethylene fractures, displaced components, and small polyethylene fragments.[107]

NERVE INJURY AND NEUROPATHY

Nerve injury may occur intraoperatively or postoperatively secondary to periprosthetic fracture or dislocation. The tibial nerve is most susceptible to saw blade injury during tibial osteotomy.[108] Tibial nerve injury range from sensory deficits to loss of motor function, with plantar muscle denervation findings on MRI, including muscle edema and atrophy.[109] Anterior TAA implantation may be associated with injury and perineural scarring of the peroneal nerves anterior to the tibiotalar joint line.

Nerve injuries may not be detected on radiographs or CT. High-resolution ultrasonography is useful for characterizing tibial and peroneal nerves but requires advanced operator skills (**Table 4**).[110] MRI is most accurate for detecting and characterizing nerve injuries and neuropathies along the entire nerve course. MRI signs of nerve injury scale with injury severity, including nerve edema, nerve thickening, perineural scarring, neuroma-in-continuity formation, and nerve discontinuity (**Fig. 15**).[14,111]

MRI has the potential to assist in the initial noninvasive identification of nerve damage, distinguish between low-grade and high-grade nerve injuries, and determine the affected nerve segment, including instances of external compression. Delayed alterations in electromyography are common, whereas MRI can detect muscle edema related to denervation effects at an earlier stage.[112,113]

The Seddon classification of nerve injuries differentiates neurapraxia, axonotmesis, and neurotmesis (see **Table 5**). Neuropraxia and axonotmesis both involve macroscopic continuity of the injured nerves. Neuropraxia refers to myelin sheath disruption with axonal continuity, whereas axonotmesis indicates axonal disruption with varying degrees of endoneurium and perineurium disruptions. In neurotmesis, the nerve is completely severed. The Sunderland classification provides a more comprehensive categorization, ranging from classes I to V. Sunderland class I corresponds to neuropraxia. Classes II to IV represent various degrees of axonotmesis, involving axonal

Table 7	
MRI terminology and MRI findings of ligamentous injuries	
Ligamentous Integrity and MRI Terminology	**MRI Findings**
Interstitial injury	Increased proton density and T2 signal inside the ligament without visualized fiber disruption
Partial-thickness tear	Mixed disrupted and intact ligament fibers
Full-thickness tear	Disruption of all ligament fibers with optional fiber retraction and displacement of torn ligament ends.

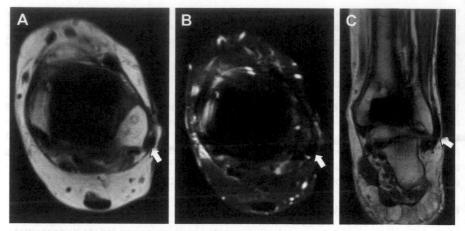

Fig. 16. MRI appearance of lateral peroneus longus dislocation after total ankle arthroplasty. Axial intermediate-weighted (*A*), axial STIR (*B*), and coronal intermediate-weighted (*C*) SEMAC MR images demonstrate lateral dislocation (*arrows*) of the peroneus longus tendon. The peroneus brevis tendon is located anatomically in the retromalleolar groove.

disruption (class II), disruption of the endoneurium (class III), and additional fascicular disruption (class IV). Class V represents neurotmesis.

Sunderland class I nerve injuries are mild and characterized by temporary clinical symptoms. MRI shows nerve edema (increased T2 signal) at the injury site, while muscle denervation effects are usually absent. These types of injuries typically have a full recovery of the affected nerves. In Sunderland class II-IV nerve injuries, motor function impairment is more common. In the acute phase, MRI shows nerve edema and enlargement with accompanying muscle edema in the distribution area of the affected nerve. Class

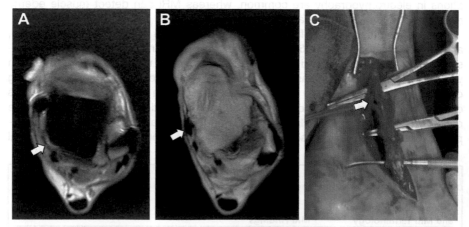

Fig. 17. MRI appearance of a partial posterior tibial tendon tear after total ankle arthroplasty. Axial intermediate-weighted (*A* and *B*) SEMAC MR images at (*A*) and below (*B*) the implant level demonstrate a segmentally attenuated posterior tibial tendon (*arrow* in *A*) near the posteromedial margin of the talar implant, indicating a partial thickness tear. The posterior tibial tendon is normal more distally (*arrow* in *B*). The surgical photo (*C*) demonstrates the focal partial thickness tear of the posterior tibial tendon (*arrow*).

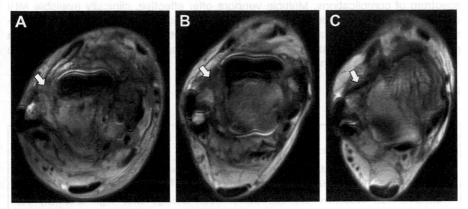

Fig. 18. MRI appearance of anterior talofibular ligament healing after total ankle arthroplasty. Axial intermediate-weighted SEMAC MR images 2 weeks (A), 3 months (B), and 9 months (C) after total ankle arthroplasty via a lateral approach demonstrate healing of the anterior talofibular ligament (arrows).

II injuries may exhibit mild muscle edema, while classes III and IV may show more pronounced edema. As axonal regeneration occurs, nerve and muscle edema may return to normal. However, the lack of regeneration indicates a Sunderland class IV injury, confirmed by MRI findings of internal nerve scarring. This scarring is evident as neuroma-in-continuity, characterized by fusiform nerve enlargement and a heterogeneous internal fascicular pattern (**Table 6**).[114] MRI is useful for distinguishing low-grade Sunderland class I-III injuries from high-grade Sunderland class IV-V injuries, with a sensitivity of 75% and a specificity of 83%. MR neurography findings such as architectural nerve distortion, fusiform enlargement, perineural fibrosis, nerve discontinuity, and skeletal muscle denervation findings are particularly valuable for differentiation.[115]

TENDON AND LIGAMENT ABNORMALITIES

The anterior approach of most ankle prosthesis systems is associated with limited visualization of the posterior tendons during implantation, including the flexor hallucis longus and posterior tibialis tendons.[116,117] Tendon injuries associated with TAA include direct iatrogenic trauma related to osteotomy and implantation and chronic repetitive contact with implant margins leading to tendon tears. On MRI, degenerative tendinopathy often presents as a cross-sectional expansion of tendon dimensions. The MRI spectrum of tendon tears ranges from interstitial to full-thickness tears (**Table 7**)[14,118,119] (**Fig. 16**). Tendon dislocation may occur secondary to retinaculum division or chronic retinaculum tearing (**Fig. 17**). MRI and ultrasonography are equally useful in demonstrating dislocated ankle tendons around TAA. MRI is the most accurate technique for assessing the medial and lateral collateral ligaments, sinus tarsi ligaments, spring ligaments, and the remainder of midfoot ligaments. Lateral TAA implantation requires the division of lateral collateral ligaments, which usually heal postoperatively (**Fig. 18**). MRI is useful for visualizing the medial and lateral collateral ligaments in suspected instability.

SUMMARY

Metal artifact reduction MRI is useful for evaluating pain and dysfunction after TAA due to its high accuracy in detecting and characterizing pain generators and a broad spectrum of complications. Multiple vendors offer effective, clinically available MRI techniques. Timely diagnosing TAA-related complications can aid management decisions, surgical planning, and prognosis. We use metal artifact reduction MRI as a problem-solving tool in patients with negative radiographs and to further characterize unclear radiographic findings.

CLINICS CARE POINTS

- Metal artifact reduction MRI after total arthroplasty has high accuracy for defining osseointegration, bone resorption, and osteolysis.
- Metal artifact reduction MRI after total arthroplasty is most accurate for diagnosing osseous stress reactions and radiographically occult nondisplaced fractures.
- Metal artifact reduction MRI can demonstrate findings with high specificity for periprosthetic joint infection after total ankle arthroplasty.
- MRI is the most accurate imaging test for evaluating tendon abnormalities, nerve injuries, and neuropathy after total ankle arthroplasty.

DISCLOSURE

A. Rashidi, C.D. Cesar Netto: Nothing to disclose. J. Fritz: Received institutional research support from Siemens AG, BTG International Ltd., United Kingdom, Zimmer Biomed, DePuy Synthes, QED, and SyntheticMR; is a scientific advisor for Siemens AG, Synthet-icMR, GE Healthcare, QED, BTG, ImageBiopsy Lab, Boston Scientific, and Mirata Pharma; and has shared patents with Siemens Healthcare, Johns Hopkins University, and NYU Grossman School of Medicine.

REFERENCES

1. Zaidi R, Cro S, Gurusamy K, et al. The outcome of total ankle replacement: a systematic review and meta-analysis. The bone & joint journal 2013;95(11): 1500–7.
2. Saltzman CL, Salamon ML, Blanchard GM, et al. Epidemiology of ankle arthritis: report of a consecutive series of 639 patients from a tertiary orthopaedic center. Iowa Orthop J 2005;25:44–6.
3. Society AOFaA. The use of total ankle replacement for the treatment of arthritic conditions of the ankle. Available at: http://wwwaofasorg/research/Documents/PositionStatement_TotalAnkleReplacement_April2018pdf Accessed April 12, 2018 April 2018.
4. Cody EA, Bejarano-Pineda L, Lachman JR, et al. Risk factors for failure of total ankle arthroplasty with a minimum five years of follow-up. Foot Ankle Int 2019; 40(3):249–58.
5. Lai WC, Arshi A, Ghorbanifarajzadeh A, et al. Incidence and predictors of early complications following primary and revision total ankle arthroplasty. Foot Ankle Surg 2019;25(6):785–9.
6. Hahn ME, Wright ES, Segal AD, et al. Comparative gait analysis of ankle arthrodesis and arthroplasty: initial findings of a prospective study. Foot Ankle Int 2012;33(4):282–9.
7. Nunley JA, Caputo AM, Easley ME, et al. Intermediate to long-term outcomes of the STAR Total Ankle Replacement: the patient perspective. JBJS 2012; 94(1):43–8.

8. Queen RM, De JB, Butler RJ, et al. J. Leonard Goldner Award 2011: changes in pain, function, and gait mechanics two years following total ankle arthroplasty performed with two modern fixed-bearing prostheses. Foot Ankle Int 2012; 33(7):535–42.

9. Lee JW, Im WY, Song SY, et al. Analysis of early failure rate and its risk factor with 2157 total ankle replacements. Sci Rep 2021;11(1):1901.

10. Mulcahy H, Chew FS. Current concepts in total ankle replacement for radiologists: complications. Am J Roentgenol 2015;205(6):1244–50.

11. Barg A, Elsner A, Chuckpaiwong B, et al. Insert position in three-component total ankle replacement. Foot Ankle Int 2010;31(9):754–9.

12. Walter SS, Fritz B, Kijowski R, et al. 2D versus 3D MRI of osteoarthritis in clinical practice and research. Skeletal Radiol 2023. https://doi.org/10.1007/s00256-023-04309-4.

13. Fritz J, Lurie B, Miller TT. Imaging of hip arthroplasty. Semin Muscoskel Radiol 2013;17(3):316–27.

14. Fritz J, Lurie B, Miller TT, et al. MR imaging of hip arthroplasty implants. Radiographics 2014;34(4):E106–32.

15. Fritz J, Lurie B, Potter HG. MR Imaging of Knee Arthroplasty Implants. Radiographics 2015;35(5):1483–501.

16. de Cesar Netto C, Fonseca LF, Fritz B, et al. Metal artifact reduction MRI of total ankle arthroplasty implants. Eur Radiol 2018;28(5):2216–27.

17. de Cesar Netto C, Schon LC, da Fonseca LF, et al. Metal artifact reduction MRI for total ankle replacement sagittal balance evaluation. Foot Ankle Surg 2019; 25(6):739–47.

18. Lu W, Pauly KB, Gold GE, et al. SEMAC: slice encoding for metal artifact correction in MRI. Magn Reson Med: An Official Journal of the International Society for Magnetic Resonance in Medicine 2009;62(1):66–76.

19. Fritz J, Lurie B, Miller TT. Imaging of hip arthroplasty. Semin Musculoskelet Radiol 2013;17(3):316–27.

20. Sofka CM. Postoperative magnetic resonance imaging of the foot and ankle. J Magn Reson Imag 2013;37(3):556–65.

21. Chen CA, Chen W, Goodman SB, et al. New MR imaging methods for metallic implants in the knee: artifact correction and clinical Impact. J Magn Reson Imag 2011;33(5):1121–7.

22. Mulcahy H, Chew FS. Current concepts in total ankle replacement for radiologists: features and imaging assessment. Am J Roentgenol 2015;205(5): 1038–47.

23. Omar IM, Abboud SF, Youngner JM. Imaging of Total Ankle Arthroplasty: Normal Imaging Findings and Hardware Complications. Semin Musculoskelet Radiol 2019;23(2):177–94.

24. Guyer AJ, Richardson EG. Current concepts review: total ankle arthroplasty. Foot Ankle Int 2008;29(2):256–64.

25. Yu J, Sheskier S. Total ankle replacement–evolution of the technology and future applications. Bull Hosp Jt Dis (2013) 2014;72(1):120–8.

26. Cracchiolo A III, DeOrio JK. Design features of current total ankle replacements: implants and instrumentation. JAAOS-Journal of the American Academy of Orthopaedic Surgeons 2008;16(9):530–40.

27. Kofoed H. Scandinavian total ankle replacement (STAR). Clin Orthop Relat Res 2004;424:73–9.

28. Mann JA, Mann RA, Horton E. STAR™ ankle: long-term results. Foot Ankle Int 2011;32(5):473–84.

29. Robati S, Salih A, Ghosh K, et al. The Scandinavian Total Ankle Replacement and the ideal biomechanical requirements of ankle replacements. J Orthop 2016;13(1):48–51.

30. Rush SM, Todd N. Salto Talaris fixed-bearing total ankle replacement system. Clin Podiatr Med Surg 2013;30(1):69–80.

31. Barg A, Bettin CC, Burstein AH, et al. Early clinical and radiographic outcomes of trabecular metal total ankle replacement using a transfibular approach. JBJS 2018;100(6):505–15.

32. Kim D-R, Choi YS, Potter HG, et al. Total ankle arthroplasty: an imaging overview. Korean J Radiol 2016;17(3):413–23.

33. Braito M, Dammerer D, Reinthaler A, et al. Effect of coronal and sagittal alignment on outcome after mobile-bearing total ankle replacement. Foot Ankle Int 2015;36(9):1029–37.

34. Low SBL, Kim M, Smith T, et al. The reliability of radiographic measures of total ankle replacement position: an analysis from the OARS cohort. Skeletal Radiol 2021;50(7):1411–7.

35. Hagen F, Fritz J, Mair A, et al. Dual-Energy Computed Tomography-Based Quantitative Bone Marrow Imaging in Non-Hematooncological Subjects: Associations with Age, Gender and Other Variables. J Clin Med 2022;11(14).

36. Ghodasara N, Yi PH, Clark K, et al. Postoperative Spinal CT: What the Radiologist Needs to Know. Radiographics 2019;39(6):1840–61.

37. Khodarahmi I, Haroun RR, Lee M, et al. Metal Artifact Reduction Computed Tomography of Arthroplasty Implants: Effects of Combined Modeled Iterative Reconstruction and Dual-Energy Virtual Monoenergetic Extrapolation at Higher Photon Energies. Invest Radiol 2018;53(12):728–35.

38. Navalkissoor S, Nowosinska E, Gnanasegaran G, et al. Single-photon emission computed tomography–computed tomography in imaging infection. Nucl Med Commun 2013;34(4):283–90.

39. Mertens J, Lootens T, Vercruysse J, et al. Bone SPECT/CT in the Evaluation of Painful Total Ankle Replacement: Validation of Localization Scheme and Preliminary Evaluation of Diagnostic Patterns. Clin Nucl Med 2021;46(5):361–8.

40. Lintz F, Mast J, Bernasconi A, et al. 3D, Weightbearing Topographical Study of Periprosthetic Cysts and Alignment in Total Ankle Replacement. Foot Ankle Int 2020;41(1):1–9.

41. Fritz B, Fritz J, Fucentese SF, et al. Three-dimensional analysis for quantification of knee joint space width with weight-bearing CT: comparison with non-weight-bearing CT and weight-bearing radiography. Osteoarthritis Cartilage 2022;30(5):671–80.

42. Jungmann PM, Agten CA, Pfirrmann CW, et al. Advances in MRI around metal. J Magn Reson Imag 2017;46(4):972–91.

43. Murthy S, Fritz J. Metal Artifact Reduction MRI in the Diagnosis of Periprosthetic Hip Joint Infection. Radiology 2023;306(3):e220134.

44. Kijowski R, Fritz J. Emerging Technology in Musculoskeletal MRI and CT. Radiology 2023;306(1):6–19.

45. Kumar NM, de Cesar Netto C, Schon LC, et al. Metal Artifact Reduction Magnetic Resonance Imaging Around Arthroplasty Implants: The Negative Effect of Long Echo Trains on the Implant-Related Artifact. Invest Radiol 2017;52(5):310–6.

46. Olsen RV, Munk PL, Lee MJ, et al. Metal artifact reduction sequence: early clinical applications. Radiographics 2000;20(3):699–712.

47. Burke CJ, Khodarahmi I, Fritz J. Postoperative MR Imaging of Joints: Technical Considerations. Magn Reson Imag Clin N Am 2022;30(4):583–600.

48. Ulbrich EJ, Sutter R, Aguiar RF, et al. STIR sequence with increased receiver bandwidth of the inversion pulse for reduction of metallic artifacts. AJR Am J Roentgenol 2012;199(6):W735–42.

49. Khodarahmi I, Fishman EK, Fritz J. Dedicated CT and MRI Techniques for the Evaluation of the Postoperative Knee. Semin Muscoskel Radiol 2018;22(4): 444–56.

50. Umans H, Cerezal L, Linklater J, et al. Postoperative MRI of the Ankle and Foot. Magn Reson Imag Clin N Am 2022;30(4):733–55.

51. Khodarahmi I, Keerthivasan MB, Brinkmann IM, et al. Modern Low-Field MRI of the Musculoskeletal System: Practice Considerations, Opportunities, and Challenges. Invest Radiol 2023;58(1):76–87.

52. Khodarahmi I, Brinkmann IM, Lin DJ, et al. New-Generation Low-Field Magnetic Resonance Imaging of Hip Arthroplasty Implants Using Slice Encoding for Metal Artifact Correction: First In Vitro Experience at 0.55 T and Comparison With 1.5 T. Invest Radiol 2022;57(8):517–26.

53. Khodarahmi I, Fritz J. The Value of 3 Tesla Field Strength for Musculoskeletal Magnetic Resonance Imaging. Invest Radiol 2021;56(11):749–63.

54. Khodarahmi I, Rajan S, Sterling R, et al. Heating of Hip Arthroplasty Implants During Metal Artifact Reduction MRI at 1.5- and 3.0-T Field Strengths. Invest Radiol 2021;56(4):232–43.

55. Khodarahmi I, Isaac A, Fishman EK, et al. Metal About the Hip and Artifact Reduction Techniques: From Basic Concepts to Advanced Imaging. Semin Musculoskelet Radiol 2019;23(3):e68–81.

56. Sutter R, Ulbrich EJ, Jellus V, et al. Reduction of metal artifacts in patients with total hip arthroplasty with slice-encoding metal artifact correction and view-angle tilting MR imaging. Radiology 2012;265(1):204–14.

57. Hayter CL, Koff MF, Shah P, et al. MRI after arthroplasty: comparison of MAVRIC and conventional fast spin-echo techniques. AJR Am J Roentgenol 2011;197(3): W405–11.

58. Fritz J, Ahlawat S, Demehri S, et al. Compressed Sensing SEMAC: 8-fold Accelerated High Resolution Metal Artifact Reduction MRI of Cobalt-Chromium Knee Arthroplasty Implants. Invest Radiol 2016;51(10):666–76.

59. Fritz J, Fritz B, Thawait GK, et al. Advanced metal artifact reduction MRI of metal-on-metal hip resurfacing arthroplasty implants: compressed sensing acceleration enables the time-neutral use of SEMAC. Skeletal Radiol 2016; 45(10):1345–56.

60. Fritz J, Guggenberger R, Del Grande F. Rapid Musculoskeletal MRI in 2021: Clinical Application of Advanced Accelerated Techniques. AJR Am J Roentgenol 2021;216(3):718–33.

61. Lin DJ, Walter SS, Fritz J. Artificial Intelligence-Driven Ultra-Fast Superresolution MRI: 10-Fold Accelerated Musculoskeletal Turbo Spin Echo MRI Within Reach. Invest Radiol 2023;58(1):28–42.

62. Fritz B, Yi PH, Kijowski R, et al. Radiomics and Deep Learning for Disease Detection in Musculoskeletal Radiology: An Overview of Novel MRI- and CT-Based Approaches. Invest Radiol 2023;58(1):3–13.

63. Fritz J, Kijowski R, Recht MP. Artificial intelligence in musculoskeletal imaging: a perspective on value propositions, clinical use, and obstacles. Skeletal Radiol 2022;51(2):239–43.

64. Del Grande F, Rashidi A, Luna R, et al. Five-Minute Five-Sequence Knee MRI Using Combined Simultaneous Multislice and Parallel Imaging Acceleration: Comparison with 10-Minute Parallel Imaging Knee MRI. Radiology 2021; 299(3):635–46.

65. Germann C, Filli L, Jungmann PM, et al. Prospective and longitudinal evolution of postoperative periprosthetic findings on metal artifact-reduced MR imaging in asymptomatic patients after uncemented total hip arthroplasty. Skeletal Radiol 2021;50(6):1177–88.

66. Khodarahmi I, Fritz J. Advanced MR Imaging after Total Hip Arthroplasty. The Clinical Impact. Semin Musculoskelet Radiol, 2017;21(5):616–29.

67. Bestic JM, Bancroft LW, Peterson JJ, et al. Postoperative imaging of the total ankle arthroplasty. Radiol Clin 2008;46(6):1003–15.

68. Bestic JM, Peterson JJ, DeOrio JK, et al. Postoperative evaluation of the total ankle arthroplasty. Am J Roentgenol 2008;190(4):1112–23.

69. Clough T, Alvi F, Majeed H. Total ankle arthroplasty: what are the risks? A Guide to Surgical Consent and a Review of the Literature. Bone Joint Lett J 2018; 100(10):1352–8.

70. Maffulli N, Longo UG, Locher J, et al. Outcome of ankle arthrodesis and ankle prosthesis: a review of the current status. Br Med Bull 2017;124(1):91–112.

71. Lawton CD, Butler BA, Dekker RG, et al. Total ankle arthroplasty versus ankle arthrodesis—a comparison of outcomes over the last decade. J Orthop Surg Res 2017;12(1):76.

72. Gadd RJ, Barwick TW, Paling E, et al. Assessment of a three-grade classification of complications in total ankle replacement. Foot Ankle Int 2014;35(5): 434–7.

73. Rippstein PF, Huber M, Coetzee JC, et al. Total ankle replacement with use of a new three-component implant. JBJS 2011;93(15):1426–35.

74. Conti SF, Wong YS. Complications of total ankle replacement. Clin Orthop Relat Res 2001;391:105–14.

75. Espinosa N, Klammer G, Wirth SH. Osteolysis in total ankle replacement: how does it work? Foot Ankle Clin 2017;22(2):267–75.

76. Singh G, Reichard T, Hameister R, et al. Ballooning osteolysis in 71 failed total ankle arthroplasties: Is hydroxyapatite a risk factor? Acta Orthop 2016;87(4): 401–5.

77. Tang H, Yang D, Guo S, et al. Digital tomosynthesis with metal artifact reduction for assessing cementless hip arthroplasty: a diagnostic cohort study of 48 patients. Skeletal Radiol 2016;45(11):1523–32.

78. Arcângelo J, Guerra-Pinto F, Pinto A, et al. Peri-prosthetic bone cysts after total ankle replacement. A systematic review and meta-analysis. Foot Ankle Surg 2019;25(2):96–105.

79. Abu-Amer Y, Darwech I, Clohisy JC. Aseptic loosening of total joint replacements: mechanisms underlying osteolysis and potential therapies. Arthritis Res Ther 2007;9(1):S6.

80. Yoon HS, Lee J, Choi WJ, et al. Periprosthetic osteolysis after total ankle arthroplasty. Foot Ankle Int 2014;35(1):14–21.

81. Walde TA, Weiland DE, Leung SB, et al. Comparison of CT, MRI, and radiographs in assessing pelvic osteolysis: a cadaveric study. Clin Orthop Relat Res 2005;437:138–44.

82. Claus AM, Engh CA Jr, Sychterz CJ, et al. Radiographic definition of pelvic osteolysis following total hip arthroplasty. JBJS 2003;85(8):1519–26.

83. Wiewiorski M, Barg A, Hoerterer H, et al. Risk factors for wound complications in patients after elective orthopedic foot and ankle surgery. Foot Ankle Int 2015; 36(5):479–87.
84. Patton D, Kiewiet N, Brage M. Infected total ankle arthroplasty: risk factors and treatment options. Foot Ankle Int 2015;36(6):626–34.
85. Kessler B, Sendi P, Graber P, et al. Risk factors for periprosthetic ankle joint infection: a case-control study. JBJS 2012;94(20):1871–6.
86. Alrashidi Y, Galhoum AE, Wiewiorski M, et al. How to diagnose and treat infection in total ankle arthroplasty. Foot Ankle Clin 2017;22(2):405–23.
87. Vaz S, Ferreira TC, Salgado L, et al. Bone scan usefulness in patients with painful hip or knee prosthesis: 10 situations that can cause pain, other than loosening and infection. Eur J Orthop Surg Traumatol 2017;27(2):147–56.
88. Plate A, Weichselbaumer V, Schüpbach R, et al. Diagnostic accuracy of (99m) Tc-antigranulocyte SPECT/CT in patients with osteomyelitis and orthopaedic device-related infections: A retrospective analysis. Int J Infect Dis 2020;91: 79–86.
89. Fritz J, Meshram P, Stern SE, et al. Diagnostic Performance of Advanced Metal Artifact Reduction MRI for Periprosthetic Shoulder Infection. J Bone Joint Surg Am 2022;104(15):1352–61.
90. Alaia EF, Chhabra A, Simpfendorfer CS, et al. MRI nomenclature for musculoskeletal infection. Skeletal Radiol 2021;50(12):2319 47.
91. Deshmukh S, Omar IM. Imaging of Hip Arthroplasties: Normal Findings and Hardware Complications. Semin Musculoskelet Radiol 2019;23(2):162–76.
92. Buechel Sr FF, Buechel FF Jr, Pappas MJ Jr. Ten-year evaluation of cementless Buechel-Pappas meniscal bearing total ankle replacement. Foot Ankle Int 2003; 24(6):462–72.
93. Labek G, Todorov S, Iovanescu L, et al. Outcome after total ankle arthroplasty— results and findings from worldwide arthroplasty registers. Int Orthop 2013; 37(9):1677–82.
94. Manegold S, Haas NP, Tsitsilonis S, et al. Periprosthetic fractures in total ankle replacement: classification system and treatment algorithm. JBJS 2013;95(9): 815–20.
95. Cadden AR. Imaging in total ankle replacement. Semin Musculoskelet Radiol 2012;16(3):205–16.
96. Glazebrook MA, Arsenault K, Dunbar M. Evidence-based classification of complications in total ankle arthroplasty. Foot Ankle Int 2009;30(10):945–9.
97. Rupp M, Kern S, Ismat A, et al. Computed tomography for managing periprosthetic femoral fractures. A retrospective analysis. BMC Muscoskel Disord 2019; 20(1):258.
98. Yi PH, Della Valle CJ, Fishman EK, et al. Imaging of Periprosthetic Fractures of the Hip and Knee. Semin Roentgenol 2021;56(1):90–105.
99. Manegold S, Springer A, Landvoigt K, et al. Heterotopic ossification after total ankle replacement: The role of prosthesis alignment. Foot Ankle Surg 2017; 23(2):122–7.
100. Brunner S, Barg A, Knupp M, et al. The Scandinavian total ankle replacement: long-term, eleven to fifteen-year, survivorship analysis of the prosthesis in seventy-two consecutive patients. JBJS 2013;95(8):711–8.
101. King CM, Schuberth JM, Christensen JC, et al. Relationship of alignment and tibial cortical coverage to hypertrophic bone formation in Salto Talaris® total ankle arthroplasty. J Foot Ankle Surg 2013;52(3):355–9.

102. Wan DD, Choi WJ, Shim DW, et al. Short-term clinical and radiographic results of the Salto mobile total ankle prosthesis. Foot Ankle Int 2018;39(2):155–65.
103. Choi W, Lee J. Heterotopic ossification after total ankle arthroplasty. Journal of bone and joint surgery British 2011;93(11):1508–12.
104. Brooker AF, Bowerman JW, Robinson RA, et al. Ectopic ossification following total hip replacement: incidence and a method of classification. JBJS 1973;55(8):1629–32.
105. Gao G-Y, Zhang X, Dai L-H, et al. Heterotopic ossification after arthroscopy for hip impingement syndrome. Chin Med J 2019;132(7):827–33.
106. Scott AT, Nunley JA. Polyethylene fracture following STAR ankle arthroplasty: a report of three cases. Foot Ankle Int 2009;30(4):375–9.
107. Li AE, Sneag DB, Miller TT, et al. MRI of polyethylene tibial inserts in total knee arthroplasty: normal and abnormal appearances. Am J Roentgenol 2016;206(6):1264–71.
108. Primadi A, Xu H-X, Yoon T-R, et al. Neurologic injuries after primary total ankle arthroplasty: prevalence and effect on outcomes. J Foot Ankle Res 2015;8(1):55.
109. Reb CW, McAlister JE, Hyer CF, et al. Posterior ankle structure injury during total ankle replacement. J Foot Ankle Surg 2016;55(5):931–4.
110. Fritz B, Fritz J. MR Imaging-Ultrasonography Correlation of Acute and Chronic Foot and Ankle Conditions. Magn Reson Imag Clin N Am 2023;31(2):321–35.
111. Chhabra A, Deshmukh SD, Lutz AM, et al. Neuropathy Score Reporting and Data System: A Reporting Guideline for MRI of Peripheral Neuropathy With a Multicenter Validation Study. AJR Am J Roentgenol 2022;219(2):279–91.
112. Kamath S, Venkatanarasimha N, Walsh MA, et al. MRI appearance of muscle denervation. Skeletal Radiol 2008;37(5):397–404.
113. Chhabra A, Deshmukh SD, Lutz AM, et al. Neuropathy Score Reporting and Data System (NS-RADS): MRI Reporting Guideline of Peripheral Neuropathy Explained and Reviewed. Skeletal Radiol 2022;51(10):1909–22.
114. Chhabra A, Ahlawat S, Belzberg A, et al. Peripheral nerve injury grading simplified on MR neurography: As referenced to Seddon and Sunderland classifications. Indian J Radiol Imag 2014;24(3):217–24.
115. Ahlawat S, Belzberg AJ, Fayad LM. Utility of Magnetic Resonance Imaging for Predicting Severity of Sciatic Nerve Injury. J Comput Assist Tomogr 2018;42(4):580–7.
116. Peters PG, Miller SD. Flexor hallucis longus tendon laceration as a complication of total ankle arthroplasty. Foot Ankle Int 2013;34(1):148–9.
117. Criswell B, Hunt K, Kim T, et al. Association of short-term complications with procedures through separate incisions during total ankle replacement. Foot Ankle Int 2016;37(10):1060–4.
118. Park EH, de Cesar Netto C, Fritz J. MRI in Acute Ankle Sprains: Should We Be More Aggressive with Indications? Foot Ankle Clin 2023;28(2):231–64.
119. Fritz B, Fritz J. MR Imaging of Acute Knee Injuries: Systematic Evaluation and Reporting. Radiol Clin 2023;61(2):261–80.
120. Khodarahmi I, Khanuja HS, Stern SE, et al. Compressed Sensing SEMAC MRI of Hip, Knee, and Ankle Arthroplasty Implants: A 1.5-T and 3-T Intrapatient Performance Comparison for Diagnosing Periprosthetic Abnormalities. AJR Am J Roentgenol 2023. https://doi.org/10.2214/AJR.23.29380.

SPECT/CT of Total Ankle Arthroplasty

Alena Richter, MD, Christina Stukenborg-Colsman, MD,
Christian Plaass, MD*

KEYWORDS

- Total ankle arthroplasty • Total ankle replacement • SPECT • Imaging
- Prosthetic loosening • Periprosthetic pain • Revision surgery

KEY POINTS

- SPECT/CT can complement clinical examination and radiological imaging in chronic pain after total ankle arthroplasty by providing metabolic information.
- High diagnostic accuracy of SPECT/CT in diagnosing gutter impingement and prosthetic loosening of total ankle arthroplasty has been shown.
- SPECT/CT can provide additional information in inconclusive diagnostic findings and can help to differentiate symptoms in painful total ankle arthroplasty.
- Evidence of diagnostic accuracy of SPECT/CT in periprosthetic joint infection of the ankle is rare but seems to provide additional information.

COMPLICATIONS FOLLOWING TOTAL ANKLE ARTHROPLASTY

With the introduction of second and third-generation total ankle arthroplasty (TAA), concomitant decreasing complication rates and prolonged implant survival there is a significant increase in total ankle replacements over the last decades.[1,2] Despite high patient satisfaction rates, up to 60% of the patients report persistent ankle pain, swelling, and stiffness.[3-5] The need for secondary procedures has been observed in up to 39%[6] and also relatively high failure rates of 10% to 20% within the first 10 years are reported in the literature.[7] Therefore, surgeons must be aware of proper diagnostic evaluation and therapeutic management particularly as the cause of persistent pain can be difficult to identify. Meticulous diagnostic workup is required to find the best conservative or operative treatment, as these reach from specific local debridement and implant retention to revision TAA, arthrodesis or even below-knee amputation.[8,9]

Department for Foot and Ankle surgery, DIAKOVERE Annastift, Orthopedic Clinic of the Hannover Medical School, Anna-von-Borries Strasse 1-7, Hannover 30625, Germany
* Corresponding author.
E-mail address: christian.plaass@diakovere.de

Foot Ankle Clin N Am 28 (2023) 493–507
https://doi.org/10.1016/j.fcl.2023.04.001
1083-7515/23/© 2023 Elsevier Inc. All rights reserved.

CAUSES OF ANKLE PAIN AFTER TOTAL ANKLE ARTHROPLASTY

Migratory complications are the most common cause of failure including aseptic loosening and subsidence occurring in 8.7% and 10.7% of primary TAA respectively.[10] Patients mostly describe a deep pain inside the joint on the initiation of weight bearing or after sedentary activity.[11] Mechanical overload or progressive cyst formation also can provoke fractures. Postoperative fractures occur in up to 4% of primary TAA and can cause significant pain.[12,13] Fatigue fractures can cause unspecific deep ankle pain and are sometimes not visible on x-ray and MRI near the joint, especially in the initial phase.[14]

Another common pathology of delayed complications following TAA is the formation of bony overgrowth observed in 63% of total ankle replacements, partially with concomitant impingement.[15] Other authors report an incidence of heterotopic ossifications of about 90%.[16,17] In a recent meta-analysis impingement was found as one of the most frequent postoperative complications occurring in approximately 6% after TAA.[18] Gutter discomfort can result in case of inadequate intraoperative gutter debridement, exacerbated by varus or valgus malalignment or developing ossifications.[19] Rippstein and colleagues also reported impingement between the talar component and the malleoli resulting presumably in medial pain.[20]

Arthrofibrosis and ankle stiffness caused by overstuffing of the ankle with too large implant components or insufficient bone resection of the distal tibia has to be included in the differential diagnosis.[8] Further explanations for persistent ankle pain comprises instability and malposition of prosthetic components.[21] Discomfort of surrounding joints and structures can also be wrongly assigned to the ankle prosthesis. In particular, stiffness of the ankle can intensify pain in the subtalar joint. Degeneration of adjacent joints can develop or become painful.[8] It is mandatory to discern adjacent etiologies of pain from TAA failure or discomfort.

Besides structural and hardware problems, periprosthetic joint infection has to be excluded. This can cause persistent ankle pain affecting 3% to 5% of patients after TAA.[22,23] Especially chronic infections generating moderate symptoms without specific signs of inflammation, normal laboratory values and negative aspirate tend to be misdiagnosed.[24]

It is often difficult to differentiate the cause of pain after TAA clinically. Therefore, imaging modalities are necessary for analysis.

IMAGING AFTER TOTAL ANKLE ARTHROPLASTY

Plain weight-bearing radiographs are the first imaging tool to evaluate prosthesis and bony alignment with special regard to loosening zones and subsidence of the tibial or the talar component. Furthermore, fractures and osteophytes suggesting gutter impingement can be depicted.[25,26]

Nevertheless, radiographs are often nonpathologic or underrate loosening signs. Hanna and colleagues[27] found 87% of periprosthetic lesions in CT were inadequately characterized in plain radiographs with osteolytic lesions being three times larger on CT than on radiography. Linear lucencies greater than 2 mm are considered to be significant.[28] Bonnin and colleagues[7] reported tibial or talar cysts of about 5 mm in 22% after TAA at an average follow-up of approximately 9 years.

MRI is used for many foot and ankle problems due to its adequate resolution and excellent soft tissue contrast. But in postoperative state with embedded metal components the value of MRI is limited, though metal-suppression mode is available.[29]

Overall, radiographic abnormalities and complications have been observed in up to 62% after TAA, even if it is not inevitably linked to prosthetic failure or clinical symptoms.[30] The common limitation of the aforementioned imaging tools is the inability to determine structural findings being symptomatic for the patient. Since revision surgery of TAA is an important psychologic and physical burden for the patient and also leads to high economic costs, unnecessary revision surgeries have to be avoided.[31,32]

BONE SCINTIGRAPHY

Bone scintigraphy enables a functional diagnostic in contrast to radiographs presenting only structural and anatomical conditions. Compared to other nuclear medicine scans such as positron emission tomography (PET), scintigraphy and its variations are cheaper and have a higher availability.[33] After injection the radiopharmaceutical accumulates in metabolically active areas of the skeleton resulting in enhancements in planar bone scintigraphy images. The choice of a specific radiopharmaceutical depends on the analyzed tissue. For Bone, mostly Tc-99-m-labeled diphosphonates are used, for example, methylene diphosphonate, hydroxymethylene diphosphonate, or hydroxyethylene diphosphonate. Binding to hydroxyapatite as part of the inorganic bone matrix, regions of enhanced vascularity and osteoblastic activity can be detected.[34-37] Even a 5% change in bone metabolism induces a corresponding signal in nuclear imaging, whereas in radiographs and CT a bone loss of 40% to 50% is warranted to be detected as lucency zones.[37,38] Therefore, scintigraphy enables early diagnosis of bone dysfunctions and has emerged to an important tool in the diagnostics of metastases with a sensitivity between 85% and 96%, though the detection of purely lytic metastases is limited.[39]

Diagnostic accuracy, especially in infections, was increased up to 70% by triple-phase bone scan. Combination of bone and gallium-67 imaging, a radiotracer accumulating in infections, showed further improved sensitivity and specificity in the diagnosis of infective bony conditions like osteomyelitis and periprosthetic joint infections reaching an accuracy up to 80%. Further improvement in diagnostic accuracy of infections was reached by labeled leukocyte imaging. Pure leukocyte imaging is limited by the natural accumulation of white blood cells in the healthy red bone marrow resulting in false positive diagnoses of osteomyelitis. Combination of leukocyte/marrow imaging finally was shown to have the highest sensitivity and specificity with an overall accuracy of about 90% in diagnosing periprosthetic joint infection compared to bone, gallium/bone, and leukocyte/bone imaging.[24,40]

Despite the relevant results of bone scintigraphy, low spatial resolution, and two-dimensional characteristics result in the inability to exactly localize pathologic enhancements and therefore to carry out a specific diagnosis in anatomically complex structures like the foot.

SPECT AND SPECT/CT

Single Positron Emission Computer Tomography (SPECT), once introduced in the 1960s and 1970s, also uses Tc-99-m-labeled diphosphonates accumulating in regions of enhanced bone metabolism. In contrast to plane scintigraphy, three-dimensional images are generated by one or several rotating gamma-cameras detecting single photons. But even with modern SPECT-cameras the resolution and accurate localization are limited by the lack of anatomical markers.[41,42]

Along with further developments in nuclear medicine, radiological assessment improved enabling high anatomical resolution by multislice CT scans. In 1999, the fusion of SPECT and CT was introduced as hybrid imaging technology joining the high sensitivity of functional imaging and the high specificity of morphologic imaging allowing the correlation of tracer uptake and anatomical landmarks.[43]

Due to the combined presentation multimodality SPECT/CT is a useful tool to precisely localize main pathologies in diffuse pain symptoms, especially in anatomically complex regions like the foot. SPECT/CT was found to provide additional information compared to planar scintigraphy and therefore can influence further management.[44] Correlation of spatial diagnostics and pain generation was confirmed by pain relief after injections guided by pathologic tracer uptake.[45,46]

Regarding the amount of radioactivity administered, SPECT has generally a lower effective dose than PET. The effective dose of bone scintigraphy for an adult is approximately 3-4 mSv. The additional CT adds less than 0.1 mSv.[33]

SPECT-CT IN ORTHOPEDIC INDICATIONS
Painful Total Hip and Knee Arthroplasty and Lower Back Pain

SPECT-CT is already an established tool in orthopedics. Its use has been shown very beneficial in low back pain and after total joint arthroplasty.[42] SPECT/CT has been established as a second-line tool in the diagnostic regime of periprosthetic disorders in hip and knee showing high diagnostic accuracy.[47] Hirschmann and colleagues[48] evaluated SPECT/CT after totoal knee arthroplasty (TKA) in a prospective study analyzing 100 patients. Findings of SPECT/CT influenced further therapy in 85% and matched intraoperative diagnoses in 97%. Particularly, femoral loosening and patella-femoral osteoarthritis have been found in SPECT/CT with a specificity of 100%. The benefit of hybrid imaging in diagnosing implant loosening and patellofemoral osteoarthritis has been confirmed by Murer and colleagues[49] reporting a sensitivity and specificity for aseptic loosening of 95% and 100% respectively. For patellofemoral osteoarthritis, a sensitivity of 96.5% and a specificity of 96.2% were found. This high diagnostic accuracy for implant loosening has been affirmed in a meta-analysis by Barnsley and colleagues comparing SPECT/CT arthrography with plane bone scintigraphy and ^{18}F-FDG-PET.[50] Based on imaging findings and assured diagnosis a standard localization scheme presenting typical pathology-related uptake patterns was described.[51] Likewise, Mathis and colleagues[52] identified special activity patterns in SPECT-CT corresponding to component-positioning of TKA, instability, and patella-related problems. Patella mal tracking based on tibial malrotation resulting in specific tracer enhancements has been described before.[53] Therefore, biomechanical malfunction can be revealed emphasizing the effect of implant position on surrounding biologic structures. In unicondylar knee arthroplasty SPECT/CT has been proven to deliver additional diagnostic findings in case of implant loosening and osteoarthritis in the other compartments of the knee.[54] Besides clinical advantages, also economic profits are described. Van der Wyngaert found that SPECT/CT is highly cost-saving and superior to standard CT or MARS-MRI (Metal Artifact Reduction Sequence) in painful TKA.[55]

Similarly, SPECT/CT in painful total hip arthroplasty (THA) has been evaluated in diagnosing aseptic loosening showing a diagnostic accuracy up to 100%[56,57] and therefore outperforming MRI.[58] Comprising a multiplicity of causes for persistent periprosthetic pain a lower diagnostic efficacy of 61% has been reported for THA[59] compared to the diagnostic accuracy of 97% in TKA.[48] This unequal diagnostic accuracy has been confirmed by Arican and colleagues.[60] Nevertheless, SPECT/CT has been proven to deliver specific imaging characteristics for several pathologies in painful THA[61] including aseptic loosening,[62] symptomatic heterotopic ossification,[63] periprosthetic fractures[64] and tendinopathies[61]

Distinction between aseptic and septic loosening is difficult as both pathologies are characterized by diffuse tracer enhancements at the bone/implant interface particularly in the first year after implantation due to an individual basic tracer acquisition.[40]

Therefore, SPECT/CT is recommended to rule out but not to confirm periprosthetic joint infection based on it's high negative predictive value. SPECT/CT using Tc-99m-labeled antigranulocyte antibody had a sensitivity of 89% and a specificity of 73% resulting in a positive predictive value of 57% and a negative predictive value of 94% in diagnosing infections in TKA and THA.[65] Nevertheless, hybrid imaging of white blood cells and bone marrow has been shown to have the highest diagnostic accuracy of about 90%.[66]

The third common application field of SPECT/CT in orthopedics is chronic lower back pain. A high incidence of asymptomatic degenerative changes can interfere with the cause of pain complicating the detection of the underlying pathology.[67] Sensitivity of SPECT/CT in detecting facet arthropathy has been confirmed by high success rates in pain relief after facet infiltrations guided by SPECT/CT imaging.[68] Accordingly, this imaging tool is also beneficial in determining segments for spine fusion.[67] Also in vertebral fractures SPECT/CT is able to reveal acute fractures in a multiply affected osteoporotic spine resulting in a significant higher satisfaction rate after vertebroplasty compared to preoperative planar bone imaging.[69] Considering enhanced basic tracer uptake up to 1 year after surgical therapy in the back area, SPECT/CT is also used to reveal causes of persistent pain comprising hardware loosening, pseudarthrosis, adjacent instability, active degeneration of facet joint, sacroiliac joints and discs. According to aseptic loosening after THA and TKA, SPECT/CT shows a high diagnostic accuracy with a sensitivity of 100% and a specificity of 89.7% in diagnosing hardware loosening after lumbar fusion.[70]

SPECT/CT IN FOOT AND ANKLE

SPECT/CT is gaining in importance in foot and ankle surgery delivering additional information in the diagnostic work up of different pathologies.[71] Recently, Eelsing and colleagues[72] systematically reviewed the added value of SPECT/CT in the management of foot and ankle pain reporting an overall improvement in diagnostics compared to clinical examination and plain radiography in 60%. Change of further management is described in 62% leading to an improvement of pain symptoms in 92%. Besides radiography and clinical evaluation, also MRI, planar bone scintigraphy and CT and SPECT only have been outperformed in diagnostic accuracy by hybrid imaging in SPECT/CT. Mohan and colleagues[44] developed a diagnostic algorithm rating SPECT/CT as a useful tool in patients with conditions of assumed bone pathology rather than soft tissue discomforts. Here, SPECT/CT has been shown to provide additional information in 80% of the patients and led to more accurate localization of pathologies in 64% of cases compared to plain scintigraphy influencing therapeutic management in about 50%. Accordingly, the most relevant applications of SPECT/CT in foot and ankle pain include osteoarthritis, malalignments, osteochondral lesions, stress fractures, symptomatic accessory bones, tarsal coalition, diabetic feet, and postoperative pain.[26,73] Since the anatomy of the midfoot is highly complex, localization of active osteoarthritis is quite difficult. Advantages of SPECT/CT in localizing symptomatic changes with high inter- and intra-rater reliabilities have been reported.[74,75] SPECT/CT-guided injections in symptomatic degenerative pathologies in the ankle, hindfoot, and midfoot resulted in pain improvement in 86% to 88%[45,46] and SPECT/CT-guided management showed symptom improvement in more than 90% of patients particularly in Lisfranc- and Chopart-joints.[75] Osteochondral lesions (OCL) are a common cause of ankle pain since both chronic ankle instability and acute ankle sprains can result in osteochondral lesions of the talus. Nevertheless, there are also asymptomatic osteochondral lesions. Like in osteoarthritic changes, also in OCL SPECT/CT shows a high correlation between tracer uptake and pain, confirmed by pain reductions after local anesthesia injection based on SPECT/CT findings.[76] Meftah and colleagues[77] compared SPECT/CT with MRI in characterizing talar OCL. They highlighted early detection of OCL and accurate assessment of lesion size in SPECT/CT resulting in an optimized preoperative planning and postoperative management in case of persistent pain.

Besides degenerative changes and sterile inflammatory pathologies, SPECT/CT was also used in diagnosing and observing progress of osteomyelitis in diabetic feet showing a high sensitivity up to 90% but a lower specificity of 56%.[78,79] Dual isotope scanning using Tc-99-m-labeled HDP and In-111-labeled white blood cells reached a higher accuracy with a sensitivity of 95% and a specificity of 94% than bone scan or leukocyte scanning alone.[80]

Though limited diagnostic value in soft tissue pathologies, the use of SPECT/CT in impingement, Achilles tendinitis, and plantar fasciitis has been reported.[81,82] Showing a similar sensitivity but a slightly higher specificity compared to MRI,[83] SPECT/CT can provide additional findings particularly in inconclusive symptoms and diagnostic results.[84]

Overall, SPECT/CT is recommended in complex ambiguous foot pathologies delivering additional information for treatment optimization.[26,71,85]

SPECT/CT IN PAINFUL TOTAL ANKLE ARTHROPLASTY

Managing chronic ankle pain after total ankle replacement is challenging since cause of pain is diverse. Limitations of radiography, CT, and MRI have been described before. Especially, imaging findings do not necessarily accord to clinical symptoms. High rates of tibial and talar cyst formations without indication for revision surgery are reported in the literature.[86,87]

Correlation of sensitive functional evaluation and specific structural imaging may help to overcome these limitations. Patients undergone prior surgery with retained metal implants and presumably suffering from bony pathologies rather than soft tissue disorders have been shown to mostly benefit from SPECT/CT.[44,88]

Accordingly, the diagnostic value of SPECT/CT in periprosthetic ankle pain has been confirmed by high congruence of imaging findings and intraoperative diagnosis. Mertens and colleagues[89] reported a concordance rate of 95.8% developing a localization scheme of periprosthetic tracer uptake according to the validated Bruderholz localization scheme for knee replacements.[51] Similarly, Gurbani and colleagues[90] found consistent findings between SPECT-CT and clinical or intraoperative findings in 89.2% and 92.9% respectively. In contrast, MRI findings were consistent with clinical findings in 36.8% and in 57.9% of the cases in which MRI and SPECT/CT were performed. The most common findings in SPECT-CT were aseptic loosening and impingement. Further diagnoses were malalignment, cyst formation, subtalar arthritis, and infection.

Nevertheless, the use of SPECT/CT after TAA is limited by the lack of information about periprosthetic tracer uptake in asymptomatic patients. A certain level of physiologic uptake after TAA is known, but the degree of this and changes over time have not been described.[90] In THA increased enhancement is described up to 2 years post-implantation depending on the use of bone cement and implant surface.[91] Some authors recommend serial imaging for detection of pathologic changes in tracer uptake, whereas persistent tracer enhancement has been reported in some segments 12 to 24 month after hip arthroplasty without any evidence of pathologic cause. Persistent tracer uptake beyond 1 year after implantation was more frequent in porous-coated hip replacement than in cemented implants reflecting a normal healing process.[92] Since total ankle replacements are mainly noncemented types having rough surfaces, prolonged periprosthetic tracer enhancement is conceivable. Equally, postsurgical tracer uptake is reported for total knee arthroplasty with individual time course.[93] Within the first 12 to 18-months differentiation between aseptic and septic loosening therefore has been proven to be difficult.[94] Because of those inconsistent periprosthetic uptake patterns a general orientation on knee and hip replacements does not seem to be reliable. Therefore, a specific evaluation of basal tracer uptake after ankle replacements is necessary. Mertens and colleagues[89] also found a persistent diffuse uptake surrounding asymptomatic total ankle prosthesis 2.5 years after implantation.

SPECT/CT IN ASEPTIC LOOSENING AND CYST FORMATION AFTER TOTAL ANKLE ARTHROPLASTY

Although being the most common cause of TAA failure, diagnosing implant loosening is often impeded by asymptomatic cyst formation or lucency lines. On the other hand, aseptic loosening may often be misdiagnosed. In a recent study, high incidences of medial talar prosthesis loosening or poor bony ongrowth not diagnosed in conventional radiographs have been identified in SPECT/CT.[21] Loosening of TAA has been described to affect the talar component in only 11%.[30] Mason and colleagues[21] found insufficient talar component integration with enhanced tracer uptake in 12 of 14 patients with negative radiograph findings. Accordingly, the authors claim that the incidence of talar loosening might be underestimated in routine diagnostics presumably due to the complex structure of the talar part of the prosthesis. As well, Gurbani and colleagues[90] found aseptic loosening in 11 of 28 patients undergoing revision surgery. In 2 patients both tibial and talar components were affected showing tracer uptake both at the tibial and the talar interface. The other 9 revisions only showed talar loosening with tracer enhancement only beneath the talar component. Nevertheless, Gurbani and colleagues also assumed loosening in 2 of 28 cases not confirmed intraoperatively resulting in a false positive rate of 15%. In a comparable study, Mertens and colleagues[89] found aseptic loosening in 25% (5 out of 22) affecting only the tibial component. They suggested a localization scheme based on the one of TKA.[51] Thereby, the tibia component was divided into 8 areas (anterior medial, anterior central, anterior lateral, posterior medial, posterior central, posterior lateral, tibia shaft, and tibia tip) and the talus into 9 areas. Activity was scored on a 5-point scale (1 = no increased uptake, 3 = moderate increased uptake, 5 = marked increased uptake). Hereby, a concordance rate between SPECT/CT imaging and intraoperative findings of 95.8% has been achieved. **Fig. 1** shows radiographs, CT-scans, and SPECT-CT images in a patient with cyst formation and subsequent fracture and prosthetic loosening. Overall, the use of hybrid imaging with SPECT/CT can increase the sensitivity of diagnosing aseptic loosening after TAA.

SPECT/CT IN GUTTER IMPINGEMENT AFTER TOTAL ANKLE ARTHROPLASTY

Gutter impingement structurally presents with talomalleolar degeneration and gutter ossification.[95] If plain radiographs or CT-scans are not conclusive, nuclear imaging with SPECT/CT can help to confirm diagnosis showing an enhanced tracer uptake at the gutters medially or laterally.[19] Mertens and colleagues[89] diagnosed gutter impingement in 12 of 22 analyzed TAA by detecting a significantly enhanced tracer uptake at the gutters. As well, Gurbani and colleagues[90] found gutter impingement with enhanced tracer uptake localized at the gutters in 7 of 28 revision surgeries. Specific treatment comprising infiltrations, debridement, and analgesics resulted in pain relief

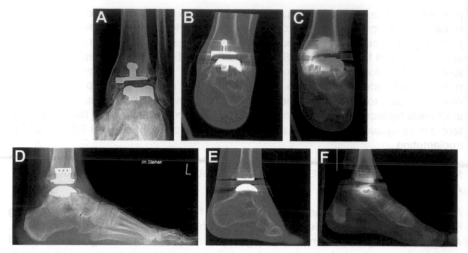

Fig. 1. Talar cyst formation and subsequent prosthetic loosening after total ankle arthroplasty. A 50-year-old man presented in our clinic with acute pain 8 years after implantation of total ankle prosthesis (Tornier Salto) and subtalar arthrodesis. (*A, D*): Conventional radiographs showed tibial stress shielding without other abnormalities. (*B, E*): CT imaging reveals talar cyst formation. (*C, F*): To exclude prosthetic loosening, SPECT/CT was performed depicting high grade osteolysis with tracer enhancement presumably in talar bone (**Fig.** 1B, C, E, F). Acute pain was likely due to acute osteolytic fracture. Therapy options comprised cyst filling and revision of the talar component or arthrodesis of the ankle joint.

in 90% to 100%. Also in other studies pain relief after appropriate debridement of the gutters is described in 84% of affected patients with symptomatic gutter impingement.[96] Therefore, using SPECT/CT can help to introduce a specific therapy and avoid unnecessary revision surgeries.

SPECT/CT IN PERIPROSTHETIC FRACTURES AFTER TOTAL ANKLE ARTHROPLASTY

Occult periprosthetic fractures after TAA affect up to 4% of patients after primary TAA.[12,13] Mertens and colleagues[89] describe diagnosing periprosthetic fractures after TAA with SPECT/CT. Diagnosis of periprosthetic fracture was met in 5 of 22 scans showing focal enhancement in SPECT/CT. Structural fracture lines were obvious in CT-scans without nuclear imaging in 3 patients. Two cases did not show any cortical abnormality and were treated as stress fractures. Generally, stress fractures are mainly diagnosed by MRI depicting the osseus edema more sensitive than other imaging modalities. Since its use is limited nearby metal implants, SPECT/CT was shown to be advantageous.[14] Most common localization of periprosthetic fractures in the ankle is the medial malleolus.[18] There is a multiplicity of differential diagnoses in this area comprising gutter impingement or tendinopathies. Nevertheless, after appropriate therapy of temporary immobilization in 4 patients and screw fixation in 1 patient pain relief is reported confirming correct diagnosis in the before mentioned study.[89]

SPECT/CT IN DIAGNOSING OSTEOARTHRITIS OF ADJACENT JOINTS AFTER TOTAL ANKLE ARTHROPLASTY

The hindfoot is anatomically and biomechanically complex since tibiotalar, subtalar, and Chopart-joints are close together and abnormalities in one of them can lead to increased load and wear in the other joints. Initial subtalar osteoarthritis can progress, especially in case of tibiotalar stiffness after TAA.[8] Gurbani and colleagues[90] evaluated the use of SPECT/CT in painful TAA and found symptomatic subtalar osteoarthritis in 2 of 33 patients. Diagnosis based on structural changes in the subtalar joint in CT scan and corresponding tracer enhancement in SPECT can identify these findings as symptomatic. Subtalar arthrodesis was performed and led to significant improvement in pain symptoms. Advantages of SPECT/CT in identifying active osteoarthritis particularly in the midfoot are described above. **Fig. 2** shows the ability to differentiate active

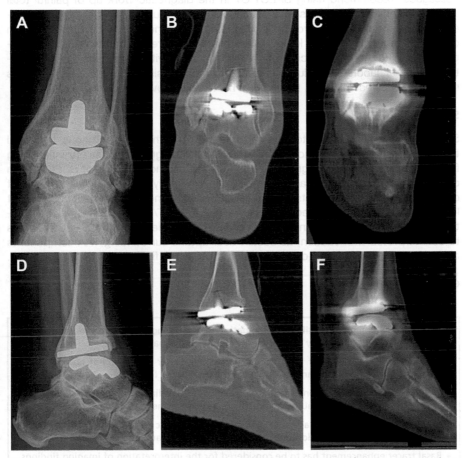

Fig. 2. Aseptic prosthetic loosening. A 56-year-old man presented with pain at rest and under stress 8 years after implantation of total ankle prosthesis. Clinical examination was inconclusive to differentiate prosthetic loosening and subtalar osteoarthritis. (*A, D*): Radiographs showed talar cyst formation assuming prosthetic loosening and incipient osteoarthritis in the posterior part of the subtalar joint. (*B, E*): Also CT-scans show both periprosthetic loosening zones and subtalar degenerative changes. For preoperative decision making regarding the need of arthrodesis both in the ankle and subtalar joint, SPECT/CT was performed. (*C, F*): Hybrid imaging showed prosthetic loosening both of the tibial and talar component with relevant tracer enhancement. There was no tracer enhancement of subtalar joint. Removal of total ankle prosthesis and arthrodesis with autologous interposition bone graft was planned.

osteoarthritis in adjacent joints structurally seen in x-ray imaging from prosthetic disadvantages like aseptic loosening.

SPECT/CT IN PERIPROSTHETIC JOINT INFECTION AFTER TOTAL ANKLE ARTHROPLASTY

Studies dealing with the use of SPECT/CT in periprosthetic joint infection of the ankle are rare and controversial. While implant infection has been confirmed by additional gallium scan by Gurbani and colleagues,[90] in another study, ankles being positive for infection in labeled white blood cell-scans proofed to be false positive.[89] Finally, Henry and colleagues[9] recommend using SPECT/CT in the diagnostic work up of painful total ankle replacement after exclusion of infection following Musculoskeletal Infection Society (MSIS) criteria[97] of periprosthetic joint infections. Since these criteria have been developed regarding hip and knee replacements, they are not optimized for ankle replacements. Furthermore, in case of chronic situations without obvious clinical symptoms, normal laboratory values, and dry arthrocentesis additional diagnostics is necessary to detect infection. Here, SPECT/CT could provide additional information.

SUMMARY

SPECT-CT has been shown to be a valuable tool for orthopedic surgeons. In painful total ankle replacements studies have shown high diagnostic accuracy influencing further management. Although information on the diagnostic value of SPECT/CT in diagnosing osteoarthritis of adjacent joints is rare, daily clinical use and confident cases show its value. While its clinical value in diagnosing impingement and implant loosening has been confirmed, the accuracy of SPECT/CT in diagnosing periprosthetic joint infection of the ankle is still controversial. Nevertheless, SPECT-CT has to be interpreted with caution, as basal tracer uptake surrounding TAA components can occur especially in high-demand patients and in the first years after implantation.

CLINICS CARE POINTS

- SPECT/CT can complement clinical examination and radiological imaging in chronic pain after total ankle arthroplasty by providing metabolic information
- High diagnostic accuracy of SPECT/CT in diagnosing gutter impingement and prosthetic loosening of total ankle arthroplasty has been shown in the literature
- SPECT/CT can provide additional information in inconclusive diagnostic findings and can help to differentiate symptoms caused by prosthesis or periprosthetic discomforts
- Evidence of diagnostic accuracy of SPECT/CT in periprosthetic joint infection of the ankle is rare but seems to provide additional information in clinical and imaging work up
- Basal tracer enhancement has to be considered for the interpretation of imaging findings

DISCLOSURE

The authors have nothing to declare regarding this study.

REFERENCES

1. Singh JA, Ramachandran R. Time trends in total ankle arthroplasty in the USA: a study of the National Inpatient Sample. Clin Rheumatol 2016;35:239–45.

2. Rushing CJ, Mckenna BJ, Zulauf EA, et al. Intermediate-term outcomes of a third-generation, 2-component total ankle prosthesis. Foot Ankle Int 2021;42:935–43.
3. Gougoulias N, Khanna A, Maffulli N. How successful are current ankle replacements?: a systematic review of the literature. Clin Orthop Relat Res 2010;468: 199–208.
4. Wood PLR, Karski MT, Watmough P. Total ankle replacement: the results of 100 mobility total ankle replacements. J Bone Joint Surg Br 2010;92:958–62.
5. Clough TM, Ring J. Total ankle arthroplasty: Seven-year survivorship of 118 consecutive Zenith ankle arthroplasties from a non-designer centre. Bone Joint Lett J 2021;103:696–703.
6. Jastifer JR, Coughlin MJ. Long-term follow-up of mobile bearing total ankle arthroplasty in the United States. Foot Ankle Int 2015;36:143–50.
7. Bonnin M, Gaudot F, Laurent J-R, et al. The Salto total ankle arthroplasty: survivorship and analysis of failures at 7 to 11 years. Clin Orthop Relat Res 2011;469: 225–36.
8. Hsu AR, Haddad SL, Myerson MS. Evaluation and management of the painful total ankle arthroplasty. JAAOS-Journal of the American Academy of Orthopaedic Surgeons 2015;23:272–82.
9. Henry JK, Rider C, Cody E, et al. Evaluating and managing the painful total ankle replacement. Foot Ankle Int 2021;42:1347–61.
10. Glazebrook MA, Arsenault K, Dunbar M. Evidence-based classification of complications in total ankle arthroplasty. Foot Ankle Int 2009;30:945–9.
11. Vulcano E, Myerson MS. The painful total ankle arthroplasty: a diagnostic and treatment algorithm. Bone Joint Lett J 2017;99:5–11.
12. Cody EA, Lachman JR, Gausden EB, et al. Lower bone density on preoperative computed tomography predicts periprosthetic fracture risk in total ankle arthroplasty. Foot Ankle Int 2019;40:1–8.
13. Manegold S, Haas NP, Tsitsilonis S, et al. Periprosthetic fractures in total ankle replacement: classification system and treatment algorithm. JBJS 2013;95: 815–20.
14. Pelletier-Galarneau M, Martineau P, Gaudreault M, et al. Review of running injuries of the foot and ankle: clinical presentation and SPECT-CT imaging patterns. Am J Nucl Med Mol Imaging 2015;5:305.
15. Valderrabano V, Hintermann B, Dick W. Scandinavian total ankle replacement: a 3.7-year average followup of 65 patients. Clin Orthop Relat Res 2004;424:47–56.
16. Haytmanek CT Jr, Gross C, Easley ME, et al. Radiographic outcomes of a mobile-bearing total ankle replacement. Foot Ankle Int 2015;36:1038–44.
17. Brunner S, Barg A, Knupp M, et al. The Scandinavian total ankle replacement: long-term, eleven to fifteen-year, survivorship analysis of the prosthesis in seventy-two consecutive patients. JBJS 2013;95:711–8.
18. Hermus JP, Voesenek JA, van Gansewinkel EHE, et al. Complications following total ankle arthroplasty: a systematic literature review and meta-analysis. Foot Ankle Surg 2022;28(8):1183–93.
19. Schuberth JM, Wood DA, Christensen JC. Gutter impingement in total ankle arthroplasty. Foot Ankle Spec 2016;9:145–58.
20. Rippstein PF. Clinical experiences with three different designs of ankle prostheses. Foot Ankle Clin 2002;7:817–31.
21. Mason LW, Wyatt J, Butcher C, et al. Single-photon-emission computed tomography in painful total ankle replacements. Foot Ankle Int 2015;36:635–40.
22. Myerson MS, Shariff R, Zonno AJ. The management of infection following total ankle replacement: demographics and treatment. Foot Ankle Int 2014;35:855–62.

23. Kessler B, Sendi P, Graber P, et al. Risk factors for periprosthetic ankle joint infection: a case-control study. JBJS 2012;94:1871–6.
24. Love C, Marwin SE, Palestro CJ. Nuclear medicine and the infected joint replacement. Semin Nucl Med 2009;39:66–78.
25. Cadden AR. Imaging in total ankle replacement. Semin Musculoskelet Radiol 2012;16:205–16.
26. Veerwal H, Meena A, Dhingra VK. Current status of bone single-photon emission computed tomography combined with computed tomography in evaluation of foot and ankle pain. Journal of Radiation Medicine in the Tropics 2022;3:1.
27. Hanna RS, Haddad SL, Lazarus ML. Evaluation of periprosthetic lucency after total ankle arthroplasty: helical CT versus conventional radiography. Foot Ankle Int 2007;28:921–6.
28. LiMarzi GM, Fursevich DM, Cole JD, et al. Imaging of ankle replacements. Semin Musculoskelet Radiol 2015;19:67–76.
29. Yoo IR. Bone SPECT/CT of the foot and ankle: potential clinical application for chronic foot pain. Nucl Med Mol Imaging 2020;54:1–8.
30. Lee AY, Ha AS, Petscavage JM, et al. Total ankle arthroplasty: a radiographic outcome study. Am J Roentgenol 2013;200:1310–6.
31. Lai WC, Arshi A, Ghorbanifarajzadeh A, et al. Incidence and predictors of early complications following primary and revision total ankle arthroplasty. Foot Ankle Surg 2019;25:785–9.
32. Law TY, Sabeh KG, Rosas S, et al. Trends in total ankle arthroplasty and revisions in the Medicare database, Ann Transl Med, 6 (7), 2018, 112. doi: 10.21037/atm.2018.02.06.
33. Crişan G, Moldovean-Cioroianu NS, Timaru D-G, et al. Radiopharmaceuticals for PET and SPECT Imaging: A literature review over the last decade. Int J Mol Sci 2022;23:5023.
34. Jødal L, Afzelius P, Alstrup AKO, et al. Radiotracers for bone marrow infection imaging. Molecules 2021;26:3159.
35. Tsubaki F, Kurata S, Nagata S, et al. Clinical spectrum and diagnostic pitfalls of multiple abnormal uptakes on bone scintigraphy. Jpn J Radiol 2016;34:771–8.
36. Serino J, Kunze KN, Jacobsen SK, et al. Nuclear medicine for the orthopedic foot and ankle surgeon. Foot Ankle Int 2020;41:612–23.
37. Brenner AI, Koshy J, Morey J, et al. The bone scan. Semin Nucl Med 2012;42:11–26.
38. Vijayanathan S, Butt S, Gnanasegaran G, et al. Advantages and limitations of imaging the musculoskeletal system by conventional radiological, radionuclide, and hybrid modalities. Semin Nucl Med 2009;39:357–68.
39. Israel O, Pellet O, Biassoni L, et al. Two decades of SPECT/CT–the coming of age of a technology: an updated review of literature evidence. Eur J Nucl Med Mol Imaging 2019;46:1990–2012.
40. Palestro CJ, Love C. Role of nuclear medicine for diagnosing infection of recently implanted lower extremity arthroplasties. Semin Nucl Med 2017;47:630–8.
41. Hutton BF. The origins of SPECT and SPECT/CT. Eur J Nucl Med Mol Imaging 2014;41:3–16.
42. Scharf S. SPECT/CT imaging in general orthopedic practice. Semin Nucl Med 2009;39:293–307.
43. Hasegawa BH, Gingold EL, Reilly SM, et al. Description of a simultaneous emission-transmission CT system. Medical Imaging IV: Image Formation 1990;1231:50–60.

44. Mohan HK, Holker PF, Gnanasegaran G, et al. The applicability of SPECT-CT in directing the management of bony foot and ankle pathology. Eur J Nucl Med Mol Imaging 2007;34:S166.
45. Parthipun A, Moser J, Mok W, et al. 99mTc-HDP SPECT-CT aids localization of joint injections in degenerative joint disease of the foot and ankle. Foot Ankle Int 2015;36:928–35.
46. Pountos I, Charpail C, Tellisi N. Evaluation of the Diagnostic Value of SPECT/CT in Defining Foot and Ankle Pathologies. Foot Ankle Orthop 2019;4. 2473011419S00062.
47. Palestro CJ. Nuclear medicine and the failed joint replacement: Past, present, and future. World J Radiol 2014;6:446.
48. Hirschmann MT, Amsler F, Rasch H. Clinical value of SPECT/CT in the painful total knee arthroplasty (TKA): a prospective study in a consecutive series of 100 TKA. Eur J Nucl Med Mol Imaging 2015;42:1869–82.
49. Murer AM, Hirschmann MT, Amsler F, et al. Bone SPECT/CT has excellent sensitivity and specificity for diagnosis of loosening and patellofemoral problems after total knee arthroplasty. Knee Surg Sports Traumatol Arthrosc 2020;28:1029–35.
50. Barnsley L, Barnsley L. Detection of aseptic loosening in total knee replacements: a systematic review and meta-analysis. Skeletal Radiol 2019;48:1565–72.
51. Hirschmann MT, Iranpour F, Konala P, et al. A novel standardized algorithm for evaluating patients with painful total knee arthroplasty using combined single photon emission tomography and conventional computerized tomography. Knee Surg Sports Traumatol Arthrosc 2010;18:939–44.
52. Mathis DT, Tschudi S, Amsler F, et al. Correlations of typical pain patterns with SPECT/CT findings in unhappy patients after total knee arthroplasty. Knee Surg Sports Traumatol Arthrosc 2022;30(9):3007–23.
53. Slevin O, Schmid FA, Schiapparelli F-F, et al. Coronal femoral TKA position significantly influences in vivo patellar loading in unresurfaced patellae after primary total knee arthroplasty. Knee Surg Sports Traumatol Arthrosc 2017;25:3605–10.
54. Suter B, Testa E, Stämpfli P, et al. A novel standardized algorithm using SPECT/CT evaluating unhappy patients after unicondylar knee arthroplasty–a combined analysis of tracer uptake distribution and component position. BMC Med Imaging 2015;15:1–8.
55. van den Wyngaert T, Palli SR, Imhoff RJ, et al. Cost-effectiveness of bone SPECT/CT in painful total knee arthroplasty. J Nucl Med 2018;59:1742–50.
56. Dobrindt O, Amthauer H, Krueger A, et al. Hybrid SPECT/CT for the assessment of a painful hip after uncemented total hip arthroplasty. BMC Med Imaging 2015;15:1–10.
57. Peng Z, Jia Y, Li J, et al. Diagnostic Performance of Single-Photon Emission Computed Tomography/Computed Tomography in Aseptic Loosening: A Systematic Review and Meta-Analysis. J Arthroplasty 2021;36:4003–12.
58. Bäcker HC, Steurer-Dober I, Beck M, et al. Magnetic resonance imaging (MRI) versus single photon emission computed tomography (SPECT/CT) in painful total hip arthroplasty: a comparative multi-institutional analysis. Br J Radiol 2020;93: 20190738.
59. Schweizer T, Schiapparelli F-F, Rotigliano N, et al. Patterns of bone tracer uptake on SPECT-CT in symptomatic and asymptomatic patients with primary total hip arthroplasty. Eur J Nucl Med Mol Imaging 2018;45:283–91.
60. Arican P, Okudan Tekin B, Şefizade R, et al. The role of bone SPECT/CT in the evaluation of painful joint prostheses. Nucl Med Commun 2015;36:931–40.

61. van den Wyngaert T, Paycha F, Strobel K, et al. SPECT/CT in postoperative pain-ful hip arthroplasty. Semin Nucl Med 2018;48:425–38.

62. Abele JT, Swami VG, Russell G, et al. The accuracy of single photon emis-sion computed tomography/computed tomography arthrography in evaluating aseptic loosening of hip and knee prostheses. J Arthroplasty 2015;30: 1647–51.

63. Ghanem MA, Dannoon S, Elgazzar AH. The added value of SPECT-CT in the detection of heterotopic ossification on bone scintigraphy. Skeletal Radiol 2020; 49:291–8.

64. Vaz S, Ferreira TC, Salgado L, et al. Bone scan usefulness in patients with painful hip or knee prosthesis: 10 situations that can cause pain, other than loosening and infection. Eur J Orthop Surg Traumatol 2017;27:147–56.

65. Graute V, Feist M, Lehner S, et al. Detection of low-grade prosthetic joint infec-tions using 99mTc-antigranulocyte SPECT/CT: initial clinical results. Eur J Nucl Med Mol Imaging 2010;37:1751–9.

66. van der Bruggen W, Bleeker-Rovers CP, Boerman OC, et al. PET and SPECT in osteomyelitis and prosthetic bone and joint infections: a systematic review. Semin Nucl Med 2010;40:3–15.

67. Waldman LE, Scharf SC. Bone SPECT/CT of the spine, foot, and ankle: Evaluation of surgical patients. Semin Nucl Med 2017;47:639–46.

68. McDonald M, Cooper R, Wang MY. Use of computed tomography–single-photon emission computed tomography fusion for diagnosing painful facet arthropathy. Neurosurg Focus 2007;22:1–4.

69. Kumar K, Halkar RK, Bartley SC, et al. Incremental benefit of SPECT+ CT bone scans over conventional planar and SPECT bone scans in vertebroplasty. Indian J Nucl Med 2011;26:181.

70. Hudyana H, Maes A, Vandenberghe T, et al. Accuracy of bone SPECT/CT for identifying hardware loosening in patients who underwent lumbar fusion with pedicle screws. Eur J Nucl Med Mol Imaging 2016;43:349–54.

71. Plaass C, Yao D, Ettinger S, et al. Einsatz des SPECT-CT in der Fuß-und Sprung-gelenkchirurgie. Fuß & Sprunggelenk 2021;19:39–50.

72. Eelsing R, Hemke R, Schepers T. The added value of SPECT/CT in the painful foot and ankle: A review of the literature. Foot Ankle Surg 2021;27:715–22.

73. Claassen L, Yao D, Ettinger S, et al. Relevance of SPECT-CT in complex cases of foot and ankle surgery: a comparison with MRI. Foot Ankle Spec 2020;13: 451–62.

74. Pagenstert GI, Barg A, Leumann AG, et al. SPECT-CT imaging in degenerative joint disease of the foot and ankle. J Bone Joint Surg Br 2009;91:1191–6.

75. Claassen L, Uden T, Ettinger M, et al. Influence on therapeutic decision making of SPECT-CT for different regions of the foot and ankle. BioMed Res Int 2014;2014.

76. Wiewiorski M, Pagenstert G, Rasch H, et al. Pain in osteochondral lesions. Foot Ankle Spec 2011;4:92–9.

77. Meftah M, Katchis SD, Scharf SC, et al. SPECT/CT in the management of osteo-chondral lesions of the talus. Foot Ankle Int 2011;32:233–8.

78. Lazaga F, van Asten SA v, Nichols A, et al. Hybrid imaging with 99mTc-WBC SPECT/CT to monitor the effect of therapy in diabetic foot osteomyelitis. Int Wound J 2016;13:1158–60.

79. Vouillarmet J, Moret M, Morelec I, et al. Application of white blood cell SPECT/CT to predict remission after a 6 or 12 week course of antibiotic treatment for diabetic foot osteomyelitis. Diabetologia 2017;60:2486–94.

80. Heiba SI, Kolker D, Mocherla B, et al. The optimized evaluation of diabetic foot infection by dual isotope SPECT/CT imaging protocol. J Foot Ankle Surg 2010; 49:529–36.
81. Nathan M, Mohan H, Vijayanathan S, et al. The role of 99mTc-diphosphonate bone SPECT/CT in the ankle and foot. Nucl Med Commun 2012;33:799–807.
82. Chicklore S, Gnanasegaran G, Vijayanathan S, et al. Potential role of multislice SPECT/CT in impingement syndrome and soft-tissue pathology of the ankle and foot. Nucl Med Commun 2013;34:130–9.
83. Ha S, Hong SH, Paeng JC, et al. Comparison of SPECT/CT and MRI in diagnosing symptomatic lesions in ankle and foot pain patients: diagnostic performance and relation to lesion type. PLoS One 2015;10:e0117583.
84. Breunung N, Barwick T, Fernando R, et al. Additional benefit of SPECT-CT in investigating heel pain. Clin Nucl Med 2008;33:705–6.
85. Claassen L, Ettinger S, Modrejewski C, et al. Das SPECT-CT in der Fuß-und Sprunggelenkschirurgie. Fuß & Sprunggelenk 2015;13:103–12.
86. Mehta N, Serino J, Hur ES, et al. Pathogenesis, evaluation, and management of osteolysis following total ankle arthroplasty. Foot Ankle Int 2021;42:230–42.
87. Rodriguez D, Bevernage BD, Maldague P, et al. Medium term follow-up of the AES ankle prosthesis: high rate of asymptomatic osteolysis. Foot Ankle Surg 2010;16:54–60.
88. Kampen WU, Westphal F, van den Wyngaert T, et al. SPECT/CT in postoperative foot and ankle pain. Semin Nucl Med 2018;48:454–68.
89. Mertens J, Lootens T, Vercruysse J, et al. Bone SPECT/CT in the Evaluation of Painful Total Ankle Replacement: Validation of Localization Scheme and Preliminary Evaluation of Diagnostic Patterns. Clin Nucl Med 2021;46:361–8.
90. Gurbani A, Demetracopoulos C, O'Malley M, et al. Correlation of single-photon emission computed tomography results with clinical and intraoperative findings in painful total ankle replacement. Foot Ankle Int 2020;41:639–46.
91. Utz JA, Lull RJ, Galvin EG. Asymptomatic total hip prosthesis: natural history determined using Tc-99m MDP bone scans. Radiology 1986;161:509–12.
92. Oswald SG, van Nostrand D, Savory CG, et al. Three-phase bone scan and indium white blood cell scintigraphy following porous coated hip arthroplasty: a prospective study of the prosthetic tip. J Nucl Med 1989;30:1321 31.
93. Hofmann AA, Wyatt RW, Daniels AU, et al. Bone scans after total knee arthroplasty in asymptomatic patients. Cemented versus cementless. Clin Orthop Relat Res 1990;183–8.
94. Thiele K, Fussi J, Perka C, et al. Berliner diagnostischer Algorithmus der schmerzhaften Knie-TEP. Orthopä 2016;45:38–46.
95. Lam HY, Lui TH. Arthroscopic Decompression for Medial Ankle Impingement After Total Ankle Arthroplasty. Arthrosc Tech 2021;10:e1383–8.
96. Gross CE, Adams SB, Easley M, et al. Surgical treatment of bony and soft-tissue impingement in total ankle arthroplasty. Foot Ankle Spec 2017;10:37–42.
97. Parvizi J, Tan TL, Goswami K, et al. The 2018 Definition of Periprosthetic Hip and Knee Infection: An Evidence-Based and Validated Criteria. J Arthroplasty 2018; 33:1309–14.e2.

Cone-Beam Weight-Bearing Computed Tomography of Ankle Arthritis and Total Ankle Arthroplasty

Kepler Alencar Mendes de Carvalho, MD[a],
Nacime Salomão Barbachan Mansur, MD, PhD[a],
Cesar de Cesar Netto, MD, PhD[a,b,*]

KEYWORDS

- Ankle • Alignment • Hindfoot • WBCT • Deformity • Osteoarthritis • Joint
- Replacement

KEY POINTS

- A complete understanding of the foot deformity in patients with ankle osteoarthritis is necessary to ensure adequate treatment.
- The three-dimensional visualization approach using weight-bearing computed tomography (WBCT) allows a more accurate assessment of foot alignment with attention to planus, cavus, varus, or valgus deformities.
- WBCT has benefited the evaluation of ankle osteoarthritis since evaluating the hindfoot axis, fibula position to the tibia, and joint space analysis.

BACKGROUND

Ankle osteoarthritis (OA) is a debilitating chronic disease affecting approximately 1% of the world's adult population. It is a growing problem in health care with an estimated prevalence of 30 cases per 100,000 inhabitants and corresponds to between 2% and 4% of all patients with OA.[1-4]

Knowing the etiology is essential to select the best treatment strategy and achieving satisfactory results in the medium and long term. Epidemiologic and clinical studies have identified prior trauma caused by severe ankle fractures or sprains as the most common source of ankle OA. Patients with post-traumatic OA are generally younger than patients with primary OA.[2,4]

[a] Department of Orthopedics and Rehabilitation, University of Iowa, Carver College of Medicine, Iowa City, IA, USA; [b] Department of Orthopedic Surgery, Division of Orthopedic Foot and Ankle Surgery, Duke University, Durham, NC, USA
* Corresponding author. Department of Orthopaedic Surgery, Duke University Medical Center, 5601 Arringdon Park Drive, Suite 300, Morrisville, NC 27560.
E-mail address: cesar-netto@uiowa.edu

Foot Ankle Clin N Am 28 (2023) 509–528
https://doi.org/10.1016/j.fcl.2023.04.002

foot.theclinics.com

Ankle sprains are one of the most common reasons for attending emergency departments with a reported incidence of between 220 and 720 per 100,000. Ankle fractures have been reported to have an incidence of between 112 and 248 per 100,000.[4–6]

Repetitive ankle sprains in sports are the leading cause of post-traumatic ligament OA of the ankle with concomitant hindfoot varus deformity.[4] It was confirmed in a study by Valderrabano and colleagues,[3] who evaluated the etiology of ankle OA in 390 consecutive patients (406 ankles) with painful end-stage ankle OA. In this study, most patients (78%) had post-traumatic OA. Malleolar fractures were the most common reason for degenerative changes in the ankle joint (157 patients), followed by ligament injuries of the ankle (post-traumatic ligament OA of the ankle; 60 patients). Only 31 patients were affected by primary OA, whereas secondary OA was considered the most common cause of terminal ankle OA (46 patients). Secondary OA has also been associated with a variety of underlying diseases or disorders, such as rheumatoid disease, hemochromatosis, hemophilia, gout, neuropathic diseases, avascular necrosis of the talus, osteochondral lesions, and postinfectious arthritis.[3,4,7]

Saltzman and colleagues,[8] in a study, designed to identify the cause of symptomatic ankle arthritis in a consecutive series of patients seen at a tertiary service evaluated 639 patients with end-stage painful ankle OA (Kellgren grade 3 or 4). In this study, 445 patients (70%) had post-traumatic OA, 76 (12%) had rheumatoid OA, and 46 (7%) had primary ankle OA. Although rotational ankle fractures were identified as the most common reason for post-traumatic ankle OA (164 patients), anterior ligament injuries also caused ankle OA in 126 patients.

The investigators concluded that patients with arthritis were more commonly associated with anterior rotational fractures of the ankle, and most of ankle arthritis is associated with previous trauma, whereas the main cause of knee or hip arthritis is idiopathic.[8]

Recently, Goldberg and colleagues,[4] a study whose objective was to verify the incidence of OA of the ankle in the United Kingdom, concluded that most of OA of the ankle is post-traumatic and estimated that at least 29,000 cases of symptomatic OA of the ankle are being referred specialist foot and ankle surgeons each year in the United Kingdom, representing a demand incidence of 47.7 per 100,000. Of these, at least 3000 cases are being treated by surgical intervention (ankle replacement and ankle arthrodesis).[4]

PREDISPOSING FACTORS

Most ankle OA cases, as mentioned above, are secondary to unresolved chronic fractures or instabilities. However, some factors, such as macro and microscopic cartilage injuries, malalignment, instability, and joint incongruity, can act independently to accelerate the ankle's OA process.[3]

Macroscopic Cartilage Injury

The direct relationship between osteochondral ankle injuries and the future development of ankle OA is controversial; however, anterolateral osteochondral lesions of the talus, posteromedial tibia, and medial malleolus have the worst prognosis.[9] Several authors have reported the presence of occult or undiagnosed osteochondral lesions after ankle fractures.17,1[8] Some studies have reported the presence of occult or undiagnosed osteochondral lesions after ankle fractures.[10,11] This may explain the findings of a 3-year follow-up study carried out by Nilsson and colleagues who found that up to 50% of patients with a fractured ankle had suboptimal functional outcomes in terms of persistent pain and decline in activities of daily living.[12]

Microscopic Cartilage Injury

Circumstances that stress the cartilage of the ankle, whether a single event (acute impact) or repetitive stress (cumulative contact stress), are known to be a potential cause of clinical OA.[3] In 2011, Tochigi and colleagues,[13] based on the analysis of cell death in seven ankle specimens collected from amputee patients, reported that chondrocyte apoptosis occurred mainly in the region of the fracture line. Moreover, it spread spontaneously from the fracture line to healthy areas within 48 hour after trauma, suggesting that intra-articular mediators of cell damage are released from injured chondrocytes and also affect healthy chondrocytes. In conclusion, cartilage damage at the cell level of whole organs in a fractured human ankle joint depends on the overall length of the fracture line. It is, therefore, closely associated with the initial severity of the injury.[13]

Joint Incongruity

It is evident that the presence of an intra-articular step favors the development of post-traumatic arthrosis in any joint, hence the importance of anatomical reduction of the fracture.[1,3,14] McKinley and colleagues,[15] who created an intra-articular step in the distal tibia of 10 ankle specimens and observed a substantial increase of up to 300% in the contact stress peak, which may be decisive in the appearance of post-traumatic OA. Studies have shown that instability associated with incongruity promotes cellular damage to the ankle cartilage; that is, incongruity is closely related to instability. In a second study, McKinley and colleagues suggested that instability associated with incongruity increases contact stress per surface area by up to 60% in ankle cartilage compared with incongruity alone.[16]

Instability

Instability itself increases the peak contact stress of the joint, resulting in cartilage deterioration. Ankle instability leads to OA.[14] The term "post-traumatic ligament OA of the ankle" was used by Valderrabano and colleagues,[17] during a study of the main characteristics of this type of ankle OA. In this study, the investigators concluded that there is evidence that the ankle joint is more susceptible to arthritic changes following severe ligament trauma than is commonly believed. Epidemiologically, sports injuries (mainly football) were the main factor leading to the development of ankle ligament OA. Single ankle sprains have a worse survival rate than chronic recurrent ligament injuries. In addition, there was an essential correlation between chronic lateral ankle instability and varus misalignment.[17]

Malalignment

In most patients, the deformity underlying the asymmetry is located close to the ankle joint, either in the inferior peritalar complex (subtalar or calcaneus) or in the supramalleolar region, or both. Ankle OA is asymmetrical in almost 70% of cases.[18] Although the origin of most cases of asymmetric ankle arthropathy is close (supramalleolar or inframalleolar), one should remember that it must be explored at the proximal level. Deformities at the level of the proximal tibia, knee, or distal femur can be causes of an asymmetric load distribution at the ankle, which in turn results in asymmetric ankle OA.[1] In a study to determine whether knee misalignment is associated with the development and progression of ankle OA in patients with end-stage knee OA, Xie and colleagues[19] concluded that tibial varus deformity of the knee is associated with the development and progression of ankle OA. In these cases, the original ankle problem or manifestation must be surgically resolved away from the ankle.[1,19]

PHYSICAL EXAMINATION AND DIAGNOSIS

Most patients with ankle OA seek medical help due to progressive joint pain. The physical examination should incorporate the history of the presenting problem. A functional impairment survey is beneficial and should be included in the initial work. The presenting symptom of OA of the ankle is most commonly pain.[20]

Patients often describe the pain as a deep ache in the tibiotalar joint. Pain may be localized (eg, anterolateral) or general with pain around the entire hindfoot complex. All patients can be divided into two main groups: those with slowly and rapidly progressive ankle OA.[2]

This pain is often exacerbated with activity and prolonged standing. Many patients complain of ankle stiffness, which is often worse in the morning. Activity and heat usually improve symptoms as do rest and the use of analgesics or anti-inflammatories.[20]

A routine physical examination includes careful inspection of the entire hindfoot and foot complex.[2] Ankle alignment should be evaluated clinically with the patient standing.[21] Frigg and colleagues[22] demonstrated that visual judgment needs to be improved to determine hindfoot alignment, as it predicts radiographic alignment in less than half of clinical cases. Substantial muscle atrophy of the lower leg can occur in patients with intermediate and end-stage ankle OA, as demonstrated by Valderrabano and colleagues.[23,24]

The ankle's active and passive range of motion (ROM) is usually decreased, although passive ROM may be expected. Contractures of the Achilles tendon complex, including the plantar fascia, should be evaluated. Crepitation, synovitis, and effusion may or may not be present.[20] The pain is usually generalized but can be located in the anterior or posterior joint line. Asking the patient to locate an area of discomfort can be helpful. The strength of the surrounding muscles may be normal, but it usually presents with a degree of weakness.[23] Peroneal tendons often show considerable weakness, especially after prolonged disability. Percussion and palpation can sometimes reveal associated neurological problems that need to be investigated before treatment. Associated subtalar arthrosis, tendinitis, or tendon rupture can confound the examination. The injection of local anesthetic into the ankle joint can help distinguish the diagnosis.[20]

Complements to the physical examination include the use of imaging, as it remains precious for diagnosing, treating, and evaluating outcomes in patients with ankle OA.[2] Available modalities include conventional radiography, fluoroscopy, computed tomography (CT), scintigraphy, single-photon emission CT, MRI, and ultrasonography. Most diagnostic imaging studies begin with conventional weight-bearing radiographs. Additional imaging may be needed to assess the underlying pathology better and guide treatment planning. Choosing the best imaging modality is usually based on several factors, including[1] reliability for the diagnosis at hand[2]; local availability[3]; security risks; and[4] cost.[25]

A recent study using conventional radiographs indicated that approximately 53% and 39% of varus and valgus arthritic ankles, respectively, show inframalleolar compensation for a supramalleolar and/or intra-articular deformity of the ankle.[26] A complete understanding of the deformity at the level of the hindfoot and midfoot in patients with ankle OA is necessary to ensure adequate treatment.[27] Conventional weight-bearing radiographs are still the gold standard in preoperative evaluation. Nonetheless, bony overlays inhibit a complete evaluation of the peritalar bones and joints. Furthermore, studies have shown that several measurements for analyzing deformities highly depend on the foot's position to the x-ray beam.[27–29]

The three-dimensional (3D) visualization approach using weight-bearing cone-beam CT technology may allow for a more accurate assessment of the hindfoot and midfoot and may allow for a more detailed analysis of the deformity.[27]

WEIGHT-BEARING COMPUTED TOMOGRAPHY

In the last decade, cone-beam CT technology with improved designs allowing flexible gantry movements has allowed both supine and standing weight-bearing imaging of the lower extremity.[25]

Cone-beam CT technology in supine and standing weight-bearing imaging of the lower extremity has several advantages, including the ability to obtain images with the patient standing, high-contrast resolution and spatial resolution, fast imaging, reduced radiation, a relatively small scanner size with a portable design, and generally lower capitalization cost than conventional CT technology.[25,30]

Cone-beam CT uses a large-area detector (typically >1000 detector rows and columns covering ~30 × 30 cm^2). In addition, a pyramid-shaped x-ray beam ("cone") obtaining fully volumetric data from multiple projections acquired in a single rotation about the patient without moving the patient through the scanner.[30,31]

The relatively simple mechanical configuration of cone-beam CT facilitates the development of novel platforms specifically suited to a variety of clinical applications, including musculoskeletal extremity imaging, image-guided radiation therapy,[32] maxillofacial imaging,[33] breast imaging,[34] and surgery/interventions.[35]

In musculoskeletal extremities, cone-beam CT imaging is potentially valuable, motivated by the need to image weight-bearing extremities, improve image quality and reduce radiation dose, enhance workflow, simplify site considerations, and reduce cost in comparison to that of multidetector CT.[30]

WEIGHT-BEARING COMPUTED TOMOGRAPHY ON NORMAL HINDFOOT

Hindfoot alignment has classically been determined using a hindfoot alignment view or a long axial view on plain radiography.[36]

However, all measurements of hindfoot alignment based on standard radiographs pose a substantial risk to the measurement due to malpositioning errors and overlapping of the skeletal structures of the foot and ankle caused by the radiographic fan.[37,38] Accurate knowledge of axial and rotational alignment is necessary to objectify the preoperative state and achieve correction of hindfoot misalignment.[39,40]

To investigate the normal anatomy and rotational dynamics of the distal tibiofibular joint under physiological conditions, Lepojärvi and colleagues[41] used the weight-bearing computed tomography (WBCT) in a study including 32 asymptomatic patients. Image acquisition was performed in three different ankle positions: neutral, internal, and external rotation. Parameters measured included tibiofibular clear space, sagittal fibular translation, fibular rotation, and anterior and posterior widths of the distal tibiofibular syndesmosis. During ankle rotation, the mean anteroposterior (AP) movement was 1.5 mm, and the mean fibular rotation was 3°. In addition, in patients with the ankle in a neutral position, the fibula was located anteriorly at the tibial notch in 88% of measurements.[41]

In a second study, the same cohort of patients to assess rotational dynamics of the talus using WBCT, Lepojärvi and colleagues[42] set anterior and posterior widths of the tibiotalar joint, medial free space, and rotation, translation, and inclination of the talus. The investigators found that when the ankle was rotated with a moment of

30 Nm, a 10° talus rotation was observed without substantial widening of the medial free space.[42]

Burssens and colleagues[36] described a reproducible method for measuring hindfoot alignment using WBCT. Sixty patients were included in the study and divided into two groups: 30 patients with varus alignment and 30 with valgus alignment.

Correlation between the anatomical axis of the tibia obtained from the entire leg or WBCT showed to be good. This suggests that the short end of the tibia can be used to determine the hindfoot angle completely on WBCT by the intersection of the talocalcaneal axis and the anatomical axis of the tibia. The investigators concluded that the WBCT could be used to measure hindfoot alignment, similar to plain films, objectively.[36]

WEIGHT-BEARING COMPUTED TOMOGRAPHY ON PATHOLOGIC HINDFOOT

Hirschmann[43] and colleagues performed a study comparing CT of the hindfoot in the supine, non-weight-bearing position versus the upright, weight-bearing position. Hindfoot alignment was measured in 22 patients with different indications for CT evaluation, including hindfoot OA ($n = 8$) and talar osteochondral defects ($n = 6$). Significant differences were found for all measurements except tibiocalcaneal distance and hindfoot alignment angle when comparing weight-bearing and non-weight-bearing images. The hindfoot alignment angle was comparable when measured with and without weight bearing. These findings suggest that impact assessment using the fibulocalcaneal distance should be performed using weight-bearing conditions.[2,43]

Cody[44] and colleagues in a study whose objective was to analyze the talar anatomy and subtalar joint alignment in patients with progressive collapsing foot deformity (PCFD) by correlating the angle between the inferior facet of the talus and the horizontal (inftal-hor) and the angle between the inferior and superior facets of the talus (inftal-suptal) measurements using WBCT with the measurements standard radiographic images of flatfoot, including talo-first metatarsal angle in AP and lateral views, talocalcaneal angle (TCA) in AP and lateral views, talonavicular coverage angle, calcaneal pitch, medial column height, and hindfoot alignment.

In total, the investigators used 45 patients with PCFD and 17 control patients. Alignment of the subtalar joint was assessed using two angles: (1) angle between the inferior and superior facets of the talus and (2) angle between the inferior facet of the talus and the horizontal line. Specifically, patients with PCFD have been shown to have more innate valgus in their talar anatomy and more valgus alignment of the subtalar joint. The PCFD group had a much higher prevalence of inftal-suptal angles greater than 17° than the control group, suggesting this number as a useful threshold for clinicians.[44]

Willey[45] and colleagues in a study whose objectives were[1] to develop a standardized technique to quantitatively measure regional joint space on a WBCT scan of the ankle in patients with tibial pilon fractures and[2] to quantify joint space in a series of ankles. Six months after tibial pilon fracture to determine whether there is significant global and regional joint space loss compared with the uninjured contralateral ankle. They prospectively studied 20 patients with intra-articular tibial pilon fractures treated surgically, and they observed that the patients had a significant loss of joint space that was reliably detected with a standardized measurement technique on WBCT 6 months after tibial pilon fracture.

Moreover, the investigators found good reliability and reproducibility in standardized sagittal WBCT reconstructions. They concluded that although WBCT should not supplant MRI as a tool to characterize cartilage pathology, it seems helpful in complex fractures of the tibial pilon. In addition, they recommended that WBCT is used to reliably quantify tibiotalar joint space after pilon fracture compared with the uninjured ankle.[45]

Lintz[46] and colleagues described a new 3D biometric tool for assessing hindfoot alignment using WBCT, the foot and ankle offset (FAO). In their study, 135 patients were included: 57 with normal hindfoot alignment, 40 with valgus hindfoot alignment, and 38 with varus hindfoot alignment. Foot and ankle displacement represents the torque lever arm generated at the ankle from the combined actions of body weight and ground reaction force. In patients with neutral hindfoot alignment, displacement was 2.3% ± 2.9%. In patients with varus alignment, the displacement was −11.6% ± 6.9%. Furthermore, in patients with valgus alignment, displacement was 11.4% ± 5.7%.

The investigators concluded that the findings of this study suggest that measurement of foot and ankle displacement can be used as a tool for assessing hindfoot alignment.[46]

WEIGHT-BEARING COMPUTED TOMOGRAPHY ON ANKLE OSTEOARTHRITIS

The 3D image with the WBCT allows an accurate analysis that is not influenced by the foot's projection and/or orientation associated with the advantage of evaluating the foot and the ankle with weight bearing. This technological evolution has benefited the evaluation of OA of the ankle.[47–49]

The hindfoot axis evaluation, the position of the fibula to the tibia, and the joint space analysis are essential for the proper evaluation of OA of the ankle and treatment planning.[50]

Degree of Ankle Osteoarthritis

Richter and colleagues[50] proposed a classification for ankle OA subdivided into four grades using the WBCT (Fig. 1).

First-degree ankle OA includes joint space narrowing but not a complete loss and osteophyte formation (see Fig. 1A). The second degree includes a partial or total loss of joint space (see Fig. 1B). Third degree includes additional subchondral cysts but remaining joint surface congruence (see Fig. 1C). The fourth degree includes additional destruction and incongruity of the articular surface (see Fig. 1D).

This new classification is important because it combines the classic signs of OA (narrowing or loss of joint space, formation of osteophytes, and subchondral cysts) in a 3D view.[50]

Allied with this, Tazegul and colleagues,[51] in a recent study, developed and described a new and promising computational method to objectively quantify the radiographic changes associated with apparent ankle OA on WBCT.

In their study, the severity of ankle OA in each patient was scored using the Kellgren–Lawrence classification using plain radiographs. A volume of interest (VOI) for each ankle was centered on the tibiotalar joint. The initial computational analysis used WBCT image intensity profiles (Hounsfield units [HU]) along lines perpendicular to the distal tibia's subchondral bone/cartilage interface extending across the VOI. Graphs of HU distributions were generated and recorded for each row. These graphs were then used to calculate joint space width (JSW) and HU contrast (Fig. 2).

According to the investigators, the proposed method is simple. It can be easily incorporated into the workflow for OA staging if the appropriate tools (ie, WBCT and analysis software) are available.[51]

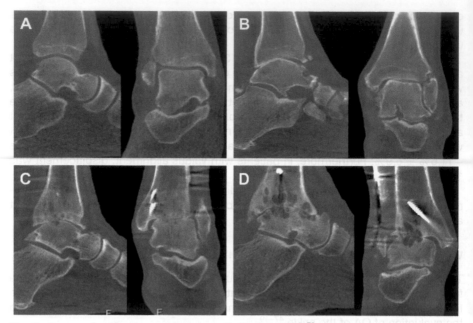

Fig. 1. Degree classification ankle osteoarthritis for WBCT[50]. (A) First degree of osteoarthritis with joint space narrowing but not complete loss and osteophyte formation. (B) Second degree of osteoarthritis with partial or complete loss of joint space. (C) Third degree of osteoarthritis with additional subchondral cysts but remaining joint surface congruency. (D) Fourth degree of osteoarthritis with additional joint surface destruction and incongruence.

Quantitative measurements and selection of objective points within each joint should improve the reliability and reproducibility of OA classification when compared with subjective classification systems described in the literature.[51]

However, we know that the classification of arthritic degeneration of the joint line based on radiolucent cartilage thickness is complex because it is in 3D and requires the development of computerized algorithms so that they can provide accurate analysis and quantifiable data.[50,52] Dibbern and colleagues[53] developed a new technique of distance mapping to objectively characterize the articular coverage in the entire peritalar surface. Including articular and nonarticular regions, if applied to the tibiotalar joint, may be of great use for a better 3D understanding of OA of the Ankle.

Alignment and Rotation Evaluation

The WBCT has shed new light on assessing and understanding alignment in ankle OA.[50]

WBCT has eliminated possible error factors present in the description of two-dimensional (2D) representations in conventional radiographs, facilitating the 3D understanding of the anatomical structures of the foot and ankle. An accurate assessment of hindfoot alignment is fundamental for surgical planning in deformity correction, hindfoot arthrodesis, and ankle arthroplasty procedures.[54–57]

In addition, multiple parameters have been previously used to assess the WBCTs hindfoot alignment angle, ankle displacement, and calcaneal displacement.[54]

Kvarda and colleagues[27] studied 72 patients treated for end-stage post-traumatic OA of the ankle. They evaluated the extent of deformities in patients with end-stage post-traumatic OA of the ankle through conventional radiographs and WBCT.

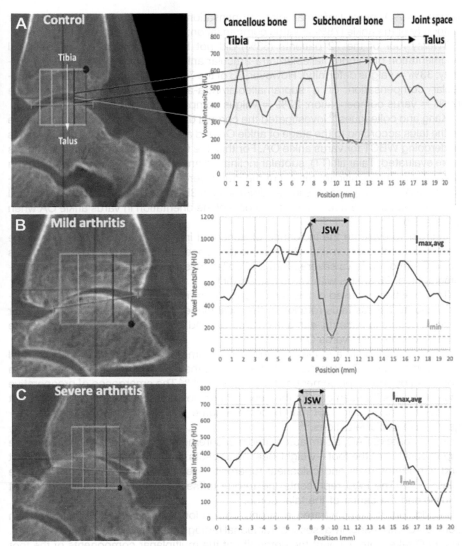

Fig. 2. Graph showing an example of intensity projection across the tibiotalar joint. The projection shows voxel intensity across tibial cancellous bone, tibial subchondral bone, joint space, talar subchondral bone, and talar cancellous bone, in that order. The joint space width (JSW) and Intensity level ($I_{max,avg}$ and I_{min}) are shown in each graph. (A) Normal ankle (Control): CT image, sagittal plane, and graphic plot. (B) Mild arthritic ankle: CT image, sagittal plane, and graphic plot. Note that the projection demonstrates narrowing of the width of the joint space. (C) Severe arthritic ankle: CT image, sagittal plane, and graphic plot. Note that the projection demonstrates narrowing of the width of the joint space (greater than in the mildly arthritic ankle).

To this end, they used the following parameters to assess osteoarthritic ankles: talar inclination, lateral tibial surface angle, hindfoot alignment angle, axial TCA, lateral TCA, medial tibiotalar angle, and medial tibial joint surface angle.

As a result, they found that the accuracy of 3D measurements taken on osteoarthritic ankles was similar to 3D measurements taken on healthy subjects. Thirty-three of the 72 patients (46%) showed inframalleolar compensation of a supramalleolar/intra-articular deformity of the ankle (78% = varus compensation; 22% = valgus compensation).

Twenty-four of the 72 patients (33%) did not have compensation or additional augmentation of a supramalleolar/intra-articular ankle deformity (67% = varus deformity; 33% = valgus deformity). However, 33 of the 72 patients (46%) showed inframalleolar compensation of a supramalleolar/intra-articular deformity of the ankle (78% = varus compensation; 22% = valgus compensation).[27]

Kang and colleagues[58] investigated the coronal orientation of the calcaneus relative to the talus according to the stage of ankle OA and a retrospective study of 132 ankles undergoing WBCT for varus ankle OA. For this, the following radiographic parameters were evaluated: Talar tilt (TT), subtalar inclination angle (SIA), and calcaneal inclination angle (CIA). The significant results of the study were that apparent subtalar compensation (SIA and CIA) was less in Takakura stages 3b and 4. In addition, the calcaneal position seems to compensate with coronal plane orientation in varus ankle OA when TT is $\leq 9.5°$.

In order to evaluate the incidence of abnormal internal rotation of the talus in the axial plane and to determine whether this incidence differs from the severity of varus ankle OA (moderate vs severe), Kim and colleagues[59] evaluated WBCT and plain radiographs of 96 ankles with varus osteoarthritis.

The investigators used a new radiographic parameter in the WBCT, the talus rotation ratio, to assess talus rotation in the axial plane. This study concluded that talar rotation occurs in patients with ankle varus OA and is more frequently seen in severe than moderate ankle varus OA.

As combined ankle and hindfoot joint misalignment should be considered in total ankle replacement (TAR) patients and assuming that intrinsic ankle deformity can be corrected by proper placement of TAR implants.[60–62] The emergence of preoperative measurements that can predict the need for additional procedures to realign the foot in patients undergoing TAR may become a game changer, helping orthopedic surgeons take decisive actions.[62]

In this context, FAO, a semiautomated measurement using WBCT, can estimate the tripod position of the foot—weight-bearing aspects of the metatarsal head of the first and fifth metatarsals and calcaneal tuberosity—relative to the center of the ankle joint.[46,63–65] The FAO represents the torque (offset) between the hindfoot–forefoot midline and the center of the talar dome.[62]

In addition, it demonstrated a strong correlation with hindfoot alignment, when compared with manually assessed traditional radiographic and WBCT measurements. The FAO takes into account the deformity of the multiplanar components of the foot and ankle.[49,65,66]

Cesar Netto and colleagues[62] retrospectively studied patients undergoing TAR to assess the ability of preoperative FAO measurements to predict the need for associated realignment procedures in patients undergoing TAR. They found a significant positive correlation between the number of bone realignment procedures required and preoperative FAO ($P = .0001$). In addition, a more significant number of auxiliary techniques ($P = .009$) were associated with preoperative valgus, and an relative risk (RR) of 6.3 for needing medial column surgery was attributed to this group of patients. The results confirmed the study hypothesis that there would be a significant correlation between the severity of preoperative FAO and the need for additional foot realignment procedures, both bone and soft tissue, that should be performed. In addition, data from this study demonstrated that FAO not only reliably distinguishes between varus and valgus hindfoot alignment preoperatively but its value can also help determine which patients may need additional intraoperative realignment procedures.[62]

They concluded that the number of necessary bone procedures was significantly higher in patients with valgus misalignment with the relative risk of valgus misalignment necessitating a medial column procedure being 6.3 times greater than a varus misalignment. Using biometrics and semiautomatic measurements that account for the relationship between the center of the ankle and the foot tripod can improve the preoperative evaluation and surgical planning of patients on TAR.[62]

WEIGHT-BEARING COMPUTED TOMOGRAPHY ON TOTAL ANKLE REPLACEMENT

Regardless of the cause, terminal OA is defined as a combination of severe and unrelenting symptoms that are sufficient to prompt the patient to consider surgical intervention. In the early stages of disease progression, most patients with ankle arthritis can respond to nonsurgical treatments (eg, analgesia, weight loss, and use of supportive orthoses). Once in the terminal stage, the main treatments of the surgical procedures for OA of the ankle are ankle arthrodesis or TAR.[67]

The most common indication for TAR is for treating advanced arthropathy resulting from end-stage primary OA, post-traumatic arthrosis, or infectious or inflammatory arthritis (after the infection has cleared).[68–70]

TAR surgery continues to grow in popularity as a viable option among end-stage ankle patients with arthritis. The ankle implant must be appropriately aligned within the ankle joint to maximize results when attempting to limit failure or revision.[71] In this sense, the WBCT has proven to be very useful in assisting orthopedic surgeons concerning preoperative planning, outcomes, and evaluation of possible complications.

Preoperative Planning Imaging Considerations

Several factors can be identified in the preoperative image: the etiology of the arthropathy, the degree of ankle misalignment, the degree of periarticular fibrosis, and the preoperative joint ROM at the ankle.[69]

In addition, the nature of ankle misalignment provides prognostic value; for example, patients with valgus angle misalignment have been shown to have a superior postoperative ROM compared with those with varus misalignment.[69,72]

WBCT should be obtained to assess foot and ankle alignment with attention to planus, cavus, varus, or valgus deformities.[69]

Preoperative hindfoot deformity is not an absolute contraindication to TAR. It is important to emphasize that these deformities must be treated when implantation of the prosthesis or the useful life of the implant may be compromised. The growing experience of surgeons in performing TAR led to an increase in attempts to treat more complex deformities.[73,74]

WBCT has been used as an imaging system to assess hindfoot and ankle alignment and pathology in ankle arthritis. In addition, it can be used in combination with other technologies under development to aid in surgical planning and execution of total ankle replacement.[50,69]

Now that WBCT can be performed down to the hip level, the 3D location of the anatomical and mechanical axis of the femur and tibia can allow the surgeon to place an implant with a more precise alignment.[50]

As observed by Pyevich and colleagues,[75] any TAR components' inconsistencies significantly impact the implants' contact pressures. Their study highlights the importance of accurate implant positioning in TAR.

To this end, WBTCs 3D imaging technology has been developing exponentially. The appearance of software and applications (eg, TALAS, CubeVue, Bonelogic) that allow surgeons to perform angular measurements in a semiautomated manner and simultaneously help as preoperative alignment and navigation guides[27,28,46,47,76–78](Fig. 3).

In addition, the similar techniques of preoperative navigation computer modeling and patient-specific instrumentation (PSI) in total knee and hip arthroplasty are being extended to TAR (eg, Prophecy/Inbone [Wright Medical])[71,77,79–81] (Fig. 4).

Alignment instruments are designed from WBCT and then manufactured for single use. They are an alternative to traditional alignment instrumentation and may reduce the number of steps required during surgery.

Thompson and colleagues,[71] comparing the accuracy and reproducibility of alignment and implant size using WBCT versus Non-WBCT, concluded that with limited deformity PSI based on WBCT has the potential for reliable postoperative alignment.

TAR Surgical Outcomes

Alignment is critical to the success and long-term survival of TAR. WBCT has previously been used to depict deformity correction and complications of residual deformities after TAR.[82–84]

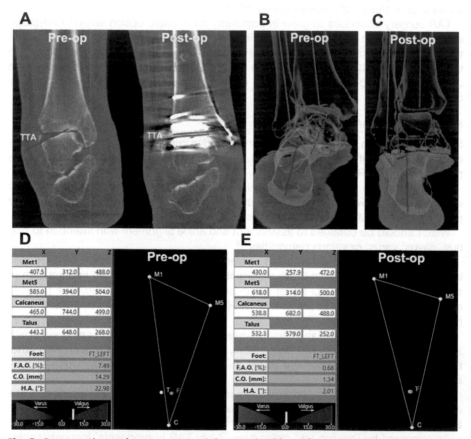

Fig. 3. Preoperative and postoperative (after total ankle replacement) WBCT images. In the images, it is possible to notice the correction of the ankle's alignment from valgus to the neutral position. (*A*) Manual measurements (talar tilt angle [TTA]). Semiautomatic measurements: (*B*) preoperative and (*C*) postoperative. Foot and ankle offset (FAO) in (*D*) preoperative and (*E*) postoperative.

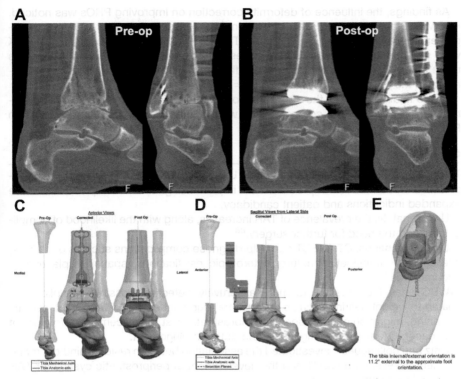

Fig. 4. Patient-specific instrumentation (PSI) in total ankle replacement with customized cutting guides and a preoperative surgical plan. (*A*) Preoperative WBCT (sagittal and coronal view), (*B*) postoperative WBCT (sagittal and coronal view), (*C*) PSI anterior view, (*D*) PSI sagittal view, and (*E*) PSI axial view showing the tibia internal/external orientation.

Several studies have demonstrated that for implant longevity, the resulting and residual hindfoot alignment is a crucial factor influencing clinical and patient-reported outcomes after TAR.[85,86]

As discussed earlier, the FAO measures the balance and alignment between the ankle joint and the foot tripod. FAO has been used in several previous studies to assess various complex foot and ankle deformities.[46,62,64,66,87]

VandeLune and colleagues[82] used WBCT measurements to address the ability of TAR to correct deformity in the coronal and sagittal planes of the ankle by correlating with patient-report outcomes (PROs) in patients with end-stage OA.

Patient-reported outcomes were evaluated and correlated with deformity correction. All deformity measures and some of the PROs were significantly improved. An association was found between these improved PROs and the correction of measured deformities.

The FAO was used to represent a measure of 3D deformity. The lateral talar station (LTS) was obtained using WBCT views in the sagittal plane to assess deformity in the sagittal plane. The hindfoot moment arm (HMA) and the talar tilt angle (TTA) were calculated to measure deformity in the coronal plane. The functional scores evaluated were: PROMIS Global Physical Health Score, the Tampa Kinesiophobia Scale (TSK), the European Foot and Ankle Society Score, the Pain Catastrophizing Scale, and Foot and Ankle Life Score Capacity Measurement Rate (FAAM).

As findings, the influence of deformity correction on improving PROs was noticed. PROMIS Global Physical Health was significantly associated (P = .0015) with improvements in FAO (P = .00065) and LTS (P = 0 .00436). Improvements in TSK were significantly associated with changes in HMA only (P = .0074). Improvements in the FAAM Daily Living Score were significantly correlated (P = .048) with improvements in the FAO (P = .023) and TTA (P = .029).

These findings confirm the study's hypothesis that significant correction of deformities in the sagittal and coronal planes would be associated with improvement in PROs.[82]

Complications

The total number of TAR performed in the United States is expanding rapidly. This increase is associated with improvements in implant design and techniques, which have expanded indications and patient candidacy.

Unfortunately, the prevalence of TAR increases, along with the likelihood of complications and the need for further surgery.[88]

Like conventional CT, WBCT can help diagnose complications such as osteolysis, infections, periprosthetic fracture, heterotopic ossifications, spacer displacement, and fractures.[69]

WBCT has the potential to more assertively detecting possible complications related to weight bearing such as residual malalignment or loss of alignment, aseptic loosening, migration of components, periprosthetic cyst, displacement or fracture of the spacer, OA of neighboring joints, and gutter impingement.

Lintz and colleagues[84] investigated the association between residual hindfoot malalignment assessed on WBCT and the development of periprosthetic cysts after TAR studied 48 patients.

The investigators found that patients with residual varus misalignment had cysts positioned in a more medial topographical location, whereas patients with residual valgus misalignment presented with cysts positioned in a more lateral location. Eighty-one percent of the patients studied had at least one periprosthetic cyst. The authors also confirmed that total cyst volume was positively correlated with the magnitude of residual deformity (assessed by FAO) and duration of follow-up. No significant correlation was found between overall cyst volume and hindfoot American Orthopaedic Foot & Ankle Society (AOFAS) scores.

The investigators concluded that periprosthetic cyst volume after primary TAR significantly correlated with postoperative hindfoot misalignment and longer follow-up. Moreover, assessing postoperative hindfoot alignment using WBCT may help identify patients at risk of developing periprosthetic cysts.[84]

Proper prosthetic alignment for TAR has been proven to improve implant survival and prevent complications.[89] However, the alignment is not restricted to the talar and tibial components of the prosthesis.[46,50,62,65,76] The behavior of the subtalar joint after TAR plays an important role and needs to be fully understood.

Carcuro and colleagues[90] evaluated the correction of subtalar joint alignment after TAR and its correlation with the correction of tibiotalar alignment using WBCT scanning. The tibiotalar axis changed in 80% of the patients, the subtalar axis in 100%, and the hindfoot axis in 80%. Changes in the upper talar platform axis were directly correlated with changes in the hindfoot axis (P < .05). The joint congruence change correlated directly with the subtalar axis (P < .01).

Finally, the investigators concluded that tibiotalar alignment is often corrected after TAR. The subtalar joint and hindfoot axes change after TAR in response to the tibiotalar axis. This change occurs in the same direction as the tibiotalar correction.[90]

Pain related to a possible subtalar impingement in an arthritic subtalar joint can become a significant complicating factor in the late postoperative period of TAR.[82,88,91,92]

In this context, Cesar de Netto and colleagues[93] compared the middle and posterior facets as markers of peritalar subluxation in patients with PCFD. They used the percentage of discovery of the middle and posterior facets in WBCT images in the coronal plane.

The model proposed by the investigators predicted 11% subluxation of the middle facet in patients with PCFD when the posterior facet is not yet subluxated. These results strongly suggest that midface subluxation provides an earlier marker of peritalar subluxation compared with current literature standards and that it can be used postoperatively as an essential marker of subtalar joint behavior after TAR.[93]

This early detection can help the surgeon, if necessary, to perform surgical interventions, such as subtalar fusion or calcaneal osteotomy, helping to preserve the alignment of the hindfoot and consequently giving more prolonged TAR survival.

SUMMARY

The 3D visualization approach using weight-bearing cone beam CT technology may allow a more accurate assessment of the hindfoot and midfoot, allowing for a more detailed analysis of the deformity.

The WBCT eliminates possible error factors present in the description of 2D representations in conventional radiographs, facilitating the 3D understanding of the foot and ankle anatomical structures.

Also, the WBCT has benefited the evaluation of ankle OA as the evaluation of the hindfoot axis, fibula position to the tibia, and the analysis of the joint space are essential for the adequate evaluation of OA of the ankle and planning the treatment.

WBCT should be obtained to assess foot and ankle alignment with attention to planus, cavus, varus, or valgus deformities.

It is important to emphasize that these deformities must be treated when implantation of the prosthesis or the useful life of the implant may be compromised.

A proper alignment is critical to the long-term success and survival of TAR. For this, the WBCT has been used to aid in correcting and assessing potential complications of residual deformities after TAR.

CLINICS CARE POINTS

- Preoperative navigation and patient-specific instrumentation are being extended to TAR and may reduce the number of steps required during surgery.
- Foot alignment is critical to long-term success and survival, influencing clinical and patient-reported outcomes after ART.
- Weight-bearing computed tomography has been used to aid in correcting and assessing potential complications of residual alignment deformities related to weight-bearing after TAR.

DISCLOSURE

K.A. Mendes de Carvalho and N.S. Barbachan Mansur have nothing to disclose. C. de Cesar Netto; Nextremity: Paid consultant; CurveBeam: Paid consultant; Paragon 28: Paid consultant. American Orthopaedic Foot and Ankle Society: Board or committee member. Weight-bearing CT International Study Group: Board or committee member. Foot and Ankle International: Editorial or governing board.

REFERENCES

1. Herrera-Pérez M, González-Martín D, Vallejo-Márquez M, et al. Ankle Osteoarthritis Aetiology. J Clin Med 2021;10(19).
2. Barg A, Pagenstert GI, Hügle T, et al. Ankle osteoarthritis: etiology, diagnostics, and classification. Foot Ankle Clin 2013;18(3):411-26.
3. Valderrabano V, Horisberger M, Russell I, et al. Etiology of ankle osteoarthritis. Clin Orthop Relat Res 2009;467(7):1800-6.
4. Goldberg AJ, MacGregor A, Dawson J, et al. The demand incidence of symptomatic ankle osteoarthritis presenting to foot & ankle surgeons in the United Kingdom. Foot 2012;22(3):163-6.
5. Bridgman SA. Population based epidemiology of ankle sprains attending accident and emergency units in the West Midlands of England, and a survey of UK practice for severe ankle sprains. Emerg Med J 2003;20(6):508-10.
6. Waterman BR, Owens BD, Davey S, et al. The epidemiology of ankle sprains in the United States. J Bone Joint Surg Am 2010;92(13):2279-84.
7. Thomas JL, Kunkel MW, Lopez R, et al. Radiographic Values of the Adult Foot in a Standardized Population. J Foot Ankle Surg 2006;45(1):3-12.
8. Saltzman CL, Salamon ML, Blanchard GM, et al. Epidemiology of ankle arthritis: report of a consecutive series of 639 patients from a tertiary orthopaedic center. Iowa Orthop J 2005;25:44-6.
9. Stufkens SA, Knupp M, Horisberger M, et al. Cartilage lesions and the development of osteoarthritis after internal fixation of ankle fractures: a prospective study. J Bone Joint Surg Am 2010;92(2):279-86.
10. Day GA, Swanson CE, Hulcombe BG. Operative treatment of ankle fractures: a minimum ten-year follow-up. Foot Ankle Int 2001;22(2):102-6.
11. Hintermann B, Regazzoni P, Lampert C, et al. Arthroscopic findings in acute fractures of the ankle. J Bone Joint Surg Br 2000;82(3):345-51.
12. Martijn HA, Lambers KTA, Dahmen J, et al. High incidence of (osteo)chondral lesions in ankle fractures. Knee Surg Sports Traumatol Arthrosc 2021;29(5):1523-34.
13. Tochigi Y, Rudert MJ, McKinley TO, et al. Correlation of dynamic cartilage contact stress aberrations with severity of instability in ankle incongruity. J Orthop Res 2008;26(9):1186-93.
14. Harrington KD. Degenerative arthritis of the ankle secondary to long-standing lateral ligament instability. J Bone Joint Surg Am 1979;61(3):354-61.
15. McKinley TO, Rudert MJ, Tochigi Y, et al. Incongruity-dependent changes of contact stress rates in human cadaveric ankles. J Orthop Trauma 2006;20(10):732-8.
16. McKinley TO, Tochigi Y, Rudert MJ, et al. The effect of incongruity and instability on contact stress directional gradients in human cadaveric ankles. Osteoarthr Cartil 2008;16(11):1363-9.
17. Valderrabano V, Hintermann B, Horisberger M, et al. Ligamentous posttraumatic ankle osteoarthritis. Am J Sports Med 2006;34(4):612-20.
18. Yi Y, Lee W. Peri-talar re-alignment osteotomy for joint preservation in asymmetrical ankle osteoarthritis. EFORT Open Rev 2017;2(7):324-31.
19. Xie K, Jiang X, Han X, et al. Association Between Knee Malalignment and Ankle Degeneration in Patients With End-Stage Knee Osteoarthritis. J Arthroplasty 2018;33(12):3694-8.e1.

20. Demetriades L, Strauss E, Gallina J. Osteoarthritis of the ankle. Clin Orthop Relat Res 1998;349:28–42.
21. Buck P, Morrey BF, Chao EY. The optimum position of arthrodesis of the ankle. A gait study of the knee and ankle. J Bone Joint Surg Am 1987;69(7):1052–62.
22. Frigg A, Nigg B, Davis E, et al. Does alignment in the hindfoot radiograph influence dynamic foot-floor pressures in ankle and tibiotalocalcaneal fusion? Clin Orthop Relat Res 2010;468(12):3362–70.
23. Valderrabano V, Nigg BM, von Tscharner V, et al. Total ankle replacement in ankle osteoarthritis: an analysis of muscle rehabilitation. Foot Ankle Int 2007;28(2):281–91.
24. Valderrabano V, Nigg BM, von Tscharner V, et al. Gait analysis in ankle osteoarthritis and total ankle replacement. Clin Biomech 2007;22(8):894–904.
25. Barg A, Bailey T, Richter M, et al. Weightbearing Computed Tomography of the Foot and Ankle: Emerging Technology Topical Review. Foot Ankle Int 2018;39(3):376–86.
26. Wang B, Saltzman CL, Chalayon O, et al. Does the subtalar joint compensate for ankle malalignment in end-stage ankle arthritis? Clin Orthop Relat Res 2015;473(1):318–25.
27. Kvarda P, Heisler L, Krähenbühl N, et al. 3D Assessment in Posttraumatic Ankle Osteoarthritis. Foot Ankle Int 2021;42(2):200–14.
28. de Carvalho KAM, Walt JS, Ehret A, et al. Comparison between Weightbearing-CT semiautomatic and manual measurements in Hallux Valgus. Foot Ankle Surg 2022;28(4):518–25.
29. Lenz AL, Krähenbühl N, Howell K, et al. Influence of the ankle position and X-ray beam angulation on the projection of the posterior facet of the subtalar joint. Skeletal Radiol 2019;48(10):1581–9.
30. Carrino JA, Al Muhit A, Zbijewski W, et al. Dedicated cone-beam CT system for extremity imaging. Radiology 2014;270(3):816–24.
31. Jaffray DA, Siewerdsen JH. Cone-beam computed tomography with a flat-panel imager: initial performance characterization. Med Phys 2000;27(6):1311–23.
32. Jaffray DA, Siewerdsen JH, Wong JW, et al. Flat-panel cone-beam computed tomography for image-guided radiation therapy. Int J Radiat Oncol Biol Phys 2002;53(5):1337–49.
33. Miracle AC, Mukherji SK. Conebeam CT of the head and neck, part 2: clinical applications. AJNR Am J Neuroradiol 2009;30(7):1285–92.
34. Boone JM, Nelson TR, Lindfors KK, et al. Dedicated breast CT: radiation dose and image quality evaluation. Radiology 2001;221(3):657–67.
35. Siewerdsen JH, Moseley DJ, Burch S, et al. Volume CT with a flat-panel detector on a mobile, isocentric C-arm: pre-clinical investigation in guidance of minimally invasive surgery. Med Phys 2005;32(1):241–54.
36. Burssens A, Peeters J, Buedts K, et al. Measuring hindfoot alignment in weight bearing CT: A novel clinical relevant measurement method. Foot Ankle Surg 2016;22(4):233–8.
37. Buck FM, Hoffmann A, Mamisch-Saupe N, et al. Hindfoot alignment measurements: rotation-stability of measurement techniques on hindfoot alignment view and long axial view radiographs. AJR Am J Roentgenol 2011;197(3):578–82.
38. Nosewicz TL, Knupp M, Bolliger L, et al. The reliability and validity of radiographic measurements for determining the three-dimensional position of the talus in varus and valgus osteoarthritic ankles. Skeletal Radiol 2012;41(12):1567–73.

39. Hintermann B, Zwicky L, Schweizer C, et al. The Use of Supramalleolar Osteotomies in Posttraumatic Deformity and Arthritis of the Ankle. JBJS Essent Surg Tech 2017;7(4):e29.

40. Becker AS, Myerson MS. The indications and technique of supramalleolar osteotomy. Foot Ankle Clin 2009;14(3):549–61.

41. Lepojärvi S, Niinimäki J, Pakarinen H, et al. Rotational Dynamics of the Normal Distal Tibiofibular Joint With Weight-Bearing Computed Tomography. Foot Ankle Int 2016;37(6):627–35.

42. Lepojärvi S, Niinimäki J, Pakarinen H, et al. Rotational Dynamics of the Talus in a Normal Tibiotalar Joint as Shown by Weight-Bearing Computed Tomography. J Bone Joint Surg Am 2016;98(7):568–75.

43. Hirschmann A, Pfirrmann CW, Klammer G, et al. Upright cone CT of the hindfoot: comparison of the non-weight-bearing with the upright weight-bearing position. Eur Radiol 2014;24(3):553–8.

44. Cody EA, Williamson ER, Burket JC, et al. Correlation of Talar Anatomy and Subtalar Joint Alignment on Weightbearing Computed Tomography With Radiographic Flatfoot Parameters. Foot Ankle Int 2016;37(8):874–81.

45. Willey MC, Compton JT, Marsh JL, et al. Weight-Bearing CT Scan After Tibial Pilon Fracture Demonstrates Significant Early Joint-Space Narrowing. J Bone Joint Surg Am 2020;102(9):796–803.

46. Lintz F, Welck M, Bernasconi A, et al. 3D Biometrics for Hindfoot Alignment Using Weightbearing CT. Foot Ankle Int 2017;38(6):684–9.

47. de Carvalho KAM, Mallavarapu V, Ehret A, et al. The Use of Advanced Semiautomated Bone Segmentation in Hallux Rigidus. Foot Ankle Orthop 2022;7(4). 24730114221137597.

48. Behrens A, Dibbern K, Lalevée M, et al. Coverage maps demonstrate 3D Chopart joint subluxation in weightbearing CT of progressive collapsing foot deformity. Sci Rep 2022;12(1):19367.

49. de Cesar Netto C, Bernasconi A, Roberts L, et al. Foot Alignment in Symptomatic National Basketball Association Players Using Weightbearing Cone Beam Computed Tomography. Orthop J Sports Med 2019;7(2). 2325967119826081.

50. Richter M, de Cesar Netto C, Lintz F, et al. The Assessment of Ankle Osteoarthritis with Weight-Bearing Computed Tomography. Foot Ankle Clin 2022;27(1):13–36.

51. Tazegul TE, Anderson DD, Barbachan Mansur NS, et al. An Objective Computational Method to Quantify Ankle Osteoarthritis From Low-Dose Weightbearing Computed Tomography. Foot Ankle Orthop 2022;7(3). 247301142211168.

52. Siegler S, Konow T, Belvedere C, et al. Analysis of surface-to-surface distance mapping during three-dimensional motion at the ankle and subtalar joints. J Biomech 2018;76:204–11.

53. Dibbern KN, Li S, Vivtcharenko V, et al. Three-Dimensional Distance and Coverage Maps in the Assessment of Peritalar Subluxation in Progressive Collapsing Foot Deformity. Foot Ankle Int 2021;42(6):757–67.

54. Arena CB, Sripanich Y, Leake R, et al. Assessment of Hindfoot Alignment Comparing Weightbearing Radiography to Weightbearing Computed Tomography. Foot Ankle Int 2021;42(11):1482–90.

55. Barg A, Harris MD, Henninger HB, et al. Medial distal tibial angle: comparison between weightbearing mortise view and hindfoot alignment view. Foot Ankle Int 2012;33(8):655–61.

56. Saltzman CL, el-Khoury GY. The hindfoot alignment view. Foot Ankle Int 1995; 16(9):572–6.

57. Krähenbühl N, Siegler L, Deforth M, et al. Subtalar joint alignment in ankle oste-oarthritis. Foot Ankle Surg 2019;25(2):143–9.
58. Kang HW, Kim DY, Park GY, et al. Coronal plane Calcaneal-Talar Orientation in Varus Ankle Osteoarthritis. Foot Ankle Int 2022;43(7):928–36.
59. Kim J-B, Park CH, Ahn J-Y, et al. Characteristics of medial gutter arthritis on weightbearing CT and plain radiograph. Skeletal Radiol 2021;50(8):1575–83.
60. Clare MP, Sanders RW. Preoperative considerations in ankle replacement surgery. Foot Ankle Clin 2002;7(4):709–20.
61. Lamm BM, Paley D. Deformity correction planning for hindfoot, ankle, and lower limb. Clin Podiatr Med Surg 2004;21(3):305–26, v.
62. de Cesar Netto C, Day J, Godoy-Santos AL, et al. The use of three-dimensional biometric Foot and Ankle Offset to predict additional realignment procedures in total ankle replacement. Foot Ankle Surg 2022;28(7):1029–34.
63. Zhang JZ, Lintz F, Bernasconi A, et al. 3D Biometrics for Hindfoot Alignment Using Weightbearing Computed Tomography. Foot Ankle Int 2019;40(6):720–6.
64. Lintz F, Barton T, Millet M, et al. Ground Reaction Force Calcaneal Offset: A new measurement of hindfoot alignment. Foot Ankle Surg 2012;18(1):9–14.
65. Lintz F, Bernasconi A, Baschet L, et al. Relationship Between Chronic Lateral Ankle Instability and Hindfoot Varus Using Weight-Bearing Cone Beam Computed Tomography. Foot Ankle Int 2019;40(10):1175–81.
66. Bernasconi A, Cooper L, Lyle S, et al. Intraobserver and interobserver reliability of cone beam weightbearing semi-automatic three-dimensional measurements in symptomatic pes cavovarus. Foot Ankle Surg 2020;26(5):564–72.
67. Goldberg AJ, Chowdhury K, Bordea E, et al. Total Ankle Replacement Versus Arthrodesis for End-Stage Ankle Osteoarthritis: A Randomized Controlled Trial. Ann Intern Med 2022;175(12):1648–57.
68. Guyer AJ, Richardson G. Current concepts review: total ankle arthroplasty. Foot Ankle Int 2008;29(2):256–64.
69. Omar IM, Abboud SF, Youngner JM. Imaging of Total Ankle Arthroplasty: Normal Imaging Findings and Hardware Complications. Semin Musculoskelet Radiol 2019;23(2):177–94.
70. Barg A, Knupp M, Hintermann B. Simultaneous bilateral versus unilateral total ankle replacement: a patient-based comparison of pain relief, quality of life and functional outcome. J Bone Joint Surg Br 2010;92(12):1659–63.
71. Thompson MJ, Consul D, Umbel BD, et al. Accuracy of Weightbearing CT Scans for Patient-Specific Instrumentation in Total Ankle Arthroplasty. Foot Ankle Orthop 2021;6(4). 247301142110614.
72. Lee WT, Myerson MS, Grosshans KT. What Variables Influence Final Range of Motion Following Total Ankle Arthroplasty. Foot Ankle Orthop 2016;1(1). 2473011416S0002.
73. Karantana A, Hobson S, Dhar S. The Scandinavian total ankle replacement: survivorship at 5 and 8 years comparable to other series. Clin Orthop Relat Res 2010;468(4):951–7.
74. Hobson SA, Karantana A, Dhar S. Total ankle replacement in patients with significant pre-operative deformity of the hindfoot. J Bone Joint Surg Br 2009;91(4):481–6.
75. Pyevich MT, Saltzman CL, Callaghan JJ, et al. Total ankle arthroplasty: a unique design. Two to twelve-year follow-up. J Bone Joint Surg Am 1998;80(10):1410–20.
76. Mallavarapu V, Jasper R, Jones M, et al. Agreement between semiautomatic and manual measurement of selected parameters on weight-bearing computed

tomography images in total ankle replacement: a retrospective study. J Foot Ankle 2022;16(1):72–8.

77. Zeitlin J, Henry J, Ellis S. Preoperative Guidance With Weight-Bearing Computed Tomography and Patient-Specific Instrumentation in Foot and Ankle Surgery. HSS J 2021;17(3):326–32.

78. Kvarda P, Krähenbühl N, Susdorf R, et al. High Reliability for Semiautomated 3D Measurements Based on Weightbearing CT Scans. Foot Ankle Int 2022; 43(1):91–5.

79. Reb CW, Berlet GC. Experience with Navigation in Total Ankle Arthroplasty. Is It Worth the Cost? Foot Ankle Clin 2017;22(2):455–63.

80. Wang C, Yu D, Xu C, et al. Simulated operation combined with patient-specific instrumentation technology is superior to conventional technology for supramalleolar osteotomy: a retrospective comparative study. Am J Transl Res 2021; 13(6):6087–97.

81. Saito GH, Sanders AE, O'Malley MJ, et al. Accuracy of patient-specific instrumentation in total ankle arthroplasty: A comparative study. Foot Ankle Surg 2019;25(3):383–9.

82. VandeLune C, Barbachan Mansur NS, Iehl C, et al. Deformity Correction in Ankle Osteoarthritis Using a Lateral Trans-Fibular Total Ankle Replacement: A Weight-Bearing CT Assessment. Iowa Orthop J 2022;42(2):36–46.

83. Hintermann B, Susdorf R, Krähenbühl N, et al. Axial Rotational Alignment in Mobile-Bearing Total Ankle Arthroplasty. Foot Ankle Int 2020;41(5):521–8.

84. Lintz F, Mast J, Bernasconi A, et al. 3D, Weightbearing Topographical Study of Periprosthetic Cysts and Alignment in Total Ankle Replacement. Foot Ankle Int 2020;41(1):1–9.

85. Dekker TJ, Hamid KS, Federer AE, et al. The Value of Motion: Patient-Reported Outcome Measures Are Correlated With Range of Motion in Total Ankle Replacement. Foot Ankle Spec 2018;11(5):451–6.

86. Frigg A, Nigg B, Hinz L, et al. Clinical relevance of hindfoot alignment view in total ankle replacement. Foot Ankle Int 2010;31(10):871–9.

87. De Cesar Netto C, Bang K, Mansur NS, et al. Multiplanar Semiautomatic Assessment of Foot and Ankle Offset in Adult Acquired Flatfoot Deformity. Foot Ankle Int 2020;41(7):839–48.

88. Henry JK, Rider C, Cody E, et al. Evaluating and Managing the Painful Total Ankle Replacement. Foot Ankle Int 2021;42(10):1347–61.

89. Zhao D, Huang D, Zhang G, et al. Positive and negative factors for the treatment outcomes following total ankle arthroplasty? A systematic review. Foot Ankle Surg 2020;26(1):1–13.

90. Carcuro GM, Avilés Espinoza C, Varela C. Subtalar Joint Behavior After Total Ankle Arthroplasty. Foot Ankle Orthop 2022.

91. Barbachan Mansur NS, Lalevee M, Maly C, et al. Association Between Middle Facet Subluxation and Foot and Ankle Offset in Progressive Collapsing Foot Deformity. Foot Ankle Int 2022;43(1):96–100.

92. Lalevée M, Barbachan Mansur NS, Rojas EO, et al. Prevalence and pattern of lateral impingements in the progressive collapsing foot deformity. Arch Orthop Trauma Surg 2023;143(1):161–8.

93. de Cesar Netto C, Silva T, Li S, et al. Assessment of Posterior and Middle Facet Subluxation of the Subtalar Joint in Progressive Flatfoot Deformity. Foot Ankle Int 2020;41(10):1190–7.

Multiaxial 3D MRI of the Ankle

Advanced High-Resolution Visualization of Ligaments, Tendons, and Articular Cartilage

Benjamin Fritz, MD, PD[a,b], Cesar de Cesar Netto, MD, PhD[c],
Jan Fritz, MD, PD, RMSK[d,*]

KEYWORDS

- MRI • 3D • 2D • Postprocessing • Multiplanar reformation
- Curved planar reformation • Ligaments • Tendons

KEY POINTS

- 3D MRI is a newer, clinically available MRI technique for high-resolution ankle MRI with isotropic voxel size and up to five times thinner image slices.
- Clinical 3D MRI of the ankle resolves the smallest anatomic ankle structures and abnormalities of ligaments, tendons, osteochondral lesions, and nerves.
- 3D MRI postprocessing permits limitless oblique planar reformations for visualizing oblique ligaments in profile and curved planner reformations for unfolding multidirectional tendons into one image plane.

INTRODUCTION

MRI is accurate for diagnosing acute and chronic ankle conditions due to its high soft tissue contrast and resolving soft structures in high spatial resolution.[1] Clinical MRI protocols typically consist of 5–6 pulse sequences in different plane orientations and with different image contrast, including proton density, T2, and T1 weightings. In addition, those pulse sequences may be acquired without or with fat suppression.

Proton density-weighted MR images provide high morphological detail and contrast resolution for detecting and characterizing structural abnormalities of cartilage, ligaments, and tendons. Fat-suppressed fluid-sensitive proton density and T2-weighted

[a] Department of Radiology, Balgrist University Hospital, Forchstrasse 340, Zurich 8008, Switzerland; [b] Faculty of Medicine, University of Zurich, Zurich, Switzerland; [c] Department of Orthopaedics and Rehabilitation, University of Iowa, 200 Hawkins Drive, Iowa City, IA 52242, USA; [d] Department of Radiology, Division of Musculoskeletal Radiology, NYU Grossman School of Medicine, 660 1st Avenue, New York, NY 10016, USA
* Corresponding author.
E-mail address: jan.fritz@nyulangone.org

Foot Ankle Clin N Am 28 (2023) 529–550
https://doi.org/10.1016/j.fcl.2023.05.008
1083-7515/23/© 2023 Elsevier Inc. All rights reserved.

MR images emphasize bone marrow and soft tissue edema, joint effusions, fluid collections, hematomas, and masses. T1-weighted MR images are fat-specific and thus predominantly used for evaluating bone marrow evaluation in cases with suspected osteomyelitis and neoplastic disease. T1-weighted MR images show non-displaced fractures; however, the combination of proton density-weighted MR images and fat-suppressed fluid-sensitive MR images demonstrate non-displaced fractures with similar accuracy.[2] T1-weighted MR images without and with fat suppression are the standard to visualize intravenous gadolinium contrast enhancement.

The most commonly employed clinical MRI technique for imaging the ankle is two-dimensional (2D) MRI (**Fig. 1**), utilizing various, separately acquired fast spin-echo or turbo spin-echo pulse sequences in standardized axial, coronal, and sagittal plane orientations. These standard orthogonal plane sequences can be supplemented with individually angulated sequences to structures of particular interest, such as the anterior inferior talofibular ligament, the calcaneofibular ligament, and the flexor and peroneal tendons to achieve single plane profile views and improve their visibility. As each pulse sequence of a 2D MRI protocol has to be acquired separately, the entire 2D MRI protocol for the ankle can be time-consuming, with total acquisition times of up to 25 minutes commonly found in clinical practice.[3–5] While new acceleration techniques and artificial intelligence-driven image reconstruction can dramatically reduce the scan times of 2D MRI,[6–11] there are limitations of 2D MRI in the ankle.

2D fast spin-echo and turbo spin-echo MRI sequences provide high signal-to-noise ratios and high in-plane and contrast resolutions. However, in clinical practice, the slice thickness of 2D MRI is inherently limited to 2–3 mm, which produces partial volume averaging of small anatomic structures resulting in blurred contours of oblique

Difference Between 2D and 3D MRI

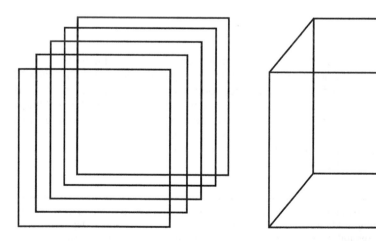

2D MRI   3D MRI

Fig. 1. Difference between two-dimensional and three-dimensional MRI. Two-dimensional MRI is acquired slice by slice, whereas 3D MRI is acquired as a single volume of small isotropic voxels. Two-dimensional MRI slices are fixated in space and may not be altered after the acquisition. As three-dimensional MRI consists of a single volume of small voxels, curved and planar slices can be created in infinite spatial orientations during postprocessing.

structures due to volume averaging effects within the image slice. This phenomenon is known as the "partial volume effect" and occurs when the size of voxel elements spans different tissues and structures, such as small ligament fibers and surrounding fat tissue or cartilage and adjacent bone (**Figs. 2** and **3**). As a result, the signals from each tissue or structure within that voxel will be mathematically combined, leading to the inability to resolve or display small anatomic structures. In some instances, this effect can also lead to the omission of subtle abnormalities in MR images.

Three-dimensional (3D) MRI is a newer, clinically available MRI technique capable of high-resolution ankle MRI, overcoming several limitations of 2D MRI.[12] While 2D MRI acquisitions are slice-by-slice, 3D MRI acquires the ankle as an entire high-resolution volume consisting of multiple voxels with symmetric edge lengths in all three spatial directions (isotropic voxels) (see **Fig. 1**). Modern clinical 3D MRI sequences allow isotropic voxels to resolve small anatomic structures and abnormalities, limit partial volume effects, and provide near-limitless multiplanar and multiaxial image reformation and postprocessing capabilities.

3D fast and turbo spin-echo MRI pulse sequences are preferable to gradient echo-based 3D MRI pulse sequences due to their better contrast resolution for bone and musculoskeletal soft tissues.[4] The primary use of gradient echo-based 3D pulse

Partial Volume Effect
2D MRI versus 3D MRI Appearances of the
Intact Anterior Talofibular Ligament

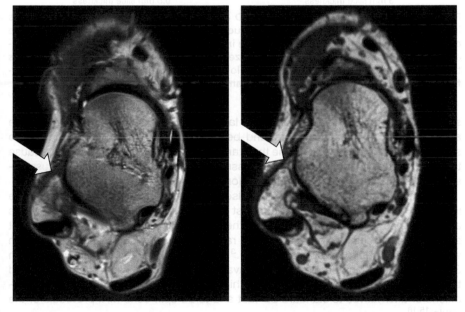

Axial Proton Density-Weighted 2D MRI   Axial Proton Density-Weighted 3D MRI
3 mm slice thickness   0.5 mm slice thickness

Fig. 2. Partial volume effect on 2D versus 3D ankle MRI. The 2D MR image (*left image*) is inherently prone to partial volume effect due to the thicker slices, which obscures fine detail of the intact anterior talofibular ligament (*arrow left image*). The 3D MR image (*right image*) minimizes such partial volume effects due to six times thinner slices, resulting in a sharply delineated ligament (*arrow right image*).

Partial Volume Effect
2D MRI versus 3D MRI Appearance of the Plantar Spring Ligaments

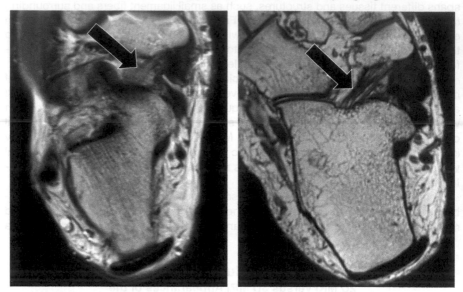

Axial Proton Density-Weighted 2D MRI
3 mm slice thickness

Axial Proton Density-Weighted 3D MRI
0.5 mm slice thickness

Fig. 3. Partial volume effect on 2D versus 3D ankle MRI. The 2D MR image (*left image*) is inherently prone to partial volume effect due to the thicker slices and stricty axial plane orientation, which obscures fine detail of the intact plantar spring ligaments (*arrow left image*). The 3D MR image (*right image*) minimizes such partial volume effects due to six times thinner slices and individually aligned slice along the axis of the ligament, resulting in perfect profile view with sharply delineated ligament fibers (*arrow right image*).

sequences is cartilage imaging since the lack of true T2-contrast often hampers the assessment of tendons, ligaments, and bone structures. Therefore, fast and turbo spin echo pulse sequences became the standard in musculoskeletal 3D MRI because they are not just limited to cartilage assessment but effectively evaluate all musculoskeletal tissues, including ligaments, tendons, bone marrow, and nerves.[13]

3D fast and turbo spin-echo MRI pulse sequences capable of producing true isotropic 3D data sets with similar contrast to 2D MRI were developed over 20 years ago.[14] Despite their technical feasibility, the time needed to acquire a single 3D fast and turbo spin-echo MRI pulse sequence ranged between 15 and 20 minutes, which was prohibitively long for clinical practice.[3] However, recent technical innovations in 3D MRI accelerations enable clinically available high-quality isotropic 3D fast and turbo spin-echo MRI pulse sequences within 5 minutes and less, providing viable additions or alternatives to standard 2D fast and turbo spin-echo MRI protocols of the ankle.[15,16]

3D fast and turbo spin-echo MRI pulse sequences can be acquired with the same MRI scanners and the same MRI coils as 2D MRI without requiring specialized equipment or scanner technology. Either 1.5 Tesla (T) or 3.0 T MRI scanners can be used; however, 3D fast and turbo spin-echo MRI pulse sequences substantially benefit from the higher signal of 3.0 T MRI regarding acquisition speed, image resolution, and tissue contrast.[13]

Multiple studies evaluated the performance of 3D fast and turbo spin-echo MRI in the ankle, typically employing a combination of proton density- and T2-weighted contrasts.[3,15,16] Five-minute non-fat-suppressed proton density-weighted 3D data sets can be acquired with an isotropic voxel size of 0.5 x 0.5 × 0.5 mm^3, providing a good balance between acquisition times and high in-plane resolution with thin slices for the display of fine anatomic details (**Table 1**).[17–19] Five-minute fat-suppressed proton density-or T2-weighted 3D data sets can be acquired with an isotropic voxel size of 0.6 x 0.6 × 0.6 mm^3 providing exquisite fluid sensitivity for detecting subtle signal abnormalities (see **Table 1**).[3,17,18]

Since fat-suppressed and non-fat-suppressed MRI pulse sequences should always be used in conjunction, a practical 3D MRI protocol includes a pair of non-fat-suppressed proton density-weighted and fat-suppressed proton density-weighted or T2-weighted 3D fast or turbo spin-echo MRI pulse sequences for a whole-ankle MRI assessment. Clinically viable scenarios also include hybrid protocols which use a single 3D fast or turbo spin-echo MRI pulse sequence in combination with 2D fast or turbo spin-echo sequences. In our experience, a 10-min isotropic 3D fast or turbo spin-echo MRI protocol that includes a fat-suppressed fluid-sensitive 3D MRI sequence for detecting soft tissue edema, fluid collections, and bone marrow edema patterns, paired with a higher resolution non-fat-suppressed 3D fast and turbo spin-echo MRI for evaluating structural abnormalities, is a powerful combination for diagnosing a wide range of orthopedic or traumatic ankle conditions.[15,16,19]

This article provides an overview of the clinical application of 3D MRI of the ankle, reviews diagnostic performances of 2D and 3D MRI for diagnosing ankle abnormalities, and illustrates clinical 3D ankle MRI applications.

TECHNICAL ASPECTS OF 3D MRI IN CLINICAL PRACTICE

When considering the practical aspects of clinical implementation, several differences exist between 2D and 3D MRI of the ankle, which primarily apply to image acquisition and diagnostic interpretation techniques (see **Fig. 1**).

Table 1
3.0 T 3D CAIPIRINHA SPACE turbo spin echo protocol for ankle MRI

	3D MRI Protocol	
Parameters	Proton Density-Weighted 3D CAIPIRINHA SPACE	T2-SPAIR 3D CAIPIRINHA SPACE
Orientation	Sagittal	Sagittal
Repetition time [ms]	1000	1100
Echo time [ms]	28	110
Echo train length	54	42
Receiver bandwidth (Hertz/pixel)	422	399
Field-of-view [mm]	160 x 160	160 x 160
Voxel dimensions [mm]	0.5 x 0.5 x 0.5	0.63 x 0.63 x 0.63
Number of Slices	176	144
In-plane frequency encoding direction	Anterior-to-posterior	Anterior-to-posterior
Acquisition time	4 min 46 s	5 min 10 s

Abbreviations: CAIPIRINHA, Controlled Aliasing In Parallel Imaging Results IN higher acceleration; SPACE, sampling perfection with application optimized contrast using different flip angle evolutions; TSE, turbo spin echo.

2D and 3D MRI of the ankle are typically performed with the patient in a supine position and the foot placed in a dedicated boot-shaped foot-and-ankle coil designed to provide a comfortable position for the patient. For ankle MRI, the images typically extend from the distal tibia and fibula to the heel and the bases of the metatarsal bones in the sagittal, axial, and coronal planes.

3D pulse sequences of the ankle are usually acquired in the sagittal plane since this is typically the most time-efficient solution. Axial and coronal images are not acquired directly but are reformatted from the isotropic sagittal MR images after the exam has ended. The isotropic geometry of the voxels with the same length in all dimensions permits the reformation of any plane orientation from the parental sagittal data set without losing image quality. 2D MRI sequences do not allow useful secondary reformations and have to be acquired separately for any desired imaging plane.

The magic angle effect is a commonly encountered artifact around the angle, which primarily occurs in structures with tightly packed parallel bundled fibers of ligaments and tendons. On MR images of pulse sequences with a short echo time of up to approximately 50 ms, such as proton density- and T1-weighted MR images, it induces an artificial signal increase in structures oriented with an angle of 55° to the z-axis of the main magnetic field (B_0), which is typically the longitudinal direction of the MR scanner. In the ankle, the strongest magic angle effect can be found at the flexor and peroneal tendons at the level of the malleoli.[20] MRI sequences with a long echo time, such as T2-weighted pulse sequences, are least prone to the magic angle effect and represent a valuable part of clinical ankle MRI protocols (**Fig. 4**). Another practical possibility to eliminate the magic angle effect is to perform ankle MRI exams with patients in the prone position; however, the boot-shaped ankle coil may no longer be used then, but open coils, such as a knee surface coil. Prone patient positioning eliminates the magic angle artifact in the long flexor and peroneal tendons, as this ankle

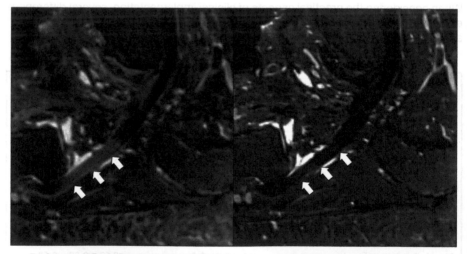

| Fat-Suppressed Proton Density-Weighted 3D MRI | Fat-Suppressed T2-Weighted 3D MRI |
| Echo Time = 35 ms | Echo Time = 105 ms |

Fig. 4. Magic angle effect of the peroneus longus tendon. Fat-suppressed proton density-weighted and T2-weighted curved planar 3D reformation images of the peroneus longus tendon (*arrows*) demonstrate the magic angle effect characterized as an increased tendon signal (*arrows* in the *left image*) with a short echo time of 35 ms. The magic angle effect (*arrows* in the *right image*) is minimized with a longer echo time of 105 ms, indicated by normal low signal intensity of the tendon segement.

position results in an almost parallel course of the tendons to the z-direction of the static magnetic B0 field. However, it should be noted that the orientation of the prone position and plantar flexion alters the medial and lateral collateral ligament orientations, potentially obscuring small tears. Furthermore, some patients will find this position uncomfortable and may induce more motion artifacts.

MRI scanner field strength, such as 1.5 T versus 3.0 T, is a critical factor for achieving high 3D MRI image quality.[3,13] In principle, 3D MRI exams of the ankle may be obtained at 1.5 T and 3.0 T; however, 3.0 T MRI scanners yield approximately twice the signal compared to 1.5 T scanners, which can be translated into higher image quality and faster scanning. While 3D MRI of the ankle may be obtained at 1.5 T with lower image resolution or substantially longer scan times, most published studies have been performed at 3.0 T. To ensure high MRI exam quality, our preferred and recommended MRI scanner choice for 3D MRI of the ankle is 3.0 T with a dedicated boot-shaped foot and ankle surface coil.[3,15,16]

Modern 3D fast and turbo spin-echo ankle MRI pulse sequences have similar contrast characteristics as 2D fast and turbo spin-echo MR images[17,18]; however, the image texture may vary depending on the sequence type, slice thickness, contrast parameter settings, acceleration technique, manufacturer, and viewing software.[10,15,16] 3D fast and turbo spin-echo MR images often appear edge-enhanced, which may need some time to get used to.

Modern viewer software is required to efficiently review and take full advantage of the capabilities of 3D ankle MRI exams. Most modern enterprise-grade PACS systems include suitable viewer software. In addition, many capable standalone DICOM viewers are commercially available for personal and Apple computers. Key capabilities to take full advantage of isotropic 3D MRI data sets include interactive and dynamic multiplanar reformation modes, adjustable slice thicknesses, maximum and minimum intensity projections, linear and curved planar reformation functions (**Fig. 5**), and synchronized zoom, panning, and rotation of linked viewports. Creating thick-slab reformations dynamically with standard signal intensity averaging from

Curved Planar 3D MRI for Unfolding of Perimalleolar Tendons

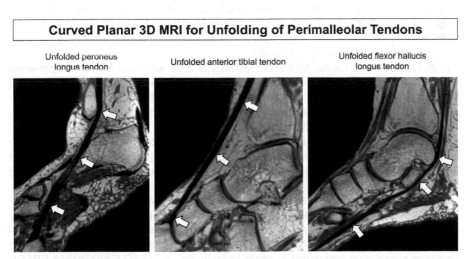

Unfolded peroneus longus tendon   Unfolded anterior tibial tendon   Unfolded flexor hallucis longus tendon

Fig. 5. 3D MRI unfolding of ankle tendons using curved planar reformation. Using a single multiaxial isotropic high-resolution 3D MRI dataset, dedicated curved multiplanar reformation images can be created for any curved tendon about the ankle. The unfolding reformation results in a planar long-axis display of double- and triple-angulated tendons (*arrows*), avoiding partial volume effects for better display and evaluation.

high-resolution isotropic thin-slice 3D fast and turbo spin-echo data sets can help reduce image noise and achieve a more 2D fast and turbo spin-echo-like image appearance, particularly for fat-suppressed data sets.[17,19,21] Reformating images with thicknesses of 1.0 to 1.5 mm may be a good balance between high-resolution thin-slice 3D MRI and 2D fast and turbo spin-echo-like image appearance for clinical interpretation.

3D MRI can also improve scan efficiency, thereby shortening ankle MRI examinations.[3,15,16] Several studies have shown that using a single 3D fast or turbo spin-echo MRI sequence instead of two or three standard 2D fast or turbo spin-echo sequences within an ankle MRI exam can shorten the total scan time.[15,16,22–24] Clinically available, modern acceleration techniques result in high-quality 3D fast and turbo spin-echo sequences in under 5 minutes,[3,10,17,18,25] saving up to 50% of the time compared to 2D fast and turbo spin-echo sequences with acquisition times of around 3 minutes each. Recent advances in artificial intelligence-based image reconstruction have substantially reduced 2D and 3D MRI scan times.[6,10,25] The time-saving potentials of 2D and 3D MRI evolve rapidly and will depend on locally available MRI sequences, surface coils, and MRI scanners.

TECHNICAL PERFORMANCE OF 3D MRI

In recent years, several studies have been conducted to compare technical image characteristics of 3D fast and turbo spin-echo MRI sequences with their 2D counterparts.[3] These studies have demonstrated that 3D fast and turbo spin-echo MRI can create comparable image signal strength (signal-to-noise ratios) and tissue contrast (contrast-to-noise ratios) and depicts anatomical structures at least as well as 2D fast and turbo spin-echo MRI.

The first results of a spin-echo-based 3D MRI sequence for the ankle were published in 2008.[22] The study found that T2-weighted 3D fast spin-echo MRI with and without fat suppression had significantly higher image signal strength than 2D fast spin-echo MRI and comparable image tissue contrast. Although image quality was judged similarly between the 2D and 3D fast spin-echo MRI exams, 3D MRI showed more blurring. The scan time for the 3D ankle MRI sequence was 5 to 6 minutes with isotropic voxels of 0.6 mm edge length.

In 2012, another 3D ankle MRI study evaluated a T2-weighted 3D turbo spin-echo MRI sequence with fat suppression.[23] 3D MRI had significantly higher image signal strength and contrast for fluid and articular cartilage than 2D turbo spin-echo MRI sequences. 3D MRI was superior for depicting articular cartilage, collateral ligaments, and the spring ligament complex.

Over the past 15 years, multiple 3.0 T studies have shown that 3D fast and turbo spin-echo MRI sequences create comparable image signal strength and contrast and depict anatomic joint structures and tissues at least, as well as 2D fast and turbo spin-echo MRI.

In 2016, a novel 4-fold accelerated 3D turbo spin-echo MRI sequence called CAIPIRINHA SPACE was introduced for 3D ankle MRI.[15] The pulse sequence was initially developed for the knee[19,21] and later adopted for the ankle.[15,16] Advantageous features included a novel bidirectional 2 x 2 parallel imaging acceleration pattern, which increases signal gain compared to older techniques.[10,13,25] 3D CAIPIRINHA SPACE MRI creates similar image characteristics to corresponding 2D MR images. The faster acceleration permits proton density-weighted 3D MRI with a voxel size of 0.5 x 0.5 × 0.5 mm^3 and fat-suppressed T2-weighted 3D MRI with a voxel size of 0.6 x 0.6 × 0.6 mm^3 at around 5 min scan time for each. 3D CAIPIRINHA SPACE MRI is our favorite technique for daily clinical practice and our recommended technique for 3D ankle MRI.

Ankle Ligaments

Ankle ligaments are important stabilizers of the syndesmosis and talocrural, subtalar, and midfoot joints. On MRI, normal ligaments appear with low signal intensity on T1-weighted, proton density-weighted, and T2-weighted MR images regardless of fat suppression. However, some ligaments have naturally occurring fatty striations interposed between intact ligament strands, appearing as alternating "zebra-like" linear bright and dark signal intensities on nonfat-suppressed high-resolution MR images (**Fig. 6**).

Ligament injuries range from low-grade interstitial injuries to complete retracted and displaced tears (**Table 2**) (**Fig. 7**). Low-grade interstitial ligamentous injuries present with edematous interstitial signal intensity on fluid-sensitive proton density-weighted and T2-weighted MR images. Due to their fluid insensitivity, the edematous signal abnormalities are typically not visible on T1-weighted MR images. In addition to the edematous signal, the injured ligaments may appear enlarged but without visible disrupted fibers. Partial-thickness tears show clearly defined disrupted and continuous fibers. The term "high-grade partial-thickness tear" is not clearly defined but might be most often applied to indicate greater than 50% fiber disruption of the cross-sectional ligament area. Full-thickness tears require the disruption of all ligament fibers. Fluid-filled gap formation indicates fiber retraction. Similar to a classic Stener

Normal Straited High-Resolution MRI Appearance
of the Anterior Inferior Tibiofibular Ligament

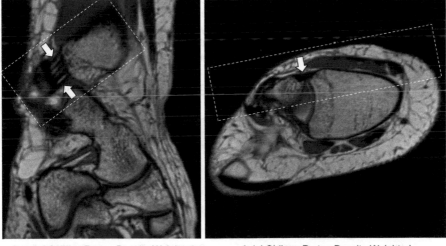

Coronal Oblique Proton Density-Weighted
3D MRI

Axial Oblique Proton Density-Weighted
3D MRI

Fig. 6. High-resolution 3D MRI appearance of striated ligaments. Coronal oblique (*left image*) and axial oblique (*right image*) program density-weighted 3D MRI reformation images demonstrate the normal striated appearance of the anterior talofibular ligament of the syndesmosis on the coronal oblique 3D MR image (*arrows* in *left image*). Upon anatomic alignment along the course of the ligament on the axial oblique 3D MR image, the ligament fibers appear continuous and with intact hypointense MRI signal (*arrow* in the *right image*). The dashed boxes indicate the slice orientations.

Table 2
MRI terminology and MRI findings of ligamentous injuries

Ligament Integrity and MRI Terminology	MRI Findings
Interstitial injury	Increased proton density and T2 signal inside the ligament without visualized fiber disruption
Partial-thickness tear	Mixed disrupted and intact ligament fibers
Full-thickness tear	Disruption of all ligament fibers with optional fiber retraction and displacement of torn ligament ends.

lesion in the thumb ulnar collateral ligament and knee medial collateral ligament,[2,26] torn ligament ends may displace, such as the calcaneofibular ligament, on top of the overlying peroneal tendons.

Lateral Collateral Ligaments

The lateral collateral ligaments are the most frequently injured ankle ligaments and are involved in about 60% to 80% of all ankle injuries.[27,28] Inversion trauma is the most common mechanism of injury. The anterior tibiofibular ligament (ATFL) is most commonly injured (see **Fig. 7; Fig. 8**), followed by the calcaneofibular ligament (CFL) and rarely the posterior tibiofibular ligament (PTFL).

Scarring and remodeling of the lateral collateral ligaments are common MRI findings in the general population, usually indicating healed ligament trauma, which may or may not corroborate a clinical diagnosis of chronic lateral ankle instability. The spectrum of scar-remodeled lateral collateral ligaments includes thinner and thicker than normal ligament diameters, irregular ligament surfaces, and higher than normal, non-edematous signal intensities on proton density-weighted, T2-weighted, and also T1-weighted MR images, which reduces to normal with increasing maturation of healing.

In 2D MRI, axial and coronal plane images are typically used to evaluate the lateral collateral ligaments. However, as the ATFL has an axial oblique and the CFL has a coronal oblique course, they are typically not visible in profile on a single standard axial,

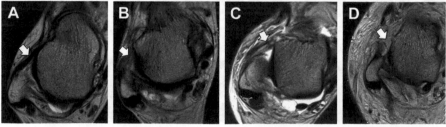

| Intact | Interstitial Injury | Partial-thickness Tear | Full-thickness Tear |

Fig. 7. MRI appearances of ligament integrity. Axial proton density-weighted MR images show the spectrum from intact (*A*) to full-thickness tear (*D*) of the anterior talofibular ligament (*arrows*). (*A*) Intact ligaments appear taut, dark, and sharply demarcated (*arrow*). (*B*) Interstitial ligament injuries appear with increased internal edema-like protein density or T2 signal and optional thickening (*arrow*), but no discrete fiber disruption. (*C*) Partial-thickness ligament tears show mixed discontinuous and continuous ligament fibers (*arrow*). (*D*) Full-thickness anterior talofibular ligament tears show the disruption of all ligament fibers (*arrow*) and often a fluid-filled gap.

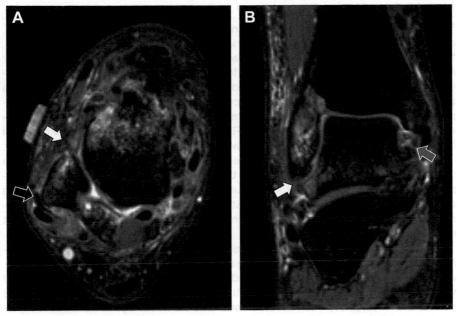

Axial Fat-Suppressed Proton Density-   Coronal Fat-Suppressed Proton Density-
Weighted 3D MRI   Weighted 3D MRI

Fig. 8. 3D MRI after ankle trauma in a 16-year-old teenager. Axial (*A*) and coronal (*B*) T2-weighted fat-suppressed 3D MRI reformations show a full-thickness anterior talofibular ligament tear (*white arrows* in *A* and *B*), full-thickness deltoid ligament complex tear (*gray arrows* in *B*), and laterally subluxated peroneal tendons (*black arrow* in *A*) due to tearing of the superior peroneal retinaculum retinaculum.

sagittal, or coronal 2D MR image but cut obliquely through multiple slices. Acquiring dedicated 2D MR images aligned individually to oblique ligaments is possible but time-consuming (see **Fig. 6**). The limitless multiplanar reformation capabilities of 3D MRI enable the alignment of long and short-axis images to oblique ligaments individually and interactively during readout.

Overall, the reported diagnostic accuracy of MRI for diagnosing ATFL tears is high, with reported sensitivities of 80%–100% and specificities of up to 100%.[29,30] Several studies showed similar diagnostic performances of 2D and 3D fast and turbo spin echo MRI techniques for detecting lateral collateral ligament injuries.[16,23,31,32] A study of 101 clinical patients found that T2-weighted 3D turbo spin echo MRI had a higher sensitivity of 96% versus 84% to 86% of 2D turbo spin echo MRI for detecting ATFL injuries.[24] The specificities were similar between 2D and 3D MRI, whereas 3D MRI had superior edge sharpness. Another study comparing 2D and 3D turbo spin echo MRI techniques found a statistically similar diagnostic performance for detecting CFL injuries, although the 3D MRI image quality was considered inferior.[33]

An anatomical morphology study applying 3D turbo spin echo MRI described a double-bundled appearance of the ATFL, with tearing of both bundles as the most common pattern in acute ankle sprains.[34] Another study evaluating the obliquely oriented CFL and peroneus tendon relationship found that the peroneal muscle-tendon unit act as a fulcrum for the deeper positioned CFL, which had a significantly lower angulation in maximum plantar flexion than in the neutral position.[35]

Medial Collateral Ligament Complex and Spring Ligament

The deltoid ligament complex, also known as the medial collateral ligament complex, comprises a superficial and deep layer. The superficial layer includes the talonavicular, tibiospring, and talocalcaneal ligaments, whereas the deep layer includes the anterior and posterior tibiotalar ligaments. Unlike lateral collateral ligament injuries, medial collateral ligament injuries are less common, accounting for only 10% to 16% of ankle injuries in athletes.[36,37] High-energy trauma with forced ankle eversion is the most commonly reported mechanism of injury. Medial collateral ligament tears often occur with lateral collateral and syndesmotic ligament injuries. MRI detects and characterizes medial collateral ligament injuries with 84% to 100% sensitivity and 93% to 100% specificity.[38,39]

The spring ligament complex comprises three parts that stabilize the medial arch connecting the calcaneus and navicular bones, including the superomedial, medioplantar oblique, and inferoplantar longitudinal components.[40] Full-thickness tearing of the spring ligament complex is rare. Still, remodeling with chronic scarring, waviness, and elongation are common MRI findings after ankle sprains with concomitant midfoot and peritalar translation injuries.

With 2D MRI, the coronal plane is typically used to evaluate the medial collateral ligament complex and superomedial spring ligament. In contrast, the plantar spring ligaments are typically evaluated on axial and sagittal plane MR images. However, partial volume effects secondary to thick slice thickness and oblique ligament orientations can result in incomplete visualization on standard 2D MR images. The limitless multiplanar reformation capabilities and much thinner slice thickness of 3D MRI data sets permit the individual alignment of imaging planes to visualize the medial collateral (see **Fig. 8**) and spring ligaments better.

Two studies compared the diagnostic performance of 2D turbo spin echo and 3D SPACE turbo spin echo MRI for detecting medial collateral and spring ligament injuries after acute ankle injuries.[16,23] The first study published in 2012 found no significant differences in detecting medial collateral ligament tears comparing axial, sagittal, and coronal fat-suppressed T2-weighted sequence with a single isotropic fat-suppressed T2-weighted 3D SPACE turbo spin echo sequence.[23] However, the other study published in 2016 found significantly more ligament tears with 3D than 2D MRI using a modern comprehensive 10-min whole-ankle 3D CAIPIRINHA SPACE MRI protocol, comprised of isotropic proton density-weighted and an isotropic fat-suppressed T2-weighted 3D MRI data sets.[16]

Syndesmosis

The syndesmosis is the primary stabilizer of the distal tibiofibular joint. The syndesmosis typically includes the anterior inferior tibiofibular ligament (see **Fig. 6**), the posterior inferior tibiofibular ligament, the interosseous ligament, and the interosseous membrane.

Multiple injury mechanisms may cause syndesmotic injuries, but the most common injury mechanism comprises dorsiflexion with external rotation on a planted foot.[41] Syndesmotic injuries occur with a 10% to 17% incidence.[42,43] Diagnosing syndesmotic injuries can be challenging, but it is crucial to prevent instability.[44–46] Treatment options range from immobilization to surgical repair and reconstruction.[5,47]

2D MRI has a 97% accuracy for detecting anterior and 100% accuracy for detecting posterior inferior tibiofibular ligaments.[48] As the syndesmotic ligaments have an oblique axial course, 45-degree angulated axial oblique 2D MR images may be obtained to improve tear detection. However, the multiplanar reformation capabilities of 3D MRI permit individual plane alignment along the syndesmotic ligament fibers for accurately detecting acute and chronic syndesmotic injuries (see **Fig. 6**; **Fig. 9**).[49] A 2017 study

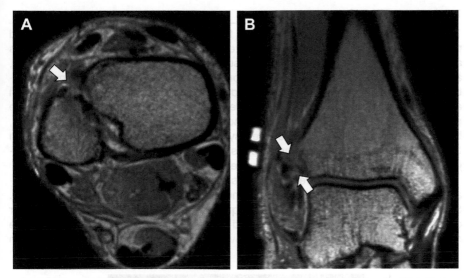

Axial Oblique Proton Density-Weighted 3D   Coronal Oblique Proton Density-Weighted
MRI   3D MRI

Fig. 9. 3D MRI after ankle trauma in a 29-year-old man. Oblique axial (*A*) and oblique coronal (*B*) proton density-weighted 3D MRI reformations show a full-thickness anterior tibiofibular ligament tear (*arrows*).

found similar accuracies in detecting anterior inferior and posterior inferior tibiofibular ligament tears using axial oblique T2-weighted 2D and proton density-weighted 3D turbo spin echo SPACE MRI reformation images, with accuracies ranging from 96% to 100%.[50]

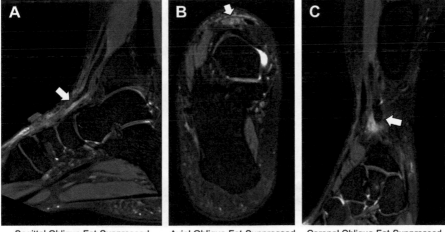

Sagittal Oblique Fat-Suppressed   Axial Oblique Fat-Suppressed   Coronal Oblique Fat-Suppressed
T2-Weighted 3D MRI   T2-Weighted 3D MRI   T2-Weighted 3D MRI

Fig. 10. 3D MRI after ankle trauma in a 44-year-old woman. Oblique sagittal (*A*), the axial (*B*), and oblique coronal (*C*) fat-suppressed T2-weighted MRI reformation images demonstrate a 6 cm retracted extensor hallucis longus tear. The proximally retracted tendon is located at the talonavicular joint line (*white arrows* in *A* and *C*). The axial oblique MRI reformation image (*B*) distal to the retracted tendon demonstrates an empty tendon sheath (*arrow* in *B*).

Tendons

The hindfoot tendons include the extensor, flexor, peroneal, and Achilles tendons and plantar fascia. In concert, the hindfoot tendons act as joint and arch stabilizers and facilitate complex ankle movements such as inversion, eversion, plantarflexion, and dorsiflexion. For example, the posterior tibial tendon is the primary dynamic stabilizer of the medial longitudinal arch, and degeneration or dysfunction can lead to an adult-acquired flatfoot deformity and progressive collapsing foot deformity.[51,52] Ankle pain may be caused by degenerative tendinopathy, tenosynovitis, and traumatic tears, but tendon abnormalities may also be asymptomatic, particularly peroneal tendon tears[53] .[54] Traumatic injuries of the tendons are much less common than ligament injuries, occurring in up to 3% of acute ankle injuries.[28,55]

Due to the complex multidirectional course of the hindfoot tendons, multiple MR imaging planes are necessary to visualize the different tendon portions appropriately. Separately acquired axial and sagittal oblique 2D MRI sequences with perpendicular orientation to the long axis of the flexor and peroneal tendons may be obtained at the medial and lateral malleolus level to improve the visualization of the different tendon

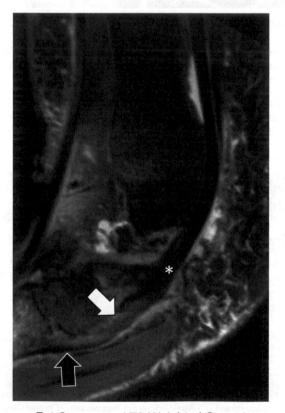

Fat-Suppressed T2-Weighted Curved
Planar 3D MRI Reformation

Fig. 11. 3D MRI of the ankle in a 58-year-old woman with chronic ankle pain. Curved planar fat-suppressed T2-weighted 3D MRI reformation image along the posterior tibial tendon (*asterisk*) shows a mildly retracted full-thickness navicular attachment tear (*white arrow*) and continuous plantar attachment fibers (*black arrow*).

segments but substantially prolong acquisition times. The multiplanar reformation capabilities of 3D MRI also include a mode called "curved planar reformation," which allows the "unfolding" of multidirectional structures, such as the extensor (**Fig. 10**), long flexor (**Fig. 11**), and peroneal (**Figs. 12 and 13**) tendons, into a single image plane (see **Fig. 5**).

The magic angle effect poses a clinically relevant challenge for 2D and 3D MRI of ankle tendons. The long flexor and peroneal tendons are especially prone to abnormally high signal intensity due to the magic angle effects around the medial and lateral malleolus. To eliminate magic angle effects, 3D MRI sequences with long echo times may be included in ankle MRI protocols, such as a T2-weighted 3D turbo spin echo MRI sequence without or with fat suppression (see **Fig. 4**). However since magic angle effects occur predictably typically affected tendon segments should be evaluated based on morphology rather than signal intensity on sequences with short echo times.

A 2019 study found around the ankle reduced magic angle effects and improved the visualization of tendons with isotropic proton density-weighted and fat-suppressed T2-weighted 3D CAIPIRINHA SPACE turbo spin echo MRI sequences.[16] Another study also applied proton density-weighted and fat-suppressed T2-weighted 3D CAIPIRINHA SPACE MRI and found improved tendon visualization and similar diagnostic performance for the detection of tears compared to a similar 2D ankle MRI protocol.[23]

Articular Cartilage

MRI has high accuracy for detecting talocrural, subtalar, talonavicular, and tarsometatarsal articular cartilage lesions, including articular cartilage defects, osteochondral lesions, chondral and osteochondral sheer injuries, and fractures (**Table 3**).[5] Osteochondral lesions are characterized by loss of cartilage integrity with or without subchondral bone fragments (**Table 4**).[56] Osteochondral lesions are commonly traumatic, in which MRI provides high accuracy for detection and predicting stability.[57,58]

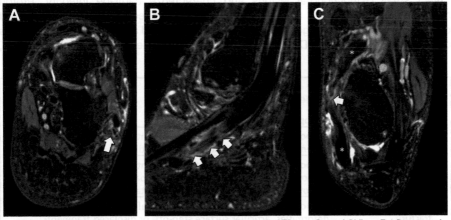

A	B	C

Axial Oblique Fat-Suppressed T2-Weighted 3D MRI   Sagittal Oblique Fat-Suppressed T2-Weighted 3D MRI   Coronal Oblique Fat-Suppressed T2-Weighted 3D MRI

Fig. 12. 3D MRI of the ankle in a 57-year-old man with chronic lateral ankle pain. Oblique axial (*A*), oblique sagittal (*B*), and oblique coronal (*C*) fat-suppressed T2-weighted MRI reformation images demonstrate a full-thickness peroneus longus tear (*white arrows*) with retracted proximal and distal tendon ends (*asterisks* in *C*).

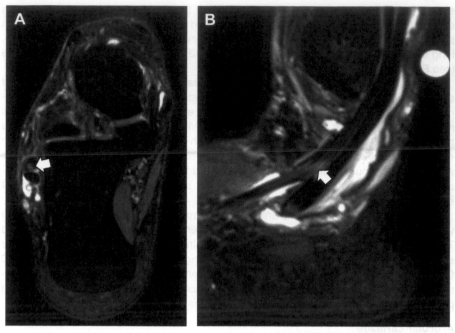

Axial Oblique Fat-Suppressed T2-Weighted 3D MRI   Sagittal Oblique Fat-Suppressed T2-Weighted 3D MRI

Fig. 13. 3D MRI of the ankle in a 37-year-old man with chronic lateral ankle pain. Oblique axial (*A*) and oblique sagittal (*B*) fat-suppressed T2-weighted MRI reformation images demonstrate a partial longitudinal peroneus brevis split tear (*arrows* in *A* and *B*).

Fluid-sensitive MRI pulse sequences with high spatial and contrast resolution help detect small osteochondral lesions and characterize cartilage integrity. Proton density-weighted fast, and turbo spin echo MRI pulse sequences provide the best contrast for articular cartilage evaluation. However, curved articular cartilage surfaces can create blind spots on 2D MRI, which 3D MRI overcomes (**Fig. 14**). Unlike 2D MRI,

Table 3	
Types of osteochondral injuries	
Type	**MRI Appearance**
Bone contusion	Focal bone marrow edema pattern. Absent cortical contour deformity. Absent fracture lines. The overlying cartilage is structurally intact.
Subchondral fracture	Focal bone marrow edema pattern. Absent cortical contour deformity. Subcortically located fracture line that parallels the articular surface. The overlying cartilage is structurally intact.
Osteochondral fracture	Focal bone marrow edema pattern. Typically presents with contour deformities, articular surface step-off, or displaced fragments. The fracture line extends through bone and articular cartilage.
Chondral fracture	Focal bone marrow edema pattern. Presents with articular cartilage contour irregularities. The separation typically occurs at the calcified-noncalcified cartilage interface near the tidemark layer. Chondral fragments may remain in situ or float in the joint cavity.

Table 4
MRI classification of osteochondral lesions of the talus

Grade	Description
1	Normal
2	Partial-thickness articular cartilage defect
3	Coapted full-thickness articular cartilage defect or exposed bone
4	Unstable but non-displaced in-situ chondral or osteochondral fragment
5	Displaced chondral or osteochondral fragment

cartilage-sensitive 3D MRI, including fast and turbo spin echo and 3D gradient-echo pulse sequences such as DESS, permits gapless thin section articular cartilage volume acquisitions for volumetry, mapping, and characterization of articular cartilage lesions.[4]

MRI has a high accuracy for detecting cartilage defects in the ankle, specifically in the talocrural joint.[59,60] Studies have shown a similar or better performance of qualitative or quantitative articular cartilage assessments with 3D than 2D fast and turbo spin echo sequences.[15,16,22,23,32,61] Fluid-sensitive MRI pulse sequences with high spatial and contrast resolution are beneficial in detecting small osteochondral lesions and characterizing cartilage integrity. A 2019 study validated the application of 3D fast and turbo spin echo MRI for detecting osteochondral lesions of the talar dome and tibial plafond. Proton density-weighted 3D MRI sequences with and without compressed sensing acceleration showed good-to-very good performance for detecting osteochondral lesions.[18,31]

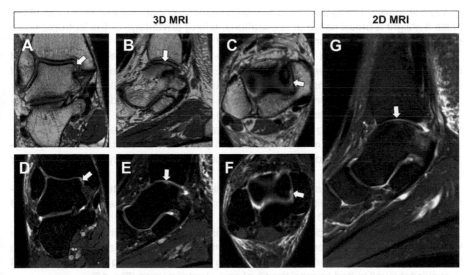

Fig. 14. 3D and 2D MRI of the ankle in a patient with recalcitrant ankle pain after trauma. Oblique coronal (*A* and *D*), oblique sagittal (*B* and *E*), and oblique axial (*C* and *F*) proton density-weighted (*A–C*) and fat-suppressed T2-weighted (*D-F*) 3D MRI reformation images demonstrate an osteochondral lesion of the medial talar dome with full-thickness articular cartilage loss and mild convex deformity of the exposed subchondral plate (*white arrows* in *A–F*). Note that on the fat-suppressed T2-weighted 2D MR image (*G*), the lesion is partially obscured and underestimated (*arrow*) due to partial volume effects.

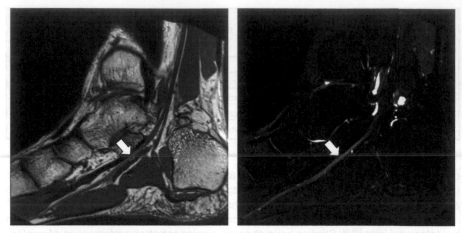

Proton Density-Weighted 3D MRI
Curved Planar Reformation Image
0.5 mm slice thickness

Fat Suppressed T2-Weighted 3D MRI
Curved Planar Reformation Image
0.5 mm slice thickness

Fig. 15. 3D MRI of medial plantar neuropathy. Curved planar reformation images along the course of the medial plantar nerves (*arrows*) of proto-density-weighted (*left image*) and fat-suppressed T2-weighted (*right image*) MR images demonstrate a thickened and edematous medial plantar nerves (*arrows*) indicating neuropathy. The fat-suppressed T2-weighted 3D MR image was acquired with an echo time greater than 100 ms to eliminate magic angle effects.

Other Structures

Multiple studies applying 3D MRI in evaluating various conditions and structures of the ankle highlight a broad range of applications, taking advantage of the isotropic voxel dimensions and thin section capabilities of 3D MRI.

A 2012 study compared the visibility of the Lisfranc ligaments of fat-suppressed isotropic proton density-weighted 3D SPACE MRI and axial, sagittal, and coronal fat-suppressed proton density-weighted 2D turbo spin echo MRI.[62] The multiplanar reformation and thin section capabilities of 3D MRI depicted the delicate Lisfranc ligament fibers to better advantage than 2D MRI.

Another study employing T2-weighted 3D fast and turbo spin echo MRI for evaluating the subtalar and sinus tarsi ligaments in patients with subtalar instability suggested that the thinning of the anterior capsular ligament may indicate subtalar instability.[63]

A study evaluating the value of 3D MRI in diagnosing anterolateral ankle impingement found higher sensitivity and specificity for contrast-enhanced T1-weighted 3D gradient-echo MRI than 2D MRI.[64]

A study applying 3D gradient-echo MRI to visualize the tibial nerve along its course through the tarsal tunnel found 3D MRI advantageous for visualizing the tibial nerve bifurcations and branches may aid in avoiding nerve injury during surgery.[65] 3D MRI is exquisitely well suited to map the tibial and plantar nerves (**Fig. 15**).

SUMMARY

3D fast and turbo spin echo MRI is a newer, clinically available multiaxial MRI technique that improves the visualization of oblique and curved ligaments, tendons, and nerves around the ankle. Multiple studies have validated the accuracy of 3D MRI.

Clinical 3D MRI of the ankle can be acquired with 0.5 mm slice thickness to resolve small anatomic structures and abnormalities, such as tendon and ligament tears, osteochondral lesions, and nerve lesions. We recommend adding 3D MRI pulse sequences to traditional 2D MRI protocols to visualize small and curved ankle structures to better advantage.

CLINICS CARE POINTS

- 3D MRI is clinically available by multiple vendors and has been validated for use in clinical practice.
- Multiplanar 3D MRI reformation postprocessing for individual image plane alignment obliquely oriented ligaments can improve the detection and characterization of ligament tears.
- The high spatial thin section resolution of 3D MRI can improve the detection, characterization, and morphological grading of osteochondral lesions.
- Curved planar 3D MRI reformation for unfolding multidirectional tendons into one image plane can improve the detection and characterization of tendon degeneration and tears.

REFERENCES

1. Fong DT, Hong Y, Chan LK, et al. A systematic review on ankle injury and ankle sprain in sports. Sports Med 2007;37(1):73–94.
2. Fritz B, Fritz J. MR Imaging of Acute Knee Injuries: Systematic Evaluation and Reporting. Radiol Clin North Am 2023;61(2):261–80.
3. Fritz B, Fritz J, Sutter R. 3D MRI of the Ankle: A Concise State-of-the-Art Review. Semin Musculoskelet Radiol 2021;25(3):514–26.
4.. Walter SS, Fritz B, Kijowski R, et al. 2D versus 3D MRI of osteoarthritis in clinical practice and research. Skeletal Radiol 2023. https://doi.org/10.1007/s00256-023-04309-4.
5. Umans H, Cerezal L, Linklater J, et al. Postoperative MRI of the Ankle and Foot. Magn Reson Imaging Clin N Am 2022;30(4).733–55.
6. Lin DJ, Walter SS, Fritz J. Artificial Intelligence-Driven Ultra-Fast Superresolution MRI: 10-Fold Accelerated Musculoskeletal Turbo Spin Echo MRI Within Reach. Invest Radiol 2023;58(1):28–42.
7. Fritz J, Kijowski R, Recht MP. Artificial intelligence in musculoskeletal imaging: a perspective on value propositions, clinical use, and obstacles. Skeletal Radiol 2022;51(2):239–43.
8. Del Grande F, Rashidi A, Luna R, et al. Five-Minute Five-Sequence Knee MRI Using Combined Simultaneous Multislice and Parallel Imaging Acceleration: Comparison with 10-Minute Parallel Imaging Knee MRI. Radiology 2021;299(3):635–46.
9. Del Grande F, Guggenberger R, Fritz J. Rapid Musculoskeletal MRI in 2021: Value and Optimized Use of Widely Accessible Techniques. AJR Am J Roentgenol 2021;216(3):704–17.
10. Fritz J, Guggenberger R, Del Grande F. Rapid Musculoskeletal MRI in 2021: Clinical Application of Advanced Accelerated Techniques. AJR Am J Roentgenol 2021;216(3):718–33.
11. Fritz J, Fritz B, Zhang J, et al. Simultaneous Multislice Accelerated Turbo Spin Echo Magnetic Resonance Imaging: Comparison and Combination With In-

Plane Parallel Imaging Acceleration for High-Resolution Magnetic Resonance Imaging of the Knee. Invest Radiol 2017;52(9):529–37.

12. Park EH, de Cesar Netto C, Fritz J. MRI in Acute Ankle Sprains: Should We Be More Aggressive with Indications? Foot Ankle Clin 2023;28(2):231–64.

13. Khodarahmi I, Fritz J. The Value of 3 Tesla Field Strength for Musculoskeletal Magnetic Resonance Imaging. Invest Radiol 2021;56(11):749–63.

14. Mugler JP 3rd. Optimized three-dimensional fast-spin-echo MRI. J Magn Reson Imaging 2014;39(4):745–67.

15. Kalia V, Fritz B, Johnson R, et al. CAIPIRINHA accelerated SPACE enables 10-min isotropic 3D TSE MRI of the ankle for optimized visualization of curved and oblique ligaments and tendons. Eur Radiol 2017;27(9):3652–61.

16. Fritz B, Bensler S, Thawait GK, et al. CAIPIRINHA-accelerated 10-min 3D TSE MRI of the ankle for the diagnosis of painful ankle conditions: Performance evaluation in 70 patients. Eur Radiol 2019;29(2):609–19.

17. Fritz J, Fritz B, Thawait GG, et al. Three-Dimensional CAIPIRINHA SPACE TSE for 5-Minute High-Resolution MRI of the Knee. Invest Radiol 2016;51(10):609–17.

18. Fritz J, Raithel E, Thawait GK, et al. Six-Fold Acceleration of High-Spatial Resolution 3D SPACE MRI of the Knee Through Incoherent k-Space Undersampling and Iterative Reconstruction-First Experience. Invest Radiol 2016;51(6):400–9.

19. Del Grande F, Delcogliano M, Guglielmi R, et al. Fully Automated 10-Minute 3D CAIPIRINHA SPACE TSE MRI of the Knee in Adults: A Multicenter, Multireader, Multifield-Strength Validation Study. Invest Radiol 2018;53(11):689–97.

20. Fritz B, Fritz J. MR Imaging-Ultrasonography Correlation of Acute and Chronic Foot and Ankle Conditions. Magn Reson Imaging Clin N Am 2023;31(2):321–35.

21. Fritz J, Ahlawat S, Fritz B, et al. 10-Min 3D Turbo Spin Echo MRI of the Knee in Children: Arthroscopy-Validated Accuracy for the Diagnosis of Internal Derangement. J Magn Reson Imaging 2019;49(7):e139–51.

22. Stevens KJ, Busse RF, Han E, et al. Ankle: isotropic MR imaging with 3D-FSE-cube–initial experience in healthy volunteers. Radiology 2008;249(3):1026–33.

23. Notohamiprodjo M, Kuschel B, Horng A, et al. 3D-MRI of the ankle with optimized 3D-SPACE. Invest Radiol 2012;47(4):231–9.

24. Park HJ, Lee SY, Park NH, et al. Three-dimensional isotropic T2-weighted fast spin-echo (VISTA) ankle MRI versus two-dimensional fast spin-echo T2-weighted sequences for the evaluation of anterior talofibular ligament injury. Clin Radiol 2016;71(4):349–55.

25. Kijowski R, Fritz J. Emerging Technology in Musculoskeletal MRI and CT. Radiology 2023;306(1):6–19.

26. Rashidi A, Haj-Mirzaian A, Dalili D, et al. Evidence-based use of clinical examination, ultrasonography, and MRI for diagnosing ulnar collateral ligament tears of the metacarpophalangeal joint of the thumb: systematic review and meta-analysis. Eur Radiol 2021;31(8):5699–712.

27. Holmer P, Sondergaard L, Konradsen L, et al. Epidemiology of sprains in the lateral ankle and foot. Foot Ankle Int 1994;15(2):72–4.

28. Roemer FW, Jomaah N, Niu J, et al. Ligamentous Injuries and the Risk of Associated Tissue Damage in Acute Ankle Sprains in Athletes: A Cross-sectional MRI Study. Am J Sports Med 2014;42(7):1549–57.

29. Joshy S, Abdulkadir U, Chaganti S, et al. Accuracy of MRI scan in the diagnosis of ligamentous and chondral pathology in the ankle. Foot Ankle Surg 2010;16(2):78–80.

30. Oae K, Takao M, Uchio Y, et al. Evaluation of anterior talofibular ligament injury with stress radiography, ultrasonography and MR imaging. Skeletal Radiol 2010;39(1):41–7.
31. Yi J, Lee YH, Hahn S, et al. Fast isotropic volumetric magnetic resonance imaging of the ankle: Acceleration of the three-dimensional fast spin echo sequence using compressed sensing combined with parallel imaging. Eur J Radiol 2019; 112:52–8.
32. Yi J, Cha JG, Lee YK, et al. MRI of the anterior talofibular ligament, talar cartilage and os subfibulare: Comparison of isotropic resolution 3D and conventional 2D T2-weighted fast spin-echo sequences at 3.0 T. Skeletal Radiol 2016;45(7): 899–908.
33. Park HJ, Lee SY, Choi YJ, et al. 3D isotropic T2-weighted fast spin echo (VISTA) versus 2D T2-weighted fast spin echo in evaluation of the calcaneofibular ligament in the oblique coronal plane. Clin Radiol 2017;72(2):176 e1–e7.
34. Choo HJ, Lee SJ, Kim DW, et al. Multibanded anterior talofibular ligaments in normal ankles and sprained ankles using 3D isotropic proton density-weighted fast spin-echo MRI sequence. AJR Am J Roentgenol 2014;202(1):W87–94.
35. Akatsuka Y, Teramoto A, Takashima H, et al. Morphological evaluation of the calcaneofibular ligament in different ankle positions using a three-dimensional MRI sequence. Surg Radiol Anat 2019;41(3):307–11.
36. Clanton TO, Porter DA. Primary care of foot and ankle injuries in the athlete. Clin Sports Med 1997;16(3):435–66.
37. Kofotolis ND, Kellis E, Vlachopoulos SP. Ankle sprain injuries and risk factors in amateur soccer players during a 2-year period. Am J Sports Med 2007;35(3): 458–66.
38. Chun KY, Choi YS, Lee SH, et al. Deltoid Ligament and Tibiofibular Syndesmosis Injury in Chronic Lateral Ankle Instability: Magnetic Resonance Imaging Evaluation at 3T and Comparison with Arthroscopy. Korean J Radiol 2015;16(5): 1096–103.
39. Crim JR, Beals TC, Nickisch F, et al. Deltoid ligament abnormalities in chronic lateral ankle instability. Foot Ankle Int 2011;32(9):873–8.
40. Mengiardi B, Zanetti M, Schottle PB, et al. Spring ligament complex: MR imaging-anatomic correlation and findings in asymptomatic subjects. Radiology 2005; 237(1):242–9.
41. Nussbaum ED, Hosea TM, Sieler SD, et al. Prospective evaluation of syndesmotic ankle sprains without diastasis. Am J Sports Med 2001;29(1):31–5.
42. Bencardino J, Rosenberg ZS, Delfaut E. MR imaging in sports injuries of the foot and ankle. Magn Reson Imaging Clin N Am 1999;7(1):131–49, ix.
43. Espinosa N, Smerek JP, Myerson MS. Acute and chronic syndesmosis injuries: pathomechanisms, diagnosis and management. Foot Ankle Clin 2006;11(3): 639–57.
44. Sman AD, Hiller CE, Refshauge KM. Diagnostic accuracy of clinical tests for diagnosis of ankle syndesmosis injury: a systematic review. Br J Sports Med 2013;47(10):620–8.
45. Rammelt S, Zwipp H, Grass R. Injuries to the distal tibiofibular syndesmosis: an evidence-based approach to acute and chronic lesions. Foot Ankle Clin 2008; 13(4):611–33, vii-viii.
46. Ogilvie-Harris DJ, Gilbart MK, Chorney K. Chronic pain following ankle sprains in athletes: the role of arthroscopic surgery. Arthroscopy 1997;13(5):564–74.
47. Czajka CM, Tran E, Cai AN, et al. Ankle sprains and instability. Med Clin North Am 2014;98(2):313–29.

48. Oae K, Takao M, Naito K, et al. Injury of the tibiofibular syndesmosis: value of MR imaging for diagnosis. Radiology 2003;227(1):155–61.
49. Hermans JJ, Ginai AZ, Wentink N, et al. The additional value of an oblique image plane for MRI of the anterior and posterior distal tibiofibular syndesmosis. Skeletal Radiol 2011;40(1):75–83.
50. Kim M, Choi YS, Jeong MS, et al. Comprehensive Assessment of Ankle Syndesmosis Injury Using 3D Isotropic Turbo Spin-Echo Sequences: Diagnostic Performance Compared With That of Conventional and Oblique 3-T MRI. AJR Am J Roentgenol 2017;208(4):827–33.
51. Myerson MS, Thordarson DB, Johnson JE, et al. Classification and Nomenclature: Progressive Collapsing Foot Deformity. Foot Ankle Int 2020;41(10):1271–6.
52. Chhabra A, Soldatos T, Chalian M, et al. 3-Tesla magnetic resonance imaging evaluation of posterior tibial tendon dysfunction with relevance to clinical staging. J Foot Ankle Surg 2011;50(3):320–8.
53. O'Neil JT, Pedowitz DI, Kerbel YE, et al. Peroneal Tendon Abnormalities on Routine Magnetic Resonance Imaging of the Foot and Ankle. Foot Ankle Int 2016;37(7):743–7.
54. Saxena A, Luhadiya A, Ewen B, et al. Magnetic resonance imaging and incidental findings of lateral ankle pathologic features with asymptomatic ankles. J Foot Ankle Surg 2011;50(4):413–5.
55. Fallat L, Grimm DJ, Saracco JA. Sprained ankle syndrome: prevalence and analysis of 639 acute injuries. J Foot Ankle Surg 1998;37(4):280–5.
56. Berndt AL, Harty M. Transchondral fractures (osteochondritis dissecans) of the talus. J Bone Joint Surg Am 1959;41-A:988–1020.
57. Rikken QGH, Kerkhoffs G. Osteochondral Lesions of the Talus: An Individualized Treatment Paradigm from the Amsterdam Perspective. Foot Ankle Clin 2021; 26(1):121–36.
58. Hannon CP, Smyth NA, Murawski CD, et al. Osteochondral lesions of the talus: aspects of current management. Bone Joint Lett J 2014;96-B(2):164–71.
59. Mintz DN, Tashjian GS, Connell DA, et al. Osteochondral lesions of the talus: a new magnetic resonance grading system with arthroscopic correlation. Arthroscopy 2003;19(4):353–9.
60. Verhagen RA, Maas M, Dijkgraaf MG, et al. Prospective study on diagnostic strategies in osteochondral lesions of the talus. Is MRI superior to helical CT? J Bone Joint Surg Br 2005;87(1):41–6.
61. Shakoor D, Guermazi A, Kijowski R, et al. Diagnostic Performance of Three-dimensional MRI for Depicting Cartilage Defects in the Knee: A Meta-Analysis. Radiology 2018;289(1):71–82.
62. Ulbrich EJ, Zubler V, Sutter R, et al. Ligaments of the Lisfranc joint in MRI: 3D-SPACE (sampling perfection with application optimized contrasts using different flip-angle evolution) sequence compared to three orthogonal proton-density fat-saturated (PD fs) sequences. Skeletal Radiol 2013;42(3):399–409.
63. Kim TH, Moon SG, Jung HG, et al. Subtalar instability: imaging features of subtalar ligaments on 3D isotropic ankle MRI. BMC Musculoskelet Disord 2017; 18(1):475.
64. Choo HJ, Suh JS, Kim SJ, et al. Ankle MRI for anterolateral soft tissue impingement: increased accuracy with the use of contrast-enhanced fat-suppressed 3D-FSPGR MRI. Korean J Radiol 2008;9(5):409–15.
65. Zhang Y, He X, Li J, et al. An MRI study of the tibial nerve in the ankle canal and its branches: a method of multiplanar reformation with 3D-FIESTA-C sequences. BMC Med Imaging 2021;21(1):51. https://doi.org/10.1186/s12880-021-00582-8.

Two-Dimensional and 3-Dimensional MRI Assessment of Progressive Collapsing Foot Deformity—Adult Acquired Flat Foot Deformity

Prajwal Gowda[a,b], Ajit Kohli, DO[a,b],
Avneesh Chhabra, MD, MBA, FACR[a,b],*

KEYWORDS

- Progressive collapsing foot deformity • Adult acquired flat foot deformity
- Pes planus • Tibialis posterior tendon dysfunction • Spring ligament • MRI • 3D MRI

KEY POINTS

- 3D MRI of ankle is excellent for finding PTT tears and outlining the gap in tendon tear.
- Knowledge of PTT staging is essential for improved diagnosis and patient management purposes.
- Spring ligament and deltoid ligament pathologies are elegantly and accurately seen on 3D MRI.

INTRODUCTION

Progressive collapsing foot deformity (PCFD), also known as adult acquired flat foot deformity (AFFD) or pes planus (flat foot), is a common developmentally acquired foot morphology characterized by the loss of the medial longitudinal arch. Subsequently, the midfoot approximates the ground and hindfoot angulates in valgus, causing reduced foot and ankle stability and awkward gait with resultant incapable arch function in supporting the weight of the body.[1] Normal stabilization of the medial longitudinal arch depends on the synergistic support of the talocalcaneal interosseus ligament, tibionavicular portion of the deltoid ligament, spring ligament, and medial talocalcaneal ligament, tibialis posterior tendon, fascia, and bones of the hind foot.[2] The condition is frequently asymptomatic until later stages.

[a] Radiology, UT Southwestern Medical Center, Dallas, TX, USA; [b] Orthopedic Surgery, UT Southwestern Medical Center, Dallas, TX, USA
* Corresponding author. UT Southwestern Medical Center, Dallas, TX 75022.
E-mail address: avneesh.chhabra@utsouthwestern.edu

Foot Ankle Clin N Am 28 (2023) 551–566
https://doi.org/10.1016/j.fcl.2023.04.009
1083-7515/23/© 2023 Elsevier Inc. All rights reserved.

However, in many patients, pain and discomfort with medial soft tissue swelling and foot and ankle malalignment are a commonplace.[3] Imaging plays an important role in confirming the clinical diagnosis, demonstrating soft tissue and bony lesions of PCFD for future management planning, and follow-ups to detect early postoperative failures. After reading this review article, the readers shall gain knowledge of PCFD/AFFD pathophysiology, relevant radiographic and MRI findings including 3-dimensional (3D) MRI assessment, and they can apply these principles in their practice for better patient managements.

EPIDEMIOLOGY OF PROGRESSIVE COLLAPSING FOOT DEFORMITY/ADULT ACQUIRED FLAT FOOT DEFORMITY

The prevalence of PCFD/AFFD is difficult to estimate due to the inconsistencies in defining PCFD/AFFD across population studies or clinical research trials, as well as increased difficulty to diagnose asymptomatic cases.[4] As of year 2020, there are an estimated 5 million adults affected by flat foot deformity in the United States alone.[5] The association between the presence of posterior tibial dysfunction and PCFD/AAFD was used to estimate the prevalence of PCFD/AAFD in the United Kingdom. In a study by Kohls-Gatzoulis and colleagues, flat foot deformity was seen among 582 women experiencing symptomatic posterior tibialis tendon (PTT) dysfunction. They found that 6.6% of the women recorded symptomatic flat foot deformity.[6] PCFD/AFFD was also 3 times more common in women than in men with a peak age of 55 years.[6,7] Other correlating demographics included white, diabetic, obese, rheumatic, and hypertensive patients.[6,8]

CLINICAL PRESENTATION OF PROGRESSIVE COLLAPSING FOOT DEFORMITY/ADULT ACQUIRED FLAT FOOT DEFORMITY

A prominent feature of most PCFD/AFFD patient's clinical history is ankle pain and/or medial ankle swelling; however, the intensity of the pain is not always correlated with increasing severity of the condition. Medial ankle pain is usually indicative of posterior tibial tendonitis/tendinopathy, and lateral hindfoot pain can develop over time, most commonly from talocalcaneal impingement and/or sinus tarsi syndrome.[9] Moreover, patients may also report foot or ankle fatigue after brief periods of activity, lack of options for well-fitting footwear, and difficulty standing on their toes.[9] On physical examination, the medial malleolus and surrounding area might present with swelling, which correlates with tenosynovitis and/or tendinopathy of the PTT.[10] Joint involvement (such as talonavicular or calcaneocuboid) and inability to perform heel rise maneuver is not uncommon, especially in the later stages of PTT dysfunction.[11] Other classic features include a significantly flattened appearance of the foot and valgus deformity of the heel.[12] In the context of these observations, the "too many toes" sign is frequently present in PCFD/AFFD; that is, more than the fourth and fifth digits are visible as observed from standing behind the patient, with a greater number of toes indicating a more severe presentation.[12] However, this sign is nonspecific to PCFD/AFFD and simply indicates forefoot abduction.

CAUSES OF PROGRESSIVE COLLAPSING FOOT DEFORMITY/ADULT ACQUIRED FLAT FOOT DEFORMITY
Posterior Tibial Tendon Insufficiency

PTT dysfunction is by far the most common cause of PCFD/AFFD. Anatomically, PTT inserts into the medial tuberosity of the navicular and continues into a second insertion in the plantar surface of the foot as multiple (4–5) slips, including a recurrent slip that attaches to the sustentaculum talus.[9] Accessory navicular, especially types II and III are associated with PTT dysfunction due to anomalous insertions. In addition, inflammation, or injury of the PTT due to trauma, arthritis, or degenerative disorders affects its ability to perform the functions of plantarflexion and inversion/stabilization of the medial longitudinal arch by locking the transverse tarsal joints.[9] Other factors that can disrupt this relationship include discontinuity of the tendon or loss of typical tendon insertion points. Overall, dysfunction of PTT often results in flatfoot ipsilateral to the affected tendon.[9] This is due to the destabilization of the transverse tarsal joint and foot abduction, eliminating counteraction against the peroneus brevis.[11] This results in increased valgus deformity of hindfoot.[11] In many cases, the spring ligament is adversely affected, which can lead to anteromedial and inferior subluxation of the talar head with respect to the navicular (aka talar fault or increased talar declination).[7,13] Other affected ligaments include the superficial deltoid ligament with attenuation or more commonly thickening of tibial spring, tibionavicular, and tibial calcaneal portions, plantar metatarsal ligament, and the naviculocuneiform ligament.[9] Midfoot-forefoot abduction and forefoot pronation also accompany the flat-footed pathologic condition.[9]

Other causes of progressive collapsing foot deformity/adult acquired flat foot deformity

Any other pathologic condition that affects the ligaments or tendons that maintain the medial longitudinal arch also results in PCFD/AFFD. This includes patients who experience trauma to portions of the midfoot and hindfoot such as fractures of navicular, first metatarsal, calcaneus, or injury to the Lis-Franc ligament complex.[14,15] Trauma resulting in bony malalignments can lead to PCFD/AFFD.[15] In addition, inflammatory disorders such as rheumatoid arthritis can disrupt above-described ligament(s) functionality cause flattening of the foot.[16] As mentioned before, diabetes patients have a higher susceptibility to developing PCFD/AFFD. This is due to the accompanying chronic sensory neuropathy, which can lead to Charcot neuroarthropathy, a condition that tends to collapse the midfoot and negative cuboid height.[17] Patients with congenital conditions such as Marfan syndrome or Ehlers Danlos or tarsal coalitions may also be present with PCFD/AFFD due to ligamentous laxity earlier in life.[18,19]

CLINICAL STAGING OF PROGRESSIVE COLLAPSING FOOT DEFORMITY/ADULT ACQUIRED FLAT FOOT DEFORMITY

The staging of *PCFD/AFFD* describes progressive foot malalignment and/or degenerations to guide future treatments and proper management. There are 4 distinct stages of PCFD/AAFD that are widely recognized as by the Bluman-Myerson classification.[20] Stage II and IV are further divided down into substages.

Stage I—Painful Medial Ankle

Stage I is characterized by the absence of pes planus but with medial ankle pain and, there may be an indication of progression toward the deformity.[21] For example, the patient may present as a medial longitudinal arch that is lower than expected with accompanying medial ankle pain.[21] Patient can still raise the heel normally. In early signs of PTT dysfuncton, there is usually PTT tenosynovitis/tendinopathy.[20]

Stage II—Flexible Foot Deformity

Progression to stage II PCFD/AAFD is defined by several qualitative and quantitative characteristics. The single-leg heel raise is decreased significantly or absent in the absent foot. Overall, there is greater deformity of the medial longitudinal arch with collapse but it can be corrected by passively inverting the talonavicular joint and hindfoot due to the flexibility of the current pathological state.[22] This flexibility, along with the measured abduction through the talonavicular joint, is the grounds on which the stage II category can be further subdivided.[12] As defined by Deland and colleagues, a stage IIa classification implies mild-to-moderate flexibility of the deformity with minimal abduction through the talonavicular joint.[22] Conversely, there is greater abduction through the talonavicular joint for stage IIb with lesser flexibility than stage IIa. The abduction magnitude is defined by the percent value of talonavicular uncoverage on a standing anteroposterior (AP) radiograph, in which 30% to 40% marks the border between stages IIa and IIb.[8] Both stage IIa and IIb can be associated with sinus tarsi (lateral hindfoot) pain. Forefoot abduction and lateral impingement at the subtalar joint/calcaneofibular joint is also characteristic of stage IIb.[12] (5) One can also divide PTT stage II dysfunction as follows: IIa, less than 40% talar uncoverage; IIb, greater than 40% uncoverage; and IIc, with forefoot abduction.

Stage III—Rigid Foot Deformity

As PCFD/AAFD worsens, the hindfoot flexibility present in stage II is no longer present. Instead, rigidity of the triple joint complex is the hallmark finding, composed of the talonavicular, subtalar, and calcaneocuboid joints.[7] Clinically, this presents as a fixed hindfoot valgus with the abduction of the midfoot and forefoot, absent single heel raise, and arch collapse.[7] There is associated severe sinus tarsi pain and subtalar arthritis.

Stage IV

The addition of ankle valgus joint deformity is typical for stage IV. This occurs due to the failure of the deltoid ligament, which can no longer support the talus appropriately, creating a lateral talar tilt.[20] It is important to distinguish the cause of ankle valgus radiographically because this finding may inform possible treatment plans. This stage is further differentiated into stage IVa and stage IVb. The differentiating factor between the 2 substages is the presence of significant ankle arthritis.[20]

MANAGEMENT OF PROGRESSIVE COLLAPSING FOOT DEFORMITY/ADULT ACQUIRED FLAT FOOT DEFORMITY
Nonsurgical Intervention

The primary initial treatment recommended for patients with PCFD/AFFD is conservative management with pain management as needed.[23] It includes physical therapy, nonsteroidal anti-inflammatory drugs (NSAIDs), corticosteroids, arch and ankle brace, and shoe modification. Up to 90% success rates can be achieved with such conservative treatments. In addition, exercise regimens that include strengthening exercises for tibialis posterior, peroneal, and gastroc-soleus muscles have produced similar rates of satisfaction among the patients. The hindrances of these conservative approaches include patient's distaste for wearing unwieldy braces and obesity/diabetes hampering the stabilization of the conditions. For this reason, counseling over treatment preferences and proper methods to manage body weight are important considerations for success of nonoperative management. Moreover, there is also a lack of comprehensive evidence that orthotic techniques can slow down the progression of PCFD/AFFD.[24,25]

Surgical Intervention

Surgery is indicated for patients with PCFD/AFFD if conservative management fails to correct the deformity during 3 to 6 months of treatments or relieve any associated pain and as per patient preferences. The specifics of surgical management procedure depend on the stage of the deformity and related causes; for example, accessory navicular or tarsal coalition may require resection of the bone or pseudoarthrosis with reattachment of PTT/tendon transfer, respectively.

Stage I

Of the 4 stages, surgery is least likely needed in stage I. Conservative management is especially indicated for low-demand and sedentary patients. However, for those who do not experience positive outcomes after 3 months of conservative therapy (NSAIDs, corticosteroid injections, calf and leg rehabilitation programs, orthotic devices leading to elevation of medial arch, and so forth), surgery may be considered.[7] The type of corrective surgery chosen will be determined by the condition of the PTT. One such procedure is a teno-synovectomy in which all or most of abnormal-appearing tenosynovium is removed in the distal leg. This may be followed with repair of any tendon tear and/or removal of fibrosis. The patient is placed in a splint and cast immobilization based on the intensiveness of the procedure (2–4+ weeks) followed by physical therapy (12 weeks).[9] More recently, PTT surgery has been supplemented with a medializing calcaneal slide osteotomy to correct the heel valgus. This is because heel valgus could be the underlying cause of future problems in the setting of a newly repaired PTT.[26] Subtalar arthroereisis is another option for stage I PCFD/AAFD but is currently under scrutiny for resulting in iatrogenic pain of the sinus tarsi.[27]

Stage II

Conservative therapy is still the first preference for those experiencing stage II PCFD/AAFD, especially for low-demand/sedentary patients; however, surgery may produce better results for high-demand patients and those with failure of conservative management. For stage IIa, one method of surgical treatment is sinus tarsi implant, especially as an alternative to the medial calcaneal osteotomy that is used for both stage I and stage II PCFD/AAFD.[27] This is due to its limitation of procedure complications, such as malunion, nonunion, and neurovascular injury. Medializing calcaneal osteotomy has the advantage over sinus tarsi implant in terms of lack of implant fracture, dislocation, new or persistent pain (most common), and foreign body reaction.[28] In the event of accessory navicular, one may resect the offending ossicle and associated adventitial bursa followed by reattachment of PTT on the naviculum (Kidner procedure). Other procedures for stage IIa PCFD/AAFD include flexor digitorum longus (FDL) transfer with PTT debridement, and a gastrocnemius recession. The former changes the insertion to navicular to compensate for the PTT insufficiency. The latter is used when the gastrocnemius is suspected cause of worsening heel valgus. The relative contraindication of FDL transfer include-rigidity of subtalar joint (<15° of motion) and fixed forefoot varus deformity (>10°–12°). For stage IIb, another option is to add a lateral column lengthening procedure to the variety of options presented for stage IIa.[11] This is to correct the talonavicular joint abduction that differentiates stages IIa and IIb. Postsurgical complications include lateral foot pain and fifth metatarsal stress fracture or stiffness.[29] Spring ligament reconstruction, typically using a peroneus longus autograft/allograft, is also considered for stage IIb surgical management.[30] It may be combined with medial column arthrodesis to correct for deformity at navicular-cuneiform joint. Finally, first tarsometatarsal arthrodesis may also be performed if there is hypermobility or significant arthritis at this joint. For all stage II presentations, splint and cast immobilization is required for 6 weeks, followed by physical therapy.[12]

Stage III

The primary goal of addressing stage III AAFD is to fuse the talonavicular and subtalar joints: 2 of the joints commonly involved in the triple-joint complex arthropathy. The third joint is avoided if possible due to increasing the risk of developing ankle arthritis.[31] If successful completion of this surgery does not eliminate heel valgus, a medializing calcaneal osteotomy can also be performed. Complications include failure of the deltoid ligament and ankle valgus due to nonunion or valgus malalignment.[32] Other risks include-lateral plantar nerve irritation and FHL impingement from long interlocking screw. After surgery, cast immobilization is warranted for 10 to 12 weeks, followed by boot immobilization and physical therapy.[12]

Stage IV

Stage IV PCFD/AAFD surgical management depends on the flexibility of the foot and ankle deformity, with stage IVa being more flexible. Stage IVb treatment is conducted with both foot and ankle correction in mind either by fusion or joint replacement. Apart from these definitions, the selection for surgical treatment of stage IV PCFD/AAFD can be algorithmic. In flexible foot deformity, flatfoot reconstruction and deltoid reconstruction are both considered. If an arthritic ankle is present, then ankle fusion or total ankle replacement (TAR) replaces the previously mentioned deltoid reconstruction. In rigid foot deformity, triple arthrodesis with deltoid reconstruction is considered. If an arthritic ankle is present, then deltoid reconstruction is not favored compared with TAR or pantalar fusion.[12]

RADIOGRAPHIC IMAGING

As with most presentations of foot or ankle instability and pain, standard radiographic imaging for PCFD/AAFD begins with AP and lateral weight-bearing views.[9] Oblique view helps in finding tarsal coalition. In stage I, pes planus can be difficult to elicit radiographically with an intact PTT or mild tenosynovitis.[9] Moreover, radiographs may be negative, despite complete PTT insufficiency even when the collapse of the medial longitudinal arch is apparent clinically. Despite such difficulties, there are several radiographic findings that can be useful in assessing PCFD/AAFD. Computed tomography (CT) and MRI imaging including 3D MRI have become useful tools with negative radiographs or if MRI cannot be obtained.[33]

On radiograph, first, the collapse of the medial longitudinal arch is assessed by measuring the talus-first metatarsal angle (Meary's angle) in weight-bearing lateral view.[9] If the angle is greater than 4°, that is, with excess talar declination, some collapse is present, whereas with 10° or more, it is implied that the medial longitudinal arch has completely collapsed. This is sometimes accompanied with depression of the talonavicular or naviculocuneiform joints, an increasingly flat angle (>170°) of the medial longitudinal arch, overlapping metatarsals, or a decrease in calcaneal pitch. Another finding in the lateral view may be the disruption of the "cyma line," which depicts a discontinuity of the otherwise congruent and smooth S-shape of the talonavicular and calcaneocuboid joints due to an anterior shift in the former (**Fig. 1**). Decreased medial cuneiform-floor height may also be seen with the loss of arch height. In the dorsoplantar view, some key radiographical findings, if present, include hindfoot valgus, medial talonavicular subluxation, increased talar-first metatarsal angle (Simmon

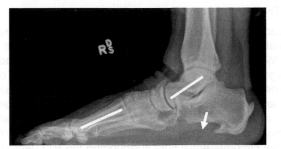

Fig. 1. Radiographic findings of PTT dysfunction. A 47-year-old woman with disrupted cyma line (*blue and green lines*) depicted in the lateral view of the foot and ankle. Other findings of note-increased Meary's angle with talar fault, obliterated sinus tarsi with reduced calcaneal pitch, plantar and calcaneal enthesophytes, thickened plantar fascia from chronic fasciitis (*arrow*), dorsal enthesophytes at talonavicular ligament attachment, and excessive overlap of metatarsals and navicular-cuboid bones.

angle), and forefoot abduction.[34–36] The axial view or mortise view can show loss of tibial-calcaneal collinearity confirming the hindfoot valgus. On lateral view, one can also observe obliteration of sinus tarsi with bony remodeling of lateral process of talus (squaring) and sclerosis of angle of Gissane suggesting chronic talocalcaneal abutment findings. These findings naturally vary from each case of PCFD/AAFD and among distinct stages of deformity. Furthermore, when evaluating a new patient, it is important to determine whether their clinically ascertained pes planus is congenital or acquired as an adult. The key to this differentiation is found when assessing the calcaneus and midtarsal joint. This is because PCFD/AAFD has a minimum calcaneal pitch of 10° to 20° and is accompanied by an overall inferiorly concave calcaneus while opposite is observed in the congenital cases. Furthermore, the talus may be anteriorly displaced in adult-acquired cases while predominantly medially displaced in those whose condition originated congenitally.[37] In addition to these general guidelines, there have been some relevant discoveries using radiographical imaging to further characterize PCFD/AAFD. Netto and colleagues found a strong association between the radiographic and clinical hindfoot alignment in patients with stage II PCFD/AAFD. Furthermore, their study suggested that clinical assessment of hindfoot alignment in these cases might not fully characterize the extent of the bony valgus deformity.[38] Lin and colleagues evaluated 100 patients in a study that assessed radiographic and MRI techniques in evaluating PCFD/AAFD. PTT insufficiency and tear, as confirmed by MRI, was found to be associated with abnormal talonavicular uncoverage, low calcaneal pitch angle, increased Meary's angle, and decreased cuneiform-to-fifth metatarsal height. Abnormal calcaneal pitch angle was also the only metric that had the best correlation with injury to structures supporting the medial longitudinal arch.[39] Finally, advanced arthropathy of subtalar and ankle joints can be easily detected on radiographs to outline the management planning.

MRI EVALUATION

MRI is the next best imaging modality following screening radiographs. Although weight-bearing radiography offers valuable insights on the alignment of the foot and ankle in the setting of PFCD/AAFD, MRI provides essential information regarding the soft tissue structures that maintain the medial longitudinal arch, including an insufficient PTT and spring ligament, other ligament injuries, and health of the articular cartilage.[40–42] These are discussed in detail in the following sections.

Posterior Tibial Tendon and Bony Findings

The PTT is located immediately posterior to the medial malleolus and adjacent to the FDL and flexor hallucis longus (FHL) tendons. It is the largest of the 3 tendons and is easily identified by its doubly large size compared with the FDL tendon. It possesses an ovoid low-signal intensity and has a measured transverse diameter of 7 to 11 mm.[42–44] It then inserts on the navicular bone with heterogeneous appearance due to interspersed fibrocartilage and other connective tissue (paratenon). There are additional slips that extend to cuneiforms, metatarsals, and the sustentaculum talus. Different abnormalities may be found in some patients with PCFD/AAFD.[45–47] Tenosynovitis seems as circumferential fluid surrounding the PTT, with or without internal septations, debris, or body (**Fig. 2**). PTT tendinopathy presents as tendon thickening (more than 2× size of FDL), surface irregularity, and heterogenous intratendinous signal intensity that is darker than the surrounding fluid. Sometimes, tendinopathy occurs only at insertional site at the navicular tuberosity, and it may be associated with surrounding increased signal of soft tissues indicating paratenonitis. Underlying bony hypertrophy of navicular tuberosity may also be present. Furthermore, these 2 former findings are usually associated with PTT tears.[43,48] There are 3 types of tears that are traditionally used to describe the PTT. Type I implicates partial thickness intrasubstance tears presenting with linear fluid in a thickened tendon, which can be difficult to differentiate from tendinopathy on 2D MRI.[42] Type II tears implicate atrophic appearance of the tendon due to chronic attritional atrophy or earlier partial tears with frank split tear creating a "4-tendon" sign, whereas type III denotes a complete tear with a fluid-filled or granulation tissue-filled gap creating a "2-tendon sign." The other 2 medial ankle tendons being the FDL and the FHL. Such type III tears typically

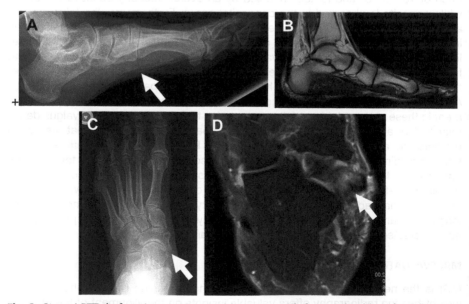

Fig. 2. Stage I PTT dysfunction. A 66-year-old woman with foot and ankle pain. (*A*) Lateral view of foot and ankle and (*B*) corresponding sagittal T1W MRI show maintained foot arch (*arrows*) and Meary's angle. (*C*) AP foot and ankle view and (*D*) corresponding coronal fsPDW image shows type II os naviculare and partial PTT split tear (*arrows*). Notice associated soft tissue edema. fsPDW, fat suppressed- proton density weighted; T1W, T1-weighted.

occur at the malleolar or in the midportion between the malleolus to the navicular attachment.[45,49] These findings, separately or synergistically, may be present in any of the stages of PCFD/AAFD while stage I typically exhibiting mild tenosynovitis or mild tendinopathy-associated bony findings include talar fault, hindfoot valgus, inferomedial uncovering of talar head, narrowing of sinus tarsi, squaring of the lateral process of talus, and sclerosis of the angle of Gissane, similar to the radiographic findings. With significant tendinopathy and/or tendon tears, retromalleolar osteophyte and/or subtendinous bone marrow edema may be seen. Uncommonly, the medial retinaculum may be deficient with medial subluxation of the PTT out of the retromalleolar groove. MRI also offers insight into health of articular cartilage with posterior subtalar joint cartilage integrity being an important determinant of type of surgery being performed-conservative to subtalar arthrodesis. Other associated findings include Achilles tendinopathy, plantar fasciitis, and calcaneal spurs. Chronic traction neuropathy changes of the medial plantar nerve may be identified. Finally, congenital coalitions, such as of the talocalcaneal or calcaneonavicular articulations may be seen, which can vary from fibro-cartilagenous to osseous coalitions (**Fig. 3**).

Accessory Navicular Bone and Its Lesions

The accessory navicular bone is a developmental ossicle that may cause midfoot pain and pes-planovalgus foot, which can precipitate PCFD/AAFD much earlier in life as compared with the typical middle-aged PTT degeneration. In this setting, PTT inserts onto the accessory navicular bone instead of the primary navicular tuberosity.[50–52] The proximally located anomalous insertions places increased stress on the tendon due to an unstable attachment.[53] Type I os naviculare is a rounded bone in the distal tendon itself, type II forms a synchondrosis, and type III is fused medially to the main navicular

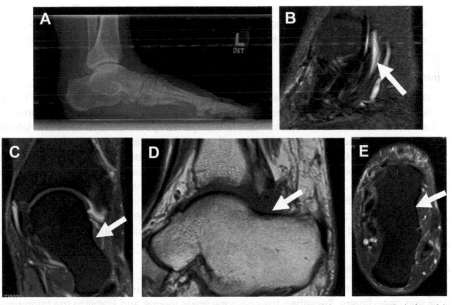

Fig. 3. Osseous coalition of the talocalcaneal joint. A 47-year-old woman with left ankle pain and peroneal spastic foot. (*A*) Lateral view of foot and ankle shows pes planus and non-visualization of sinus tarsi. (*B*) Tenosynovitis of PTT on sagittal STIR MRI (*arrow*). (*C–E*) Hindfoot valgus with solid osseous talocalcaneal fusion present on coronal fsPDW, sagittal PDW, and axial fsPDW images (*arrows*). STIR, short tau inversion recovery.

bone, aka cornuate process. Type II and III are most associated with PTT dysfunction. On MRI, one can find the accessory ossicle exhibiting marrow signal with or without associated bone marrow and soft tissue edema. Widening and/or fluid of the synchondrosis confirm clinically suspected instability. PTT tendinopathy and/or tear are associated with symptomatic ossicle. Additional bony hypertrophy of ossicle and navicular tuberosity, and superimposed adventitial bursitis are not uncommonly seen in the clinically symptomatic cases.[48] Finally, postoperative follow-up imaging using MRI is invaluable in assessing the integrity of the reconstructed PTT, FDL transfer, and spring ligament repair/reconstruction. Progressive hindfoot/midfoot joint degeneration may be present with reconstruction failures with return of the foot malalignments.

Spring Ligament Pathology

The plantar calcaneonavicular ligament, also known as the spring ligament, functionally maintains the medial longitudinal arch in addition to the PTT, the dynamic stabilizer. The spring ligament being the static stabilizer prevents excessive talar head descent and abuts the surrounding connective tissue at the medial navicular bone. It is composed of 3 segments, superomedial (SM) band, medial plantar oblique (MPO) band, and the inferoplantar (IP) band, of which the SM bundle is the most important in stabilizing the talar head and talonavicular joint. The SM band is separated from the PTT by a fibrocartilage gliding zone. PTT degeneration or tearing frequently leads to spring ligament degeneration and tearing or thickening from chronic remodeling.[54,55] The coronal and axial oblique planes are most useful in evaluating the SM bundle. This presents as a 2 to 4 mm smooth low-signal-intensity band that is continuous with the superficial deltoid-tibial spring ligament. Apart from abnormal thinning or thickening of the spring ligament, full-thickness defects may be identified, especially in more acute cases of PTT injury or insufficiency. Other abnormal findings include increased signal intensity, ligament elongation, thickening of the gliding zone, MPO/IP bands, periligamentous ganglion, and periligamentous edema (**Fig. 4**).[48]

Sinus Tarsi

Sinus tarsi is a fat-filled canal located between the calcaneus and talus, anterior to the posterior subtalar joint. It contributes to hindfoot stability.[56] The sinus tarsi ligaments include the medial interosseous talocalcaneal ligament, cervical ligament, and lateral interosseous talocalcaneal ligament from medial to lateral. These are respectively anteriorly bounded by the medial, intermediate, and lateral bands of the deep extensor retinaculum. Instability in the hindfoot, such as unstable heel valgus found in PCFD/AAFD, can lead to strain on the sinus tarsi ligaments. This results in alterations of normal fat signal, distortion/tearing of the sinus tarsi ligaments, synovitis, sinus tarsi ganglion, and interosseus ganglion cysts. However, these changes are not unique to PCFD/AAFD and can be seen in isolation as well, especially as a sequel to earlier ankle sprains.[48]

Deltoid Ligament Pathology

The deltoid ligament originates from the medial malleolus and is composed of superficial and deep layers. Together, they oppose ankle valgus and stabilize the talonavicular joint. Specifically, the tibionavicular, tibiospring, and tibiocalcaneal ligaments are the structures of interest when identifying a deltoid ligament abnormality that is affected in PCFD/AAFD.[57] MRI is an ideal imaging modality for deltoid ligament visualization. Axial and coronal views display low or intermediate signal intensity bands

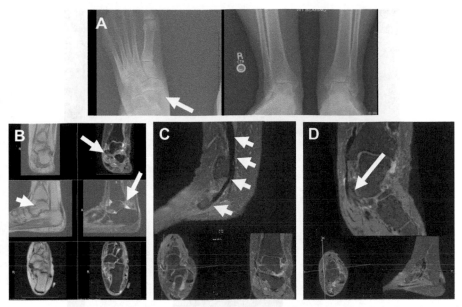

Fig. 4. Stage IIA PTT dysfunction. A 75-year-old man with suspected PTT dysfunction and flexible foot deformity. (*A*). AP foot view shows no talonavicular uncovering and possible tiny type I os naviculare. Bilateral hindfoot valgus is however present on AP ankle view consistent with commonly encountered increased frequency of bilateral PTT disease. (*B*). From top to bottom, the coronal, sagittal, and axial in-phase and water maps show presentation of stage IIA PTT insufficiency, that is, hindfoot valgus, SM spring ligament thickening (*medium arrow*), sinus tarsi edema, talar fault (*small arrow*), posterior talar disuse edema, and thickened intermalleolar ligament (*large arrow*), insertional PTT tendinopathy with type I os naviculare. (*C, D*). Three-dimensional MPR show full length of the PTT with insertional tendinopathy (small *arrows*) as well as (*D*) abnormal thickening of the spring ligament and gliding zone (*large arrow*). MPR, multiplanar reconstructions.

that broaden distally.[48] If this signal is heterogeneous, it is not always indicative of abnormality due to it being normally present with increasing age in many cases. Abnormal findings that are visible on MRI include loss of fatty striations, fluid-like signal intensity heterogeneity, chronic thickening, fibrosis, and tearing.[57]

Plantar Fascia

Plantar fascia is a triangular structure that originates at the calcaneal tuberosity and attaches at the proximal phalanges as 3 separate cords-medial, central, and lateral. It opposes plantar foot elongation and helps maintain the medial arch alignment, which is integral to the pathophysiology of PCFD/AAFD. Abnormalities in plantar fascia on MRI include thickening of the fascia (>4 mm), signal intensity heterogeneity of the fascia, partial tears, and perifascial and/or marrow edema.[48]

Tarsometatarsal Joints

The tarsometatarsal joints compose the transverse arch that supports the midfoot during standing position. The distal PTT attaches to the plantar tarsal and metatarsal surfaces.[58] These connections are susceptible to overload and can lead to transverse arch flattening. These changes are difficult to delineate; however, fractures of the metatarsals at PTT insertions can sometimes be seen with the PTT slip tears attached

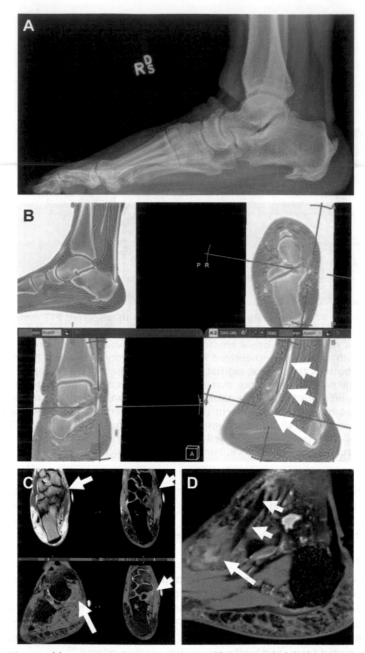

Fig. 5. A 47-year-old woman with stage II PTT insufficiency with full-thickness PTT tear. (*A*) Lateral view of disrupted cyma line of talonavicular and calcaneocuboid joints as also shown in **Fig. 1** (*arrow*). (*B*) Virtually constructed CT images from star vibe MRI image with window scale inversion depicting talar fault, and full-thickness tear (crosshairs, *large arrow*) of PTT (*small arrows*). (*C*) Axial in-phase and water, and 3D coronal and axial fsPDW images confirm PTT complete tear at distal attachment at the site patient marker (*small arrows*) and complete SM band spring ligament disruption (*large arrow*). (*D*) Sagittal oblique reconstruction along the course of PTT on 3D imaging confirms the distal full-thickness tear (large *arrow*) of PTT (*small arrows*).

to the bony fragments.[59] This finding is mostly commonly seen in acute injuries and is rare in the classic PCFD/AAFD presentation. More commonly, one can find the degenerative changes and cartilage loss in the midfoot. Finally, bony erosive changes with or without pannus may be seen in underlying inflammatory condition causing PCFD, such as rheumatoid arthritis or gout.

ROLE OF 3D COMPUTED TOMOGRAPHY AND MRI

Three-dimensional CT performed in the setting of trauma or using a cone beam weight-bearing CT incidentally may show the bony malalignments of PTT dysfunction, especially on multiplanar reconstructions and with volume rendered imaging. One can also detect the bony avulsive changes of the retromalleolar groove with medial subluxation of PTT from the retromalleolar groove in the acute–subacute setting while bony hypertrophy and/or cystic changes at the navicular tuberosity insertion are not uncommonly seen in the chronic setting. Other relevant findings on CT include improved identification of the os naviculare and bony hypertrophy of the degenerated hindfoot and midtarsal joints. Soft tissue pathologic findings on CT include the loss of normal hyperdense PTT signal, abnormal thickening/thinning or full-thickness PTT tear, or tendon entrapment at the fracture site in a traumatic condition. If performed on a dual energy scanner, bone marrow edema can be seen at the site of PTT stress/strain and bony fracture sites. Finally, osseous coalitions can be confirmed on 3D CT multiplanar reconstructions and displayed for presurgical planning and education.[42]

Three-dimensional joint MRI is becoming common with wider availability of 3Tesla (T) and newer 1.5T scanners and fast imaging. Isotropic spin-echo type volume imaging similar to 3D CT is feasible in 3 to 5 minutes of scanning times depending on the software acceleration methods available on newer machines, for example, compressed sense, and so forth. These isotropic images allow multiplanar tendon-specific and ligament-specific reconstructions to assess and demonstrate such structures in their long-axis. In addition, due to better fluid contrast on 3D imaging and lack of partial voluming effects with smaller voxels, the intrasubstance tears/split tears of PTT and other regional tendons are identified with much more conspicuity and the exact tendon gap can be outlined in full-thickness disruptions. Finally, spring ligament injuries and cartilage defects are more distinctly seen on 3D MRI for appropriate preoperative planning (see **Fig. 4**; **Fig. 5**). Postoperative imaging is also facilitated with improved identification of the above-described lesions.[60]

To conclude, this review article discusses relevant pathophysiology, demographics, cause, conservative and surgical treatments, and unique imaging features of PCFD/AAFD. Three-dimensional CT and MRI allow improved identification of bony and soft tissue lesions of this condition. The readers may apply the gained knowledge to improve management of their patients with PCFD/AAFD.

DISCLOSURES

A. Chhabra receives royalties from Jaypee and Wolters. A. Chhabra also serves as a consultant with ICON Medical and Treace Medical Concepts, Inc. A. Chhabra is a speaker for Siemens. A. Chhabra is medical advisor and has research grant from Image biopsy lab Inc. The authors do not report any conflict of interest.

REFERENCES

1. Michaudet C, Edenfield KM, Nicolette GW, et al. Foot and ankle conditions: pes planus. FP Essent 2018;465:18–23.

2. Kitaoka HB, Ahn TK, Luo ZP, et al. Stability of the arch of the foot. Foot Ankle Int 1997;18(10):644–8.

3. Aenumulapalli A, Kulkarni MM, Gandotra AR. Prevalence of flexible flat foot in adults: a cross-sectional study. J Clin Diagn Res 2017;11(6):AC17–20.

4. Godoy-Santos AL, Schmidt EL, Chaparro F. What are the updates on epidemiology of progressive collapsing foot deformity? Foot Ankle Clin 2021;26(3): 407–15.

5. Hadfield MH, Snyder JW, Liacouras PC, et al. Effects of medializing calcaneal osteotomy on Achilles tendon lengthening and plantar foot pressures. Foot Ankle Int 2003;24(7):523–9.

6. Kohls-Gatzoulis J, Woods B, Angel JC, et al. The prevalence of symptomatic posterior tibialis tendon dysfunction in women over the age of 40 in England. Foot Ankle Surg 2009;15(2):75–81.

7. Deland JT. Adult-acquired flatfoot deformity. J Am Acad Orthop Surg 2008;16: 399–406.

8. Deland JT, de Asla RJ, Sung IH, et al. Posterior tibial tendon insufficiency: which ligaments are involved? Foot Ankle Int 2005;26(6):427–35.

9. Canale ST, Beaty JH, Campbell WC. Campbell's operative orthopaedics. Philadelphia, PA: Elsevier/Mosby; 2008.

10. DeOrio JK, Shapiro SA, McNeil RB, et al. Validity of posterior tibial edema sign in posterior tibial tendon dysfunction. Foot Ankle Int 2011;32:189–92.

11. Mann RA. Flatfoot in adults. In: Mann RA, Coughlin MJ, editors. Surgery of the foot and ankle. 7. St. Louis: Mosby; 1999. p. 733–67.

12. Vulcano E, Deland JT, Ellis SJ. Approach and treatment of the adult acquired flatfoot deformity. Curr Rev Musculoskelet Med 2013;6(4):294–303.

13. Abousayed MM, Alley MC, Shakked R, et al. Adult-acquired flatfoot deformity: etiology, diagnosis, and management. JBJS Rev 2017 Aug;5(8):e7.

14. Gajendran VK, Yoo BJ, Hunter JC. Unusual variant of the nutcracker fracture of the calcaneus and tarsal navicular. Radiol Case Rep 2008;3(3):208.

15. Penner MJ. Late reconstruction after navicular fracture. Foot Ankle Clin 2006; 11(1):105–19, ix.

16. Myerson M, Solomon G, Shereff M. Posterior tibial tendon dysfunction: its association with seronegative inflammatory disease. Foot Ankle 1989;9(5):219–25.

17. Schade VL, Andersen CA. A literature-based guide to the conservative and surgical management of the acute Charcot foot and ankle. Diabet Foot Ankle 2015;6: 26627.

18. Perotti LR, Abousamra O, Del Pilar Duque Orozco M, et al. Foot and ankle deformities in children with Down syndrome. J Child Orthop 2018;12(3):218–26.

19. Lindsey JM, Michelson JD, MacWilliams BA, et al. The foot in Marfan syndrome: clinical findings and weight-distribution patterns. J Pediatr Orthop 1998;18(6): 755–9.

20. Bluman EM, Title CI, Myerson MS. Posterior tibial tendon rupture: a refined classification system. Foot Ankle Clin 2007;12(2):233–49, v.

21. Johnson KA, Strom DE. Tibialis posterior tendon dysfunction. Clin Orthop Relat Res 1989;239:196–206.

22. Deland JT, Page A, Sung I-H, et al. Posterior tibial tendon insufficiency results at different stages. HSS J 2006;2:157–60.

23. Nielsen MD, Dodson EE, Shadrick DL, et al. Nonoperative care for the treatment of adult-acquired flatfoot deformity. J Foot Ankle Surg 2011;50:311–4.

24. Chao W, Wapner KL, Lee TH, et al. Nonoperative management of posterior tibial tendon dysfunction. Foot Ankle Int 1996;17:736–41.

25. Alvarez RG, Marini A, Schmitt C, et al. Stage I and II posterior tibial tendon dysfunction treated by structured nonoperative management protocol: an orthosis and exercise program. Foot Ankle Int 2006;27:2e8.

26. Myerson MS, Badekas A, Schon LC. Treatment of stage II posterior tibial tendon deficiency with flexor digitorum longus tendon transfer and calcaneal osteotomy. Foot Ankle Int 2004;25:445–50.

27. A surgical approach for flexible flatfeet in adults including a subtalar arthroereisis with the MBA sinus tarsi implant. Foot Ankle Int 2006;27:9–18.

28. Needleman RL. Current topic review: subtalar arthroereisis for correction of flexible flatfoot. Foot Ankle Int 2005;26:336–46.

29. Ellis SJ, Williams BR, Garg R, et al. Incidence of plantar lateral foot pain before and after the use of trial metal wedges in lateral column lengthening. Foot Ankle Int 2011;32:665–73.

30. Astion DJ, Deland JT, Otis JC, et al. Motion of the hindfoot after simulated arthrodesis. J Bone Joint Surg Am 1997;79:241–6.

31. Sammarco VJ, Magur EG, Sammarco GJ, et al. Arthrodesis of the subtalar and talonavicular joints for correction of symptomatic hindfoot malalignment. Foot Ankle Int 2006;27:661–6.

32. Funk DA, Cass JR, Johnson KA. Acquired adult flatfoot secondary to posterior tibial-tendon pathology. J Bone Joint Surg Am 1986;68(1):95–102.

33. Donovan A, Rosenberg ZS. Extraarticular lateral hindfoot impingement with posterior tibial tendon tear: MRI correlation. AJR Am J Roentgenol 2009;193(3): 672–8.

34. Flores D, Mejía Gómez C, Fernández Hernando M, et al. adult acquired flatfoot deformity: anatomy, biomechanics, staging, and imaging findings. Radiographics 2019;39(5):1437–60.

35. Meyr A, Sansosti L, Ali S. A pictorial review of reconstructive foot and ankle surgery: evaluation and intervention of the flatfoot deformity. J Radiol Case Rep 2017;11(6):26–36.

36. Arunakul M, Amendola A, Gao Y, et al. Tripod Index. Foot Ankle Int 2013;34(10): 1411–20.

37. Burgener FA, Kormano M, Pudas T. Bone and joint disorders. Differential diagnosis in conventional radiology. AJNR Am J Neuroradiol 2006;33(2):125.

38. de Cesar Netto C, Kunas GC, Soukup D, et al. Correlation of clinical evaluation and radiographic hindfoot alignment in stage II adult-acquired flatfoot deformity. Foot Ankle Int 2018;39(7):771–9.

39. Lin YC, Mhuircheartaigh JN, Lamb J, et al. Imaging of adult flatfoot: correlation of radiographic measurements with MRI. AJR Am J Roentgenol 2015;204(2):354–9.

40. Conti S, Michelson J, Jahss M. Clinical significance of magnetic resonance imaging in preoperative planning for reconstruction of posterior tibial tendon ruptures. Foot Ankle 1992;13(4):208–14.

41. Arnoldner MA, Gruber M, Syré S, et al. Imaging of posterior tibial tendon dysfunction–Comparison of high-resolution ultrasound and 3T MRI. Eur J Radiol 2015; 84(9):1777–81.

42. Rosenberg ZS, Cheung Y, Jahss MH, et al. Rupture of posterior tibial tendon: CT and MR imaging with surgical correlation. Radiology 1988;169(1):229–35.

43. Schweitzer ME, Karasick D. MR imaging of disorders of the posterior tibialis tendon. AJR Am J Roentgenol 2000;175(3):627–35.

44. Premkumar A, Perry MB, Dwyer AJ, et al. Sonography and MR imaging of posterior tibial tendinopathy. AJR Am J Roentgenol 2002;178(1):223–32.

45. Chhabra A, Soldatos T, Chalian M, et al. 3-Tesla magnetic resonance imaging evaluation of posterior tibial tendon dysfunction with relevance to clinical staging. J Foot Ankle Surg 2011;50(3):320–8.
46. Khoury NJ, el-Khoury GY, Saltzman CL, et al. MR imaging of posterior tibial tendon dysfunction. AJR Am J Roentgenol 1996;167(3):675–82.
47. Delfaut EM, Demondion X, Bieganski A, et al. The fibrocartilaginous sesamoid: a cause of size and signal variation in the normal distal posterior tibial tendon. Eur Radiol 2003;13(12):2642–9.
48. Flores DV, Mejía Gómez C, Fernández Hernando M, et al. Adult Acquired Flatfoot Deformity: Anatomy, Biomechanics, Staging, and Imaging Findings. Radiographics 2019;39(5):1437–60.
49. Kong A, Van Der Vliet A. Imaging of tibialis posterior dysfunction. Br J Radiol 2008;81(970):826–36.
50. Popko J, Guszczyn T, Kwiatkowski M, et al. Pediatric flat feet. Pol J Appl Sci 2017; 3(1):20–5.
51. Ribbans WJ, Garde A. Tibialis posterior tendon and deltoid and spring ligament injuries in the elite athlete. Foot Ankle Clin 2013;18(2):255–91.
52. Miller TT, Staron RB, Feldman F, et al. The symptomatic accessory tarsal navicular bone: assessment with MR imaging. Radiology 1995;195(3):849–53.
53. Bernaerts A, Vanhoenacker FM, Van de Perre S, et al. Accessory navicular bone: not such a normal variant. J Belge Radiol 2004;87(5):250–2.
54. Taniguchi A, Tanaka Y, Takakura Y, et al. Anatomy of the spring ligament. J Bone Joint Surg Am 2003;85(11):2174–8.
55. Mengiardi B, Zanetti M, Schöttle PB, et al. Spring ligament complex: MR imaging-anatomic correlation and findings in asymptomatic subjects. Radiology 2005; 237(1):242–9.
56. Stella SM, Ciampi B, Orsitto E, et al. Sonographic visibility of the sinus tarsi with a 12 MHz transducer. J Ultrasound 2014;19(2):107–13.
57. Mengiardi B, Pfirrmann CW, Vienne P, et al. Medial collateral ligament complex of the ankle: MR appearance in asymptomatic subjects. Radiology 2007;242(3): 817–24.
58. Yao L, Gentili A, Cracchiolo A. MR imaging findings in spring ligament insufficiency. Skeletal Radiol 1999;28(5):245–50.
59. Desai KR, Beltran LS, Bencardino JT, et al. The spring ligament recess of the talocalcaneonavicular joint: depiction on MR images with cadaveric and histologic correlation. AJR Am J Roentgenol 2011;196(5):1145–50.
60. Fritz B, Fritz J, Sutter R. 3D MRI of the Ankle: A Concise State-of-the-Art Review. Semin Musculoskelet Radiol 2021;25(3):514–26.

Magnetic Resonance Neurography of the Foot and Ankle

Patrick Debs, MD[a], Laura M. Fayad, MS, MD[a],
Shivani Ahlawat, MD[a],*

KEYWORDS

- Magnetic resonance neurography • Foot and ankle • Peripheral nerves
- Tarsal tunnel syndrome • Neuropathy

KEY POINTS

- MRN provides an important information that can assist in the diagnostic and therapeutic workup of peripheral nerve lesions of the foot and ankle.
- On MRN, a normal peripheral nerve of the foot and ankle exhibit iso- to slightly hyperintense signal to skeletal muscle on fluid sensitive sequences, preserved fascicular architecture and taper in caliber as the course distally.
- Elevated T2 signal in a peripheral nerve, particularly the medial plantar nerve in the distal tarsal tunnel, is a non-specific finding and often due to magic angle.

INTRODUCTION

Foot and ankle disorders are commonly encountered in routine clinical practice,[1] with the incidence of foot injuries as high as 10% of all trauma cases at tertiary hospitals.[2] Imaging of the foot and ankle remains an integral part of any musculoskeletal practice. Because of its soft-tissue contrast resolution, high spatial resolution, and multiplanar capabilities, MRI is an invaluable tool for the evaluation of foot and ankle injuries, and[1] MR neurography (MRN) is an advanced MRI technique that is optimized for the assessment of peripheral nerves.[3] In addition, MRN can noninvasively assess skeletal muscles in the imaged field of view for acute, subacute, or chronic denervation. Several indications for MRN exist in the foot and ankle, including tarsal tunnel syndrome, the diabetic foot, and entrapment syndromes.[4–6] The aim of this article is to review the normal anatomy and pertinent pathologic conditions of the peripheral nerves of the foot and ankle, highlighting the role that MRN plays in their evaluation.

[a] The Russell H. Morgan Department of Radiology & Radiological Science, The Johns Hopkins Medical Institutions, 600 North Wolfe Street, Baltimore, MD 21287, USA
* Corresponding author.
E-mail address: sahlawa1@jhmi.edu

Foot Ankle Clin N Am 28 (2023) 567–587
https://doi.org/10.1016/j.fcl.2023.04.003
1083-7515/23/© 2023 Elsevier Inc. All rights reserved.

Table 1
Anatomy, sensorimotor innervation and common pathology of the foot and ankle peripheral nerves

	Origin	Motor Innervation	Sensory Innervation	Common Sites of Pathology
Tibial nerve (TN)	Sciatic nerve	Gastrocnemius, soleus, tibialis posterior, flexor digitorum longus, flexor hallucis longus, and other muscles through the MPN and LPN	Most of the posterior leg and foot	Tarsal tunnel
Medial plantar nerve (MPN)	TN	Abductor hallucis, flexor digitorum brevis	Medial side of the sole	Jogger's foot at master Knot Henry
Medial hallucal nerve	MPN	Flexor hallucis brevis and first lumbrical	Medial aspect of the hallux	Medial aspect of the hallux (bunions, osteophytes, or tophi)
First through the third common digital nerves	MPN		Medial 3 toes and the medial aspect of the fourth toe	Under the intermetatarsal ligament, particularly at the second and third intermetatarsal spaces
Lateral plantar nerve (LPN)	TN	Quadratus plantae, abductor digiti minimi, flexor digiti minimi brevis, adductor hallucis, dorsal and plantar interossei, and second, third, and fourth lumbricals	Lateral one-third of the sole of the foot	Between the abductor hallucis and the quadratus planus
Fourth common digital nerve	LPN		Fifth toe and lateral aspect of the fourth toe	Between the plantar aspect of the foot and the transverse intermetatarsal ligament

Nerve	Origin	Muscle innervated	Sensory distribution	Clinical notes
Medial calcaneal nerve	TN or LPN	Proximal abductor hallucis	Skin covering the medial aspect of the Achilles tendon, the posteromedial aspect of the heel, and the plantar fat pad	Variable depending on origin, mimics plantar fasciitis
Inferior calcaneal nerve	LPN	Abductor digiti minimi	Anterior aspect of the calcaneus and plantar lateral foot	Calcaneal spur/Baxter neuropathy
Sural nerve	TN (medial sural nerve) and CPN (lateral sural nerve)	—	Lateral border of the ankle and foot	Fifth metatarsal base (fifth metatarsal base, peroneal, calcaneal, or cuboid fracture)
Deep peroneal nerve	Common peroneal nerve (CPN)	Extensor digitorum brevis and extensor hallucis brevis	Dorsal first interspace	Anterior tarsal tunnel (compression at the inferior extensor retinaculum)
Superficial peroneal nerve	CPN	Peroneal brevis and peroneal longus muscles	Dorsolateral aspect of the foot (including second through fourth interspaces) and ankle	In front of the lateral malleolus
Saphenous nerve	Femoral nerve	—	Medial foot up to the first metatarsophalangeal joint	Medial malleolus (ankle eversion or extension, arthroscopy)

PERIPHERAL NERVES OF THE FOOT AND ANKLE: NORMAL ANATOMY

The foot receives its nerve supply from 5 main peripheral nerves: the tibial nerve,[7–12] the sural nerve, the deep peroneal nerve, the superficial peroneal nerve, and the saphenous nerve. Most of these nerves originate from the sciatic nerve, which is made up of the L4 to S3 nerve roots.[7] **Table 1** shows the sensory and motor innervations of the foot and ankle nerves.

The tibial nerve (**Fig. 1**) originates in the popliteal fossa as 1 of the 2 terminal branches of the sciatic nerve.[8] It gives off the medial calcaneal nerve proximal to the tarsal tunnel and bifurcates into the medial and lateral plantar nerves just proximal to the medial malleolus. This anatomy makes the posterior medial malleolus an excellent landmark for visualizing the tibial nerve on MRN, between the flexor digitorum longus and flexor hallucis longus tendons.[7] The medial plantar nerve travels lateral to the posterior tibial artery and anterior to the medial plantar artery; it then continues its course medial to the flexor digitorum brevis muscle, ultimately dividing into the medial proper digital plantar nerve and 3 common digital plantar nerves.[7,8] The lateral plantar nerve travels between the quadratus plantae and flexor digitorum brevis muscles, continues laterally to the flexor digitorum brevis muscle, and subsequently divides into superficial and deep branches.[7,8] Baxter nerve, also known as the inferior calcaneal nerve, typically originates as the first branch of the lateral plantar nerve and courses anterior to the anterior tubercle of the calcaneus, another anatomical landmark on MRN.[7]

The common peroneal nerve is the second major branch off the sciatic nerve and travels through the anterior and lateral compartments of the leg and foot before bifurcating into the superficial and deep peroneal nerves.[9] The superficial peroneal nerve courses within the peroneus longus muscle, emerges through its anterolateral aspect about 12 cm above the ankle joint, and then divides into the medial and intermediate dorsal cutaneous nerves.[7,9,10] The deep peroneal nerve descends lateral to the anterior tibial artery, anterior to the interosseous membrane, and divides into medial and lateral branches above the ankle joint.[9,10] The anterior tibial artery and the region where the extensor hallucis brevis tendon crosses over the medial branch both make excellent landmarks for identifying the deep peroneal nerve on MRN.[11]

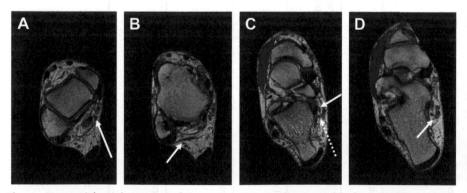

Fig. 1. Sequential axial anatomic fat-sensitive intermediate-weighted images through the hindfoot show normal tibial nerve at the tarsal tunnel (*arrow* on *A*), sural nerve posterior to the peroneal tendons (*arrow* on *B*), lateral (*dashed arrow* on *C*) and medial plantar nerves (*solid arrow* on *C*), and inferior calcaneal nerve (*arrow*) on (*D*). Normal peripheral nerves are isointense to skeletal muscle on fat-sensitive and fluid-sensitive sequences and taper in caliber as they travel distally in the body.

The sural nerve is a cutaneous nerve formed by terminal branches from both the tibial (medial sural nerve) and common peroneal (lateral sural nerve) nerves that join together in the superficial aspect of the distal third of the leg.[12] It courses subcutaneously along the posterolateral aspect of the lower leg lateral to the Achilles tendon and lies close to the lesser saphenous vein, an anatomical landmark for the sural nerve on MRN.[7,11,12] The saphenous nerve originates from the femoral nerve, courses medially within the adductor canal, exits distally between the sartorius and gracilis muscles, and continues its descent within the subcutaneous fat along the medial aspect of the lower leg adjacent to the great saphenous vein, an anatomical landmark for the saphenous nerve.[7,11]

MR NEUROGRAPHY

MRN provides an important information that can assist in the diagnostic and therapeutic workup of peripheral nerve lesions of the foot and ankle; it has the ability to delineate peripheral nerve anatomy and is increasingly being implemented into routine clinical practices.[13,14] With MRN, alterations in nerve signal intensity and morphology are sought, necessitating a combination of sequences that provides high spatial resolution and sensitivity to mobile water.[1] Acquiring a high-quality MRN study that is clinically helpful requires time and attention to detail, and protocols should be planned with all available clinical and electrodiagnostic information. The field of view might have to be tailored to cover a broader area for initial screening, followed by smaller field of view imaging targeted at areas of identified abnormalities.[1]

The high-resolution MRN examination can include two-dimensional (2D) and/or three-dimensional (3D) techniques, and protocols with a combination of T2 and diffusion-weighted imaging (DWI) neurography sequences have been recommended.[13–15] Potential sequences include T1W fast spin-echo, T2W spectrally adiabatic inversion recovery (SPAIR), proton density (PD), 3D inversion recovery, and 3D diffusion-weighted reversed fast imaging with steady-state precession hybrid pulse sequences (DW-PSIF).[13–17] T2 SPAIR imaging provides a higher signal-to-noise ratio, less pulsation artifacts, and more favorable specific absorption rate than Shor Tau Inversion Recovery (STIR) imaging while maintaining better fat suppression than fat-suppressed T2W imaging.[13,17]

Three-dimensional imaging is more advantageous than 2D imaging on 3T MRI because it avoids magnetization transfer effects between adjacent slices, and thinner axial slices can be nicely reconstructed using isotropic imaging.[18] The high-definition and high-contrast 3D images can be reconstructed in any desired plane without compromising the ability to visualize nerves as small as 2 to 3 mm with sub 1-mm voxels; moreover, 3D images can be used to produce maximum intensity projection of the nerves for longitudinal display of anatomy and pathology and thus lead to a better understanding of the lesions (**Fig. 2**).[13,17,19,20] The use of intravenous contrast is generally restricted to cases of suspected infections, inflammation, diffuse nerve lesions, and tumors; injured and entrapped nerves and posttraumatic neuromas generally show abnormal T2 hyperintensity on unenhanced images; and contrast-enhanced images do not add much value except in showing enhancement in the denervated muscles.[14,20] Of note, traumatic neuromas may enhance following contrast administration, a feature that cannot be used to distinguish tumor from neuroma.[21]

Using MRN sequences, individual fascicular enlargement, abnormal T2 hyperintensity, and disruption or effacement of the nerve fascicular appearance can be easily depicted.[13] DW-PSIF hybrid pulse sequences provide nerve-selective images and suppress adjacent vascular structures, which can be particularly helpful in the foot

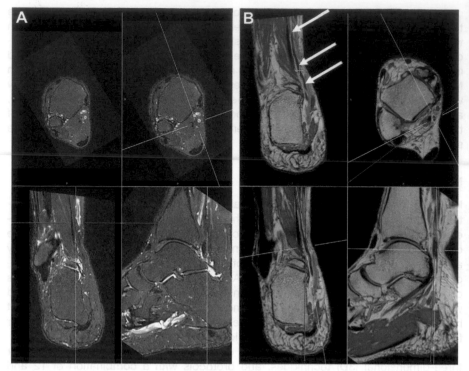

Fig. 2. Three-dimensional fluid-sensitive (*A*) and fat-sensitive (*B*) sequences are a key part of an MRN protocol. Three-dimensional T2-Fat suppressed (FS) and PD non-FS sequences were acquired in the sagittal plane and reformatted in the axial and coronal planes. The main advantage of these 3D sequences is the ability to reformat in any desired plane. Note the longitudinal anatomy of a normal tibial nerve (*arrow*).

and ankle.[1] The sequence can be implemented readily but requires optimal shimming; off-isocenter imaging or imaging of large areas may suffer from ghosting artifacts or poor fat suppression, and postprocessing image reformatting is also required.[15] Another technique that has been implemented in peripheral nerve evaluation is diffusion tensor imaging (DTI), which exploits the anisotropic properties of axonal fiber tracts and allows fiber tract mapping as well as the calculation of quantitative parameters such as the absolute diffusion coefficient (ADC).[4] Even though this technique is technically demanding and has not been broadly adapted for clinical use, it shows great promise for lesion characterization.[13,22] The mean diffusivity quantifies the average displacement of water molecules, and fractional anisotropy measures the directional preference of the diffusion of the water molecules. Neuropathic conditions often result in a decreased fractional anisotropy and an increased ADC, whereas recovering axons often exhibit increased fractional anisotropy and a decreased ADC.[4]

On current high-resolution MRN techniques, the normal peripheral nerves (more than 2–3 mm) are easily distinguished from the surrounding vessels because of their unique fascicular appearance, nonbranching, relatively straight course in most parts, and lack of flow voids. Good surface coils can depict the fascicles in normal nerves that are 3 mm or larger, and the thin epineurium can also be seen forming the outer covering of the nerve in large nerves.[5,13] Normal peripheral nerves seem isointense to skeletal muscle on T1W and T2W sequences, isointense to minimally hyperintense on STIR/fat-suppressed T2W, and uniform and symmetrically hyperintense on 3D turbo spin echo. They display a uniform fascicular pattern and a smooth course without focal deviations; enhancement is usually absent, and perineural fat appears clean. Moreover, DTI tracts seem normal, with symmetric brightness of the nerves on tensor images and normal fractional anisotropy values of greater than 0.4 to 0.5.[17]

MRN is not without its disadvantages. First, MRN may show false-positive findings, and a mildly increased T2 signal intensity of nerves can merely represent a magic angle artifact and should be reported as a nonspecific finding.[23,24] Additionally, mild hyperintensity can be observed in asymptomatic patients in nerves that are predisposed to subclinical traction or friction neuropathy because of their superficial location (such as the medial plantar nerve in the hindfoot).[17] Finally, close communication with referring physicians and correlation with available electrodiagnostic findings are essential for an accurate diagnosis and clarification of minimally abnormal findings, which in isolation should be reported as nonspecific findings.[17]

SPECTRUM OF PATHOLOGY AND ROLE OF MR NEUROGRAPHY IN PATIENTS WITH FOOT AND ANKLE NEUROPATHY

Peripheral neuropathies in the ankle and foot may be the cause of chronic pain and disability but are frequently underdiagnosed. Clinical symptoms are often subtle and subjective in the nerve territory, and physicians may have difficulty distinguishing neuropathy from other clinical entities.[25] The most frequent mechanisms of nerve injury in the ankle and foot are nerve entrapment; however, peripheral neuropathies can also be inherited or precipitated by trauma, inflammation, and neoplasms.[26,27]

Abnormal peripheral nerves show focal or diffuse enlargement that is larger than the adjacent artery. The nerves seem hyperintense on T2W, becoming similar to adjacent veins. Single or multiple fascicles, depending on the extent of the injury, may seem enlarged or disrupted, and the fascicular pattern may be lost. The nerve course is no longer smooth but may appear discontinuous with focal or diffuse deviations, and enhancement can be seen in the case of tumors or infections where the blood–nerve barrier becomes disrupted. In contrast to the preserved fat planes seen with normal peripheral nerves, the perineural fat exhibits strand-like T1 and T2 hypointensities encasing the abnormal nerve. DTI may be abnormal: tracts are disrupted or displaced, and the nerve seems asymmetrically hyperintense on tensor images with abnormal fractional anisotropy values of less than 0.4 to 0.5.[17] Grading of nerve injury by MRI has been described for larger nerves, and some of the features described can be extrapolated to characterizing pathologic condition in smaller nerves.[28]

ENTRAPMENT

Entrapment neuropathies typically occur in osteo-fibrous tunnels or when nerves travel superficially and close to the bony surfaces of the foot. The clinical presentation differs depending on the entrapped nerve but entrapment is generally well recognized on imaging and presents with detectable abnormalities in the affected nerve, such as displacement and focal swelling.[29] Nerve entrapment occurs when increased pressure within a tunnel or a space-occupying lesion leads to the blockade of axoplasmic flow, venous congestion, hyperemia, epineurial edema at and proximal to the site of entrapment, and distal Wallerian degeneration.[17] These pathologic abnormalities lead to hyperintensity on T2W images, and signal intensity approaching the signal intensity to adjacent vessels can be seen with neuropathy; moreover, the signal abnormality is maximum at and just proximal to the site of entrapment with distal fading/resolution to normal signal intensity.[17,19,30] Both proximal and distal nerve enlargement may be seen with entrapment on MRN; the proximal enlargement is much more common and pronounced than the distal enlargement, which is usually observed in more severe cases of entrapment.[17] Finally, space-occupying lesions can be classified as intraneural or perineural: intraneural lesions lead to nerve enlargement and/or fascicular involvement, whereas perineurial lesions cause nerve encasement and displacement.[17]

Tarsal tunnel syndrome is a painful condition in which either the tibial nerve or its divisional branches become entrapped as they travel through the tarsal tunnel; its true incidence is unknown, with a specific cause identified in only 60% to 80% of patients.[27,31] Onset is often insidious, manifesting clinically by paresthesia or burning pain at the plantar aspect of the foot. Depending on the compression site and the nerve branch involved, clinical symptoms can be focal, localizing to the medial plantar aspect of the heel, or radiating proximally to the tunnel or distally into the toes. Weakness and loss in volume of intrinsic foot muscles is a late and uncommon finding.[25,27] The major causes of tarsal tunnel syndrome are bone and joint disorders (**Fig. 3**), space-occupying lesions (**Fig. 4**), and congenital varus or valgus deformities of the foot.[32–37] Diagnosis of the neuropathy typically relies on the detection of a soft tissue mass or bone abnormality impinging the nerve in the tarsal tunnel on imaging; the tibial nerve may seem displaced by the mass and, despite its compressive state, most often retains a normal size and fascicular pattern.[25,38] However, MRN may also be able to detect an increase in size, T2 hyperintensity, denervation signs in the plantar muscles, and enhancement of the tarsal tunnel on gadolinium-enhanced images in chronic long-standing disease or in the case of direct bone impingement.[35]

Anterior tarsal tunnel syndrome is another syndrome that manifests clinically as weakness of the extensor digitorum brevis muscle and numbness between the first and second digits; it can occur when the deep peroneal nerve becomes entrapped

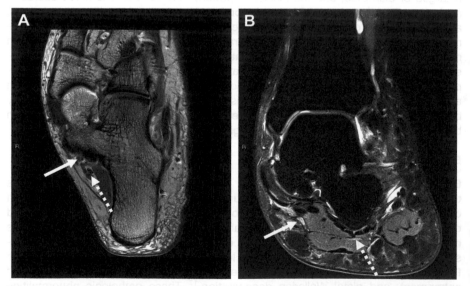

Fig. 3. A 23-year-old woman with talocalcaneal coalition and MPN neuropathy. Axial intermediate-weighted (*A*) and coronal T2-FS (*B*) images through the hindfoot show osseous talocalcaneal coalition and apparent hindfoot valgus. Note the medial plantar nerve (*solid arrows* on A and B) is disproportionately hyperintense and enlarged relative to the lateral plantar nerve (*dashed arrows* on A and B).

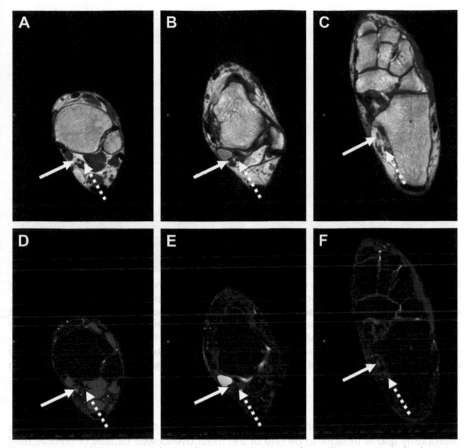

Fig. 4. 45-year-old woman with ganglion cyst originating from the posterior subtalar joint. Sequential axial fat-sensitive intermediate-weighted (*A–C*) and fluid-sensitive (*D–F*) images through the tarsal tunnel show a high division of the tibial nerve into the medial (*solid arrow*) and lateral (*dashed arrow*) plantar nerves (*A* and *D*). A ganglion cyst originating from the posterior subtalar joint protrudes into the tarsal tunnel (*B* and *E*) and flattens the medial plantar nerve (*solid arrow*). Caudal to the extrinsic compression, the medial plantar nerve (*solid arrow* on *C* and *F*) is disproportionately hyperintense and enlarged relative to the lateral plantar nerve (*dashed arrow* on *C* and *F*).

between the superior and inferior extensor retinacula or compressed by midfoot osteophytes.[39] The nerve may also be compressed by external pressure on the dorsum of the foot (eg, tight-fitting footwear worn by dancers or skiers), and the medial branch may become entrapped at its crossover point with the extensor hallucis brevis tendon, resulting in a focal neuroma.[4,29,38,40,41] An os intermetatarseum in the proximal first intermetatarsal space may also cause nerve disturbances and result in a sensory syndrome involving the first web space; however, the involvement of the motor branch may seldom occur because this branch travels deep to the inferior extensor retinaculum.[11,25] Detecting anterior tarsal tunnel syndrome on MRN may be challenging due to the small size of the nerve involved and the difficulty of distinguishing it from adjacent small vessels.[25] The major role of MRN in patients with anterior tarsal tunnel syndrome is the detection of masses (**Fig. 5**) or extrinsic compressions by a ganglion or osteophyte.

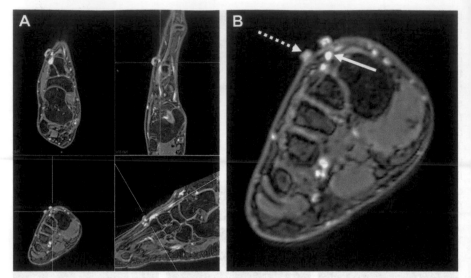

Fig. 5. A 34-year-old man with schwannomatosis and tenderness on the dorsum of the foot exacerbated while wearing shoes. Three-dimensional T1-FS postcontrast sequence (*A*) was acquired in the sagittal plane and reformatted in the axial and coronal planes. On the short axis coronal image through the midfoot (*B*), a solid enhancing mass (*solid arrow*) is visible deep to the MR (*dashed arrow*) clinical marker compatible with a small superficial schwannoma originating from the deep peroneal nerve. In patients with peripheral neuropathy and a Tinel sign, placement of an MR compatible marker can be useful for the detection of very small lesions.

Compression of the inferior calcaneal nerve results in a condition known as Baxter's neuropathy and is thought to be one of the most overlooked causes of chronic heel pain, responsible for up to 20% of patients presenting with this clinical picture.[26] Nerve compression may occur at various sites and can be caused by calcaneal enthesophytes, plantar fasciitis, and varicosities.[11] On imaging, denervation edema or fatty atrophy selectively involving the abductor digiti minimi may suggest the clinical diagnosis. Interestingly, a high prevalence of atrophic changes in this muscle has been found in patients with plantar fasciitis, supporting the notion of a possible etiologic role for plantar fasciitis in the progression to Baxter's neuropathy.[25,42–44]

Compression of the medial plantar nerve is known as "Jogger's foot" and results in burning heel pain, aching in the medial arch, and sensory disturbances in the sole of the foot behind the greater toe as well as the plantar aspect of the first and second toes.[25] The nerve is typically compressed because it passes deep to the flexor retinaculum, at the master knot of Henry; moreover, heel valgus, excessive pronation of the foot while running, and a high medial longitudinal arch seem to be predisposing factors.[11,29,38,40,41] Imaging of this condition typically relies on the detection of denervation changes in the muscles supplied by the medial plantar nerve.[25] Often, MRN can depict flexor tenosynovitis with mass effect on the medial plantar nerve as well. It is interesting to note that the compression of the medial calcaneal nerve results in a syndrome that also causes heel pain and may mimic "Jogger's foot."

Finally, the compression of the interdigital nerves originating from the medial plantar nerve and the lateral plantar nerve can also occur, and repetitive microtraumas and chronic impingement against the flexor retinaculum are thought to cause histopathological changes that result in what is commonly known as a "Morton neu-roma."[11,25] People with this condition complain of paroxysmal intermetatarsal pain and numbness exacerbated by standing and walking and relieved by rest and shoe removal. The lesion is usually unilateral with female predominance, possibly relating to the more flexible state of the female foot and the habit of wearing high heels, and the third webspace is typically involved.[25,45] On imaging, a Morton neuroma typically seems as a teardrop-shaped soft tissue masse emerging plantarly from the interme-tatarsal space and exhibits low signal intensity on both T1W and T2W sequences, although with variable signal hyperintensity on fluid-sensitive sequences (**Fig. 6**). The lesion may also show gadolinium enhancement, and T2W images may be useful to distinguish Morton neuroma from an adjacent fluid-filled intermetatarsal bursa.[46–49] In the absence of Morton's neuroma or interdigital perineural fibrosis, MRN can also depict metatarsophalangeal plantar plate tears with coexistent nonneuromatous le-sions at second or third interspace (**Fig. 7**).[50]

TRAUMA

Trauma to the foot may result in local nerve injuries, and the resulting symptoms depend on the compromised nerve. Traumatic nerve injuries can be divided into stretch injuries, high-grade nerve injuries with neuroma in continuity (**Fig. 8**), and nerve transection with end-bulb neuroma formation (**Fig. 9**).[17,19] Stretch injuries can be mild, showing an abnormally hyperintense nerve in continuity and with nearly similar size to adjacent vessels or contralateral nerves, or moderate, showing diffuse nerve enlarge-ment greater than the size of the adjacent vessels or contralateral nerves due to axonal degeneration and expansion of fluid space within the nerve. High-grade nerve injuries display an abrupt change in nerve caliber with focal nerve enlargement and fascicular effacement, and nerve transection shows complete discontinuity of the nerve in ques-tion.[17] This distinction becomes important when considering how different injuries warrant different treatment approaches: Stretch injuries usually require conservative management and rehabilitation, whereas operative management is commonly per-formed in high-grade nerve injuries for functional recovery to occur.[14,17,51] Regional muscle changes can also serve as an important key indicator of neuropathy: edema-like T2 signal abnormalities can be seen in the acute stages and fatty

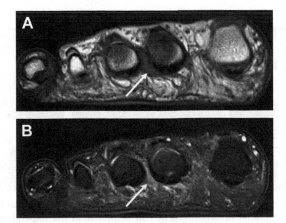

Fig. 6. Short axial coronal intermediate-weighted fat-sensitive (*A*) and fluid-sensitive (*B*) im-ages through the forefoot reveal a focal interdigital (Morton's) neuroma/perineural fibrosis (*arrow*) at the second webspace.

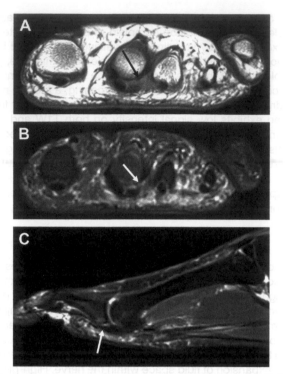

Fig. 7. Short axial coronal intermediate-weighted fat-sensitive (*A*) and fluid-sensitive (*B*) images through the forefoot reveal partial tear of the second lesser metatarsophalangeal plantar plate at its distal attachment (*arrow*) with bone marrow edema at the base of the proximal phalanx best seen on sagittal T2-FS image (*C*). In this patient, pain is concentrated at the plantar base of the space between her second and third toe and feels like walking on a large "rock." MRN enables distinction between interdigital (Morton's) neuroma/perineural fibrosis and adjacent plantar plate injury with a nonneuromatous lesion in the second interspace; both conditions can clinically overlap.

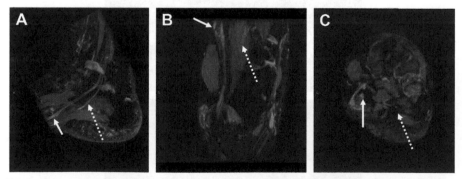

Fig. 8. A 41-year-old woman with chronic left foot pain after cyst removal from her midfoot plantar aspect. Multiplanar reformations of PSIF sequence in the sagittal (*A*), axial/long-axis (*B*), and coronal/short axis (*C*) images through the hindfoot show an enlarged distal medial plantar nerve in continuity (*solid arrow*), which is compatible with a neuroma-in-continuity. Note a normal lateral plantar nerve (*dashed arrow*) included in the field of view.

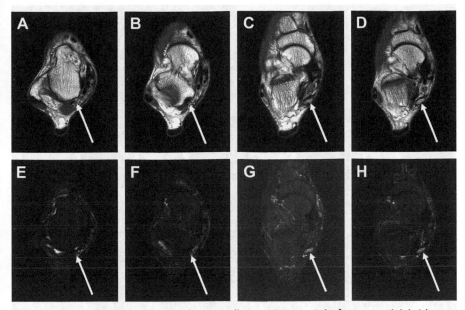

Fig. 9. A 17-year-old male patient with a propeller accident s/p right foot wound debridement, posterior tibialis tendon repair, tibial nerve neuroplasty, and repair with allograft. Sequential axial fat-sensitive intermediate-weighted (*A–D*) and fluid-sensitive (*E–H*) images shows a focal tibial nerve end-bulb neuroma (*arrow*) in the caudal aspect of the tarsal tunnel.

infiltration and atrophy can be seen in subacute or chronic stages of denervation. Additionally, muscle involvement is usually diffuse with no associated perimuscular edema, hemorrhage, or nearby fascial involvement.[30]

Sural neuropathy is one of the neuropathies that can be precipitated by trauma and typically presents with pain and sensory disturbances along the lateral border of the ankle and foot (**Fig. 10**).[52,53] It can be secondary to fractures of the lateral malleolus, the base of the fifth metatarsal, and the cuboid bone, where local soft tissue edema, hematomas, or direct nerve impingement by fracture fragments can cause nerve dysfunction.[25,27,38] Traumatic injury to the sural nerve may also occur during ankle sprains because of tension neuropathy or during open and arthroscopic ankle surgery performed with a posterolateral approach to treat conditions such as posterior impingement syndrome and peroneal tendon instability.[25] Moreover, sural neuropathy is a well-recognized complication of minimally invasive techniques for both saphenectomy and Achilles tendon repair: the nerve may be lacerated due to its close proximity to the vein during lesser saphenous stripping, and sutures used in percutaneous Achilles tendon repairs can inadvertently result in nerve entrapment.[54,55] Even with proper suturing techniques, an incidence of up to 14% of sural nerve injury has been reported in the literature.[55] Owing to the small size and sensory nature of the nerve, MRN might be limited in detecting sural nerve abnormalities in the ankle and foot. However, knowledge of the sural nerve anatomy at the hindfoot allows for the detection of subtle abnormalities of the nerve itself and the adjacent osseous and soft tissue structures.

Superficial peroneal neuropathy is another traumatic neuropathy that is most often encountered in patients with a history of inversion ankle sprains or plantar flexion injuries in whom trauma leads to persistent tingling and paresthesia along the distribution of the nerve.[25] It is related to a tension mechanism occurring at the point where the nerve is tethered because it pierces the deep fascia of the leg and has been reported in athletes (eg,

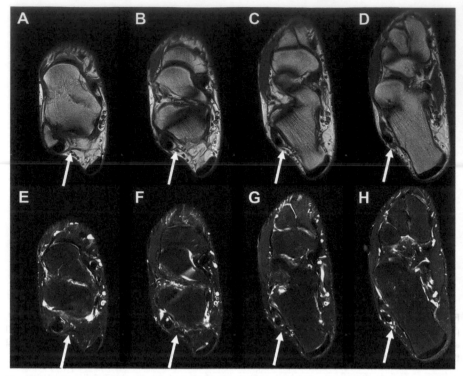

Fig. 10. A 49-year-old man with pain in lateral right calf extending to the ankle and foot. Sequential axial fat-sensitive intermediate-weighted (*A–D*) and fluid-sensitive (*E–H*) images through the hindfoot show a moderately hyperintense and enlarged sural nerve (*arrow*) posterior to the peroneal tendons compatible with stretch-related injury based on the clinical context. No intrinsic mass, discontinuity, or extrinsic compression was detected.

runners, soccer players, jockeys, bodybuilders, tennis players, and dancers).[56] More distally, the medial and intermediate dorsal cutaneous branches of the nerve may be at risk for iatrogenic injury during ankle arthroscopic procedures (particularly with anterolateral portal placement) or surgical repair for lateral malleolus fractures.[57] Clinical symptoms derive from tension neuropathy, perineural fibrosis, and local impingement: point tenderness and a positive Tinel sign can be felt, and imaging can reveal fascial thickening and fusiform swelling of either the nerve or one of its divisional branches.[25]

Other nerves that are susceptible to traumatic injury include the proper branch of the medial plantar nerve, which can be injured during a tibial sesamoidectomy performed using a medial-plantar approach, and the saphenous nerve, which can uncommonly be injured by local acute traumas, displaced fractures, ankle joint dislocations, and tarsal tunnel surgery.[25,58] Injury to the saphenous nerve can also occur during surgery for varices or with the use of an anteromedial portal for ankle arthroscopy.[11]

Finally, the tibial nerve may be injured at any point from the distal thigh to the foot. The most common causes of nerve injury are bone fractures, knee and ankle dislocations, wounds, compartment syndrome, and iatrogenic injuries.[59]

CHRONIC INFLAMMATORY DEMYELINATING POLYRADICULONEUROPATHY

Chronic inflammatory demyelinating polyradiculoneuropathy (CIDP) is an immune-mediated disease that leads to muscle weakness and sensory symptoms.[60] CIDP involves both T cell-mediated and humoral immune mechanisms that target the myelin of peripheral nerves and can disrupt innervation to the foot and ankle. The classical presentation includes symmetric proximal and distal sensory and motor involvement that leads to foot drop.[61] MRN has been used to directly assess axonal and myelin integrity with biomarkers acquired from DTI parameters.[62] More routinely, MRN may show evidence of T2 alterations or nerve enlargement.[63,64] MRN is not typically performed for establishing the diagnosis of CIDP. Its main role is to exclude structural lesions or entrapment.

HEREDITARY PERIPHERAL NEUROPATHIES

Hereditary peripheral neuropathies (HPNs) present with a chronic progressive course of muscle weakness caused by mutations in genes involved in preserving the structure and function of Schwann cells, the myelinating cells of the peripheral nervous system.[65] HPNs typically present with slowly progressive distal weakness and atrophy of the intrinsic foot and calf muscles leading to foot drop, pes cavus, hammer toes, and a stork leg deformity; pain is not a predominant complaint but sensory loss can often be present.[65] Nerve conduction studies and genetic testing are typically the gold standard for evaluating HPNs but imaging can document enlarged peripheral nerves with increased connective tissue in the epineurium.[20] Moreover, MRN with DTI can provide qualitative and quantitative information regarding the severity of neuropathy and any anatomical disruption to the nerve fascicles.[66] Similar to CIDP, MRN is not typically performed to establish the diagnosis of HPNs but enables detection of superimposed entrapment or other disorders.

NEOPLASMS

Peripheral nerve sheath tumors (PNSTs) are soft-tissue neoplasms that can be associated with neuropathy. PNSTs develop in close association with a peripheral nerve, display histological characteristics reminiscent of nerve sheath connective tissue, and can be classified into different subtypes, most notably neurofibromas, schwannomas, and plexiform PNSTs.[67] PNSTs in the foot and ankle are rare but still account for approximately 10% of all soft tissue tumors.[68] The most common presenting symptoms include pain, a noticeable mass, numbness, paresthesia, and weakness of the foot; however, the lesions' innocuous appearance and insidious growth often lead to misdiagnosis and suboptimal treatment, and patients with a foot or ankle PNST generally present later in the course of the disease.[67,69]

Schwannomas and neurofibromas are benign entities that share many similar features on MRN and usually seem as well-defined lesions measuring less than 5 cm. Lesions are typically isointense or slightly hyperintense to muscle on T1W and markedly hyperintense to fat on fluid-sensitive sequences.[70] Classic MRN findings of benign lesions include the split-fat sign, the target sign, the fascicular pattern, visualization of the entering and exiting nerve, and a thin hyperintense rim.[70] Plexiform neurofibromas are a distinctive variant associated with peripheral nerve syndromes that, although benign, carry a risk of malignant transformation. They display similar imaging characteristics to schwannomas and neurofibromas, typically with a tortuous mass of irregularly expanded nerve branches.[70] Importantly, features of benign and malignant PNSTs can overlap with conventional imaging, and MRN, when performed with DWI mapping, can characterize a PNST for malignancy based on anatomic imaging features such as growth, necrosis, perilesional edema size, and ADC values derived from DWI (**Fig. 11**).[71–75]

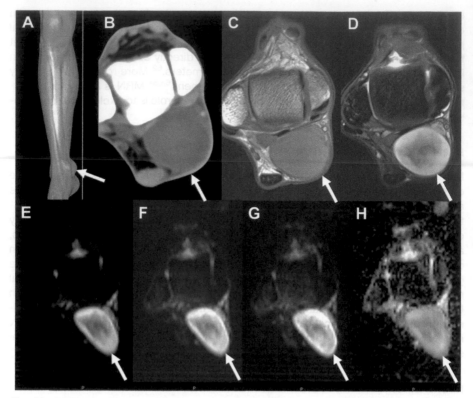

Fig. 11. A 31-year-old man with NF1 and growing ankle mass. A protuberant mass is visible along the medial hindfoot on volume rendered CT images (A) and contrast-enhanced axial CT images through the ankle (B). Axial T1-weighted (C) and T2-FS (D) weighted images through the tarsal tunnel show a large mass in the tarsal tunnel with a target sign typical of a peripheral nerve sheath tumor. Axial DWI performed using increasing b-values (E–G) and apparent diffusion coefficient (ADC) mapping (H) show persistent target sign and lack of restricted diffusion compatible with a benign peripheral nerve sheath tumor, likely a neuro-fibroma in the context of NF1. People with NF1 have a high lifetime risk of malignant trans-formation, and DWI enables accurate characterization of tumors in this patient population.

SUMMARY

To conclude, MRN is an excellent imaging modality for depicting the anatomy and pathologic condition of the peripheral nerves of the foot and ankle. Optimal imaging technique, including knowledge of the utility of DWI, is essential for MRN interpretation of the various peripheral neuropathies encountered in the foot and ankle. Further tech-nical developments in diffusion-based nerve imaging and nerve-specific contrast agents will likely play a major role in advancing our ability to identify the different nerve pathologic conditions of the foot and ankle.

CLINICS CARE POINTS

- Knowledge of nerve anatomy and pathophysiology is important for precise MRN interpretation.

- MRN can assist clinicians in differentiating between the different peripheral neuropathies of the foot and ankle.
- In routine clinical practice, standard high-resolution MRN sequences combined with DWI and ADC mapping are useful for detecting and characterizing peripheral nerve lesions.
- Imaging abnormalities may be detected in asymptomatic patients, and other clinical and/or imaging features should be sought to increase specificity.

DECLARATIONS OF INTEREST

None.

ACKNOWLEDGMENTS

None.

REFERENCES

1. Bae WC, Ruangchaijatuporn T, Chung CB. New techniques in MR imaging of the ankle and foot. Magn Reson Imaging Clin N Am 2017;25(1). https://doi.org/10.1016/j.mric.2016.08.009.
2. Sharma GK, Dhillon MS, Dhatt SS. The influence of foot and ankle injury patterns and treatment delays on outcomes in a tertiary hospital; a one-year prospective observation. Foot 2016;26. https://doi.org/10.1016/j.foot.2015.12.001.
3. Chhabra A, Madhuranthakam AJ, Andreisek G. Magnetic resonance neurography: current perspectives and literature review. Eur Radiol 2018;28(2). https://doi.org/10.1007/s00330-017-4976-8.
4. Burge AJ, Gold SL, Kuong S, et al. High-resolution magnetic resonance imaging of the lower extremity nerves. Neuroimaging Clin N Am 2014;24(1). https://doi.org/10.1016/j.nic.2013.03.027.
5. Chhabra A, Subhawong TK, Williams EH, et al. High-resolution MR neurography: evaluation before repeat tarsal tunnel surgery. Am J Roentgenol 2011;197(1). https://doi.org/10.2214/AJR.10.5763.
6. Pham M, Oikonomou D, Hornung B, et al. Magnetic resonance neurography detects diabetic neuropathy early and with Proximal Predominance. Ann Neurol 2015;78(6). https://doi.org/10.1002/ana.24524.
7. Tang A, Bordoni B. Anatomy, bony pelvis and lower limb. Foot Nerves; 2022.
8. Desai SS, Cohen-Levy WB. Anatomy, bony pelvis and lower limb. Tibial Nerve; 2022.
9. Hardin JM, Devendra S. Anatomy, Bony Pelvis and Lower Limb: Calf Common Peroneal Nerve (Common Fibular Nerve). 2022. In: StatPearls [Internet]. FL): StatPearls: Treasure Island; 2023.
10. Giuffre BA, Jeanmonod R. Anatomy. Sciatic Nerve.; 2022.
11. de Maeseneer M, Madani H, Lenchik L, et al. Normal anatomy and compression areas of nerves of the foot and ankle: US and MR imaging with anatomic correlation. Radiographics 2015;35(5). https://doi.org/10.1148/rg.2015150028.
12. Miniato MA, Nedeff N. Anatomy, bony pelvis and lower limb. Sural Nerve.; 2022.
13. Chhabra A, Andreisek G, Soldatos T, et al. MR neurography: Past, present, and future. Am J Roentgenol 2011;197(3). https://doi.org/10.2214/AJR.10.6012.
14. Chhabra A, Williams EH, Wang KC, et al. MR neurography of neuromas related to nerve injury and entrapment with surgical correlation. Am J Neuroradiol 2010; 31(8). https://doi.org/10.3174/ajnr.A2002.

15. Siriwanarangsun P, Bae WC, Statum S, et al. Advanced MRI techniques for the ankle. Am J Roentgenol 2017;209(3). https://doi.org/10.2214/AJR.17.18057.
16. Chhabra A, Belzberg AJ, Rosson GD, et al. Impact of high resolution 3 tesla MR neurography (MRN) on diagnostic thinking and therapeutic patient management. Eur Radiol 2016;26(5). https://doi.org/10.1007/s00330-015-3958-y.
17. Chhabra A. Peripheral MR neurography. Approach to interpretation. Neuroimaging Clin N Am 2014;24(1). https://doi.org/10.1016/j.nic.2013.03.033.
18. Khalilzadeh O, Fayad LM, Ahlawat S. 3D MR neurography. Semin Muscoskel Radiol 2021;25(3). https://doi.org/10.1055/s-0041-1730909.
19. Chhabra A, Lee PP, Bizzell C, et al. 3 Tesla MR neurography - Technique, interpretation, and pitfalls. Skeletal Radiol 2011;40(10). https://doi.org/10.1007/s00256-011-1183-6.
20. Thawait SK, Chaudhry V, Thawait GK, et al. High-resolution MR neurography of diffuse peripheral nerve lesions. Am J Neuroradiol 2011;32(8). https://doi.org/10.3174/ajnr.A2257.
21. Ahlawat S, Belzberg AJ, Montgomery E A, et al. MRI features of peripheral traumatic neuromas. Eur Radiol 2016;26(4). https://doi.org/10.1007/s00330-015-3907-9.
22. Simon NG, Lagopoulos J, Gallagher T, et al. Peripheral nerve diffusion tensor imaging is reliable and reproducible. J Magn Reson Imaging 2016;43(4). https://doi.org/10.1002/jmri.25056.
23. Chappell KE, Robson MD, Stonebridge-Foster A, et al. Magic angle effects in MR neurography. Am J Neuroradiol 2004;25(3). https://doi.org/10.1016/s0513-5117(08)70339-9.
24. Kästel T, Heiland S, Bäumer P, et al. Magic angle effect: a relevant artifact in MR neurography at 3T? Am J Neuroradiol 2011;32(5). https://doi.org/10.3174/ajnr.A2402.
25. Martinoli C, Court-Payen M, Michaud J, et al. Imaging of neuropathies about the ankle and foot. Semin Muscoskel Radiol 2010;14(3). https://doi.org/10.1055/s-0030-1254523.
26. Schon LC, Baxter DE. Neuropathies of the foot and ankle in athletes. Clin Sports Med 1990;9(2). https://doi.org/10.1016/s0278-5919(20)30743-2.
27. Schon LC. Nerve entrapment, neuropathy, and nerve dysfunction in athletes. Orthop Clin North Am 1994;25(1). https://doi.org/10.1016/s0030-5898(20)31866-6.
28. Ahlawat S, Belzberg AJ, Fayad LM. Utility of magnetic resonance imaging for predicting severity of sciatic nerve injury. J Comput Assist Tomogr 2018;42(4). https://doi.org/10.1097/rct.0000000000000730.
29. Allen JM, Greer BJ, Sorge DG, et al. MR imaging of neuropathies of the leg, ankle, and foot. Magn Reson Imaging Clin N Am 2008;16(1). https://doi.org/10.1016/j.mric.2008.02.006.
30. Filler AG, Maravilla KR, Tsuruda JS. MR neurography and muscle MR imaging for image diagnosis of disorders affecting the peripheral nerves and musculature. Neurol Clin 2004;22(3). https://doi.org/10.1016/j.ncl.2004.03.005.
31. Lau JTC, Daniels TR. Tarsal tunnel syndrome: a review of the literature. Foot Ankle Int 1999;20(3). https://doi.org/10.1177/107110079902000312.
32. Hochman MG, Zilberfarb JL. Nerves in a pinch: imaging of nerve compression syndromes. Radiol Clin North Am 2004;42(1). https://doi.org/10.1016/S0033-8389(03)00162-3.
33. Nagaoka M, Matsuzaki H. Ultrasonography in tarsal tunnel syndrome. J Ultrasound Med 2005;24(8). https://doi.org/10.7863/jum.2005.24.8.1035.

34. Spinner RJ, Dellon AL, Rosson GD, et al. Tibial intraneural ganglia in the tarsal tunnel: is there a joint connection? J Foot Ankle Surg 2007;46(1). https://doi.org/10.1053/j.jfas.2006.10.002.
35. Martinoli C, Bianchi S, Gandolfo N, et al. US of nerve entrapments in osteofibrous tunnels of the upper and lower limbs. Radiographics 2000;20(SPEC.ISS). https://doi.org/10.1148/radiographics.20.suppl_1.g00oc08s199.
36. Erickson SJ, Quinn SF, Kneeland JB, et al. MR imaging of the tarsal tunnel and related spaces: normal and abnormal findings with anatomic correlation. Am J Roentgenol 1990;155(2). https://doi.org/10.2214/ajr.155.2.2115260.
37. Alaia EFG, Rosenberg ZS, Bencardino JT, et al. Tarsal tunnel disease and talocalcaneal coalition: MRI features. Skeletal Radiol 2016;45(11). https://doi.org/10.1007/s00256-016-2461-0.
38. Delfaut EM, Demondion X, Bieganski A, et al. Imaging of foot and ankle nerve entrapment syndromes: from well-demonstrated to unfamiliar sites. Radiographics 2003;23(3). https://doi.org/10.1148/rg.233025053.
39. Ng JM, Rosenberg ZS, Bencardino JT, et al. US and MR imaging of the extensor compartment of the ankle. Radiographics 2013;33(7). https://doi.org/10.1148/rg.337125182.
40. Lopez-Ben R. Imaging of nerve entrapment in the foot and ankle. Foot Ankle Clin 2011;16(2). https://doi.org/10.1016/j.fcl.2011.04.001.
41. Flanigan RM, DiGiovanni BF. Peripheral nerve entrapments of the lower leg, ankle, and foot. Foot Ankle Clin 2011;16(2). https://doi.org/10.1016/j.fcl.2011.01.006.
42. Schmid DT, Hodler J, Mengiardi B, et al. Fatty muscle atrophy: prevalence in the hindfoot muscles on MR images of asymptomatic volunteers and patients with foot pain. Radiology 2009;253(1). https://doi.org/10.1148/radiol.2531090035.
43. Recht MP, Grooff P, Ilaslan H, et al. Selective atrophy of the abductor digiti quinti: an MRI study. AJR Am J Roentgenol 2007;189(3). https://doi.org/10.2214/AJR.07.2229.
44. Chundru U, Liebeskind A, Seidelmann F, et al. Plantar fasciitis and calcaneal spur formation are associated with abductor digiti minimi atrophy on MRI of the foot. Skeletal Radiol 2008;37(6). https://doi.org/10.1007/s00256-008-0455-2.
45. Shereff MJ, Grande DA. Electron microscopic analysis of the interdigital neuroma. Clin Orthop Relat Res 1991;271. https://doi.org/10.1097/00003086-199110000-00040.
46. Zanetti M, Strehle JK, Zollinger H, et al. Morton neuroma and fluid in the intermetatarsal bursae on MR images of 70 asymptomatic volunteers. Radiology 1997;203(2). https://doi.org/10.1148/radiology.203.2.9114115.
47. Zanetti M, Ledermann T, Zollinger H, et al. Efficacy of MR imaging in patients suspected of having Morton's neuroma. Am J Roentgenol 1997;168(2). https://doi.org/10.2214/ajr.168.2.9016241.
48. Zanetti M, Strehle JK, Kundert HP, et al. Morton neuroma: effect of MR imaging findings on diagnostic thinking and therapeutic decisions. Radiology 1999;213(2). https://doi.org/10.1148/radiology.213.2.r99nv06583.
49. Zanetti M, Weishaupt D. MR imaging of the forefoot: morton neuroma and differential diagnoses. Semin Muscoskel Radiol 2005;9(3). https://doi.org/10.1055/s-2005-921938.
50. Umans H, Srinivasan R, Elsinger E, et al. MRI of lesser metatarsophalangeal joint plantar plate tears and associated adjacent interspace lesions. Skeletal Radiol 2014;43(10). https://doi.org/10.1007/s00256-014-1920-8.

51. Thawait SK, Wang K, Subhawong TK, et al. Peripheral nerve surgery: the role of high-resolution MR neurography. Am J Neuroradiol 2012;33(2). https://doi.org/10.3174/ajnr.A2465.
52. Lawrence SJ, Botte MJ. The sural nerve in the foot and ankle: an anatomic study with clinical and surgical implications. Foot Ankle Int 1994;15(9). https://doi.org/10.1177/107110079401500906.
53. Fabre T, Montero C, Gaujard E, et al. Chronic calf pain in athletes due to sural nerve entrapment: a report of 18 cases. Am J Sports Med 2000;28(5). https://doi.org/10.1177/03635465000280051001.
54. Simonetti S, Bianchi S, Martinoli C. Neurophysiological and ultrasound findings in sural nerve lesions following stripping of the small saphenous vein. Muscle Nerve 1999;22(12). https://doi.org/10.1002/(SICI)1097-4598(199912)22:12<1724::AID-MUS18>3.0.CO;2-Q.
55. Majewski M, Rohrbach M, Czaja S, et al. Avoiding sural nerve injuries during percutaneous achilles tendon repair. Am J Sports Med 2006;34(5). https://doi.org/10.1177/0363546505283266.
56. Johnston EC, Howell SJ, Dusek J. Tension neuropathy of the superficial peroneal nerve: associated conditions and results of release. Foot Ankle Int 1999;20(9). https://doi.org/10.1177/107110079902000907.
57. Saito A, Kikuchi S. Anatomic relations between ankle arthroscopic portal sites and the superficial peroneal and saphenous nerves. Foot Ankle Int 1998;19(11). https://doi.org/10.1177/107110079801901107.
58. Sims AL, Kurup H v. Painful sesamoid of the great toe. World J Orthop 2014;5(2). https://doi.org/10.5312/wjo.v5.i2.146.
59. Gosk J, Rutowski R. Traumatic injuries of the tibial nerve: etiopathogenesis and surgical outcome. Ortop Traumatol Rehabil 2005;7(4).
60. Ali A, Char G, Hanchard B. Chronic inflammatory demyelinating polyneuropathy in a patient infected with human T lymphotropic virus type I. BMJ Case Rep 2009. https://doi.org/10.1136/bcr.03.2009.1680.
61. Shije J, Brannagan TH. Chronic inflammatory demyelinating polyradiculoneuropathy. Semin Neurol 2019;39(5). https://doi.org/10.1055/s-0039-1693008.
62. Pitarokoili K, Kronlage M, Bäumer P, et al. High-resolution nerve ultrasound and magnetic resonance neurography as complementary neuroimaging tools for chronic inflammatory demyelinating polyneuropathy. Ther Adv Neurol Disord 2018;11. https://doi.org/10.1177/1756286418759974.
63. Pitarokoili K, Schlamann M, Kerasnoudis A, et al. Comparison of clinical, electrophysiological, sonographic and MRI features in CIDP. J Neurol Sci 2015;357(1–2). https://doi.org/10.1016/j.jns.2015.07.030.
64. Shibuya K, Sugiyama A, Ito SI, et al. Reconstruction magnetic resonance neurography in chronic inflammatory demyelinating polyneuropathy. Ann Neurol 2015;77(2). https://doi.org/10.1002/ana.24314.
65. Pareyson D, Saveri P, Pisciotta C. New developments in Charcot-Marie-Tooth neuropathy and related diseases. Curr Opin Neurol 2017;30(5). https://doi.org/10.1097/WCO.0000000000000474.
66. Vaeggemose M, Vaeth S, Pham M, et al. Magnetic resonance neurography and diffusion tensor imaging of the peripheral nerves in patients with Charcot-Marie-Tooth Type 1A. Muscle Nerve 2017;56(6). https://doi.org/10.1002/mus.25691.
67. Carvajal JA, Cuartas E, Qadir R, et al. Peripheral nerve sheath tumors of the foot and ankle. Foot Ankle Int 2011;32(2). https://doi.org/10.3113/FAI.2011.0163.

68. Kransdorf MJ. Benign soft-tissue tumors in a large referral population: distribution of specific diagnoses by age, sex, and location. Am J Roentgenol 1995;164(2). https://doi.org/10.2214/ajr.164.2.7839977.

69. Bos GD, Esther RJ, Woll TS. Foot tumors: diagnosis and treatment. J Am Acad Orthop Surg 2002;10(4). https://doi.org/10.5435/00124635-200207000-00004.

70. Debs P, Fayad LM, Ahlawat S. MR neurography of peripheral nerve tumors and tumor-mimics. Semin Roentgenol 2022. https://doi.org/10.1053/J.RO.2022.01.008.

71. Demehri S, Belzberg A, Blakeley J, et al. Conventional and functional MR imaging of peripheral nerve sheath tumors: Initial experience. Am J Neuroradiol 2014; 35(8). https://doi.org/10.3174/ajnr.A3910.

72. Ahlawat S, Blakeley JO, Rodriguez FJ, et al. Imaging biomarkers for malignant peripheral nerve sheath tumors in neurofibromatosis type 1. Neurology 2019; 93(11). https://doi.org/10.1212/WNL.0000000000008092.

73. Ahlawat S, Fayad LM. Imaging cellularity in benign and malignant peripheral nerve sheath tumors: Utility of the "target sign" by diffusion weighted imaging. Eur J Radiol 2018;102. https://doi.org/10.1016/j.ejrad.2018.03.018.

74. Ahlawat S, Baig A, Blakeley JO, et al. Multiparametric whole-body anatomic, functional, and metabolic imaging characteristics of peripheral lesions in patients with schwannomatosis. J Magn Reson Imaging 2016;44(4). https://doi.org/10.1002/jmri.25236.

75. Ahlawat S, Blakeley JO, Langmead S, et al. Current status and recommendations for imaging in neurofibromatosis type 1, neurofibromatosis type 2, and schwannomatosis. Skeletal Radiol 2020;49(2). https://doi.org/10.1007/s00256-019-03290-1.

Osteomyelitis and Septic Arthritis of the Foot and Ankle: Imaging Update

Islam Zaki, MBBCh[a], William B. Morrison, MD[b],*

KEYWORDS

- Diabetic foot • Osteomyelitis • Septic arthritis • MRI • Neuropathic osteoarthropathy

KEY POINTS

- MRI is the modality of choice for diagnosis of osteomyelitis and septic arthritis and for the evaluation of the extent of involvement.
- Secondary MRI findings including superficial ulcer, sinus tract, soft tissue infection, and abscess adjacent to a bone marrow abnormality strongly favor osteomyelitis.
- The terms "osteitis" and "reactive arthritis" are nebulous and should be avoided.
- Gadolinium contrast can be useful for the evaluation of soft tissue extent and to identify areas of devitalization prior to surgical management; however, renal function should be taken into account.

INTRODUCTION

Osteomyelitis and septic arthritis can arise from hematogenous spread of infection, spread from soft tissue infection, or direct inoculation from penetrating injury or surgery.[1,2] Poor glycemic control in advanced diabetes mellitus (DM), trauma, intravenous drug abuse, and immunodeficiency are risk factors for developing musculoskeletal infection.[3] A foot ulcer is a common complication in patients with advanced diabetes with peripheral neuropathy and vascular disease. Previous studies reported that up to 15% of patients with diabetes will develop foot ulcers.[4,5] The majority of diabetic ulcers heal with aggressive conservative management; however, many patients with DM are of lower socioeconomic status and may not have access to high-quality healthcare, depending on location.

Up to 60% of diabetic foot ulcers are associated with the deep infection of the foot.[6] Subsequent osteomyelitis and/or septic arthritis is common in patients with DM and chronic nonhealing ulcers.[7,8] Common locations for osteomyelitis of the foot include

[a] Department of Radiology, Benha University Hospital, El-Shaheed Farid Nada, Qism Banha, Al Qalyubia Governorate, Banha, Egypt; [b] Division of Musculoskeletal Imaging and Intervention, Department of Radiology, Thomas Jefferson University Hospital, 1079a Main Building 132 South 10th Street, Philadelphia, PA 19107, USA
* Corresponding author.
E-mail address: william.morrison@jefferson.edu
Twitter: @MorrisonMSK (W.B.M.)

Foot Ankle Clin N Am 28 (2023) 589–602
https://doi.org/10.1016/j.fcl.2023.05.009
1083-7515/23/© 2023 Elsevier Inc. All rights reserved.

foot.theclinics.com

the metatarsal heads (especially the first and fifth), the toes (at the distal tuft, or over the dorsal aspect in patients with clawtoe deformity) and the calcaneus and malleoli (especially in bedridden patients).[1,9,10] Ulceration and osteomyelitis is also common at the plantar aspect of the midfoot in patients with Charcot arthropathy and "rocker-bottom" deformity secondary to collapse of the arch. Amputation is a common eventuality; this can shift weightbearing to the contralateral foot, leading to an increased complication rate on the other side.[11,12] Early diagnosis and management of osteomyelitis is critical to prevent poor prognoses such as amputation and disability from excessive deep infection, osteonecrosis, and bone destruction associated with advanced diabetic foot osteomyelitis.[13–15]

Infectious arthritis and pyogenic arthritis are synonyms used interchangeably with septic arthritis. In the foot and ankle, it is usually associated with contiguous spread from ulceration and deep infection near joint spaces. In general, around the body septic arthritis and osteomyelitis is commonly due to hematogenous spread. However, in the foot/ankle it is by far most commonly associated with contiguous spread from skin ulceration or breakdown in patients with diabetes. Distribution of septic arthritis mirrors the distribution of pedal ulceration and osteomyelitis, with metatarsophalangeal joints and interphalangeal joints most commonly involved.[1,16]

CLINICAL FINDINGS

Swelling and erythema are general signs of osteomyelitis, but the clinical picture is similar to other conditions such as neuropathic osteoarthropathy, gout, and fracture.[17] Inflammatory signs may be absent in patients with advanced DM with peripheral neuropathy and ischemic vascular disease.[18] The presence of nonhealing diabetic foot ulcers should raise clinical suspicion of osteomyelitis and generally require further laboratory and imaging investigation.[19] Drainage from a skin ulcer can be a sign of underlying sinus tract and septic arthritis or osteomyelitis.[20] Systemic symptoms and signs such as fever, chills, and lethargy are less common in cases of diabetic pedal infection.[21] As a result patients with diabetes may present later with bone destruction, osteonecrosis, soft abscess, and systemic infection.[22]

DIAGNOSIS

Diagnosis of osteomyelitis requires a combination of physical exam findings, laboratory investigation, and imaging evaluation.

PHYSICAL EXAM

As noted above, physical exam findings are often nonspecific for osteomyelitis and can mimic other conditions. Nonhealing ulceration and wound drainage in a diabetic patient warrants further investigation. Size of the ulcer (ie, >3 cm² area) has been associated with osteomyelitis.[19,23,24] A probe-to-bone (PTB) test is also used to detect the deep extension of the ulcer; a positive test suggests underlying osteomyelitis (although with low positive predictive value), but a negative PTB test does not exclude bone infection.[18,25,26] A recent study shows that these clinical tests have low value for the diagnosis of deep infection.[27]

LABORATORY DIAGNOSIS

The laboratory findings in osteomyelitis and septic arthritis may be leukocytosis, and increased erythrocyte sedimentation rate (ESR) and C-reactive protein (CRP). WBC count can be normal in bone infection.[28] Elevated ESR and CRP combined with deep ulcer and sinus tract suggest osteomyelitis.[29] CRP is better than ESR in posttreatment follow-up of osteomyelitis because ESR takes up 3 months to return to the baseline while CRP takes 7 days to normalize.[29,30] Blood culture could be positive for the causative organism in the hematogenous spread of infection but usually negative in the contiguous spread of infection via diabetic foot ulcers.[31]

IMAGING

Osteomyelitis can be difficult to diagnose by physical exam and laboratory testing alone. Imaging provides sensitivity and specificity as well as structural analysis of the extent of infection and tissues involved.,[16,27,32,33] Neuropathic osteoarthropathy is a common complication of DM and can mimic osteomyelitis; in addition, as noted above other conditions including fracture and gout can clinically simulate deep infection.[24,34] Early diagnosis is important in order to initiate antibiotic treatment and to evaluate the need for surgical intervention.

Radiography

Radiography is the standard screening exam for questioned osteomyelitis, although infected bone is typically normal on radiographs in the first 2 weeks; it is available, inexpensive, and fast in comparison to other modalities. For suspected septic arthritis, effusion can be seen on radiographs in various joints.[35,36]

Radiographic findings of osteomyelitis include soft tissue swelling, soft tissue air or gas, obliteration of the fat planes, lucency or "rarefaction" of the affected bone, periosteal reaction, bone erosion or destruction, and intraosseous abscess with focal radiolucency and sclerotic margin (**Fig. 1**).[36–40] Ulcers can often be seen on radiographs if the view is tangential to the skin surface involved. Negative radiographs should not give a false sense of security; lack of radiographic findings does not exclude osteomyelitis and further imaging is required if clinically suspected.

Joint effusion is the early radiographic finding of septic arthritis but obviously joint effusion is seen in a wide variety of conditions; in addition, depending on the location of the joint, effusion may be difficult to detect. In septic arthritis, more advanced findings include periarticular osteopenia, diffuse narrowing joint space related to chondrolysis, articular erosion and destruction, periarticular bone sclerosis, and periostitis. Osteomyelitis and septic arthritis commonly coexist in patients with diabetes with foot ulcers and deep infection.

Ultrasound

Ultrasound evaluation is limited for diagnosis of deep musculoskeletal infection, since it lacks the capability of visualizing a large field of view and capability of assessing the intramedullary space. Nevertheless, US can be useful in answering specific questions such as whether there are fluid collections or joint effusions. Power Doppler can assess vascularity and has the potential to detect inflammation associated with infection (**Fig. 2**). Ultrasound is also commonly used to measure blood flow to the feet relative to the arms in patients with diabetes (ankle brachial index, ABI).

Computed Tomography

CT has better tissue contrast resolution than radiography but lower spatial resolution. It is superior for the detection of fluid collections, joint effusion, and osseous changes

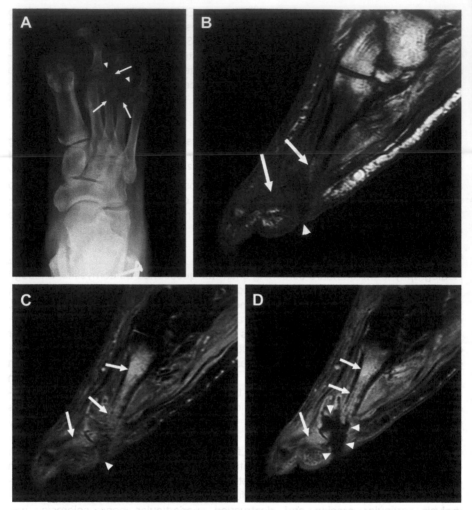

Fig. 1. 56-year-old male with diabetic foot infection. (A) AP radiograph of the foot shows the destruction of the third/fourth metatarsal bones and third proximal phalanx (*arrows*). Note air in the soft tissues (*arrowheads*) related to skin ulceration. (B) Sagittal T1-weighted MR image shows ulceration (*arrowhead*) at the plantar aspect of the fore-foot with the destruction of the third metatarsal and proximal phalanx (*arrows*) associated with the replacement of normal marrow signal. (C) Sagittal STIR image shows the plantar ulcer (*arrowhead*) with marrow edema (*arrows*) consistent with osteomye-litis. (D) Sagittal T1-weighted fat-suppressed post-contrast image shows marrow enhancement (*arrows*) consistent with osteomyelitis. Contrast outlines the destruction of the metatarsophalangeal joint (*arrowheads*) related to septic arthritis with rim-enhancement.

as described above for radiographs due to contrast resolution and cross-sectional nature (**Fig. 3**).[35,41–43] Classically CT has limited capability to detect bone marrow alteration associated with osteomyelitis; however, dual-energy CT techniques may allow the assessment of marrow infiltration and may be an option in the future for patients with a contraindication for MRI. Overall, standard CT offers similar sensitivity and

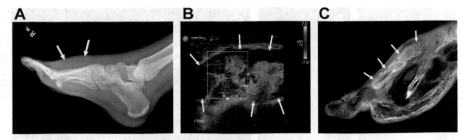

Fig. 2. Septic tenosynovitis in a 23-year-old female. (*A*) Lateral radiograph shows diffuse dorsal soft tissue swelling (*arrows*) at the forefoot. (*B*) Ultrasound of the dorsal foot with power Doppler shows marked extensor tenosynovitis with tendon sheath fluid (*arrows*) and hyperemia evident on Doppler. (*C*) Sagittal STIR MR image shows complex fluid within the extensor digitorum longus sheath (*arrows*) representing septic tenosynovitis.

specificity for osteomyelitis as radiography; negative CT examination does not exclude osteomyelitis or septic arthritis.[43,44] Intravenous contrast can provide additional benefit for the detection of abscess formation and other manifestations of soft tissue infection but must be balanced against potential for renal toxicity in patients with diabetes.

Magnetic Resonance Imaging

MRI is the modality of choice for diagnosis of septic arthritis and osteomyelitis (see **Fig. 1**). The average sensitivity and specificity of MRI for the diagnosis of osteomyelitis is 80% and 90%, respectively.[9,45] In terms of sequences, T1-weighted spin echo images have the highest specificity and fluid-sensitive sequences (ie, STIR and fat-suppressed T2w images) are more sensitive. The classic MR imaging appearance of osteomyelitis is marrow hyperintensity on fluid-sensitive sequences and replacement of fat signal (ie, low signal) on T1-weighted images (**Fig. 4**). Marrow edema itself is nonspecific and can be seen in neuropathic disease, fracture, gout, and many other conditions. However, if there is adjacent ulceration and cellulitis, sinus tract, or soft tissue abscess, any underlying bone marrow edema signal should be considered suspicious for osteomyelitis. In this regard, hyperemia is a very early finding in osteomyelitis on MRI, preceding marrow fat replacement on T1-weighted images. If T1 marrow signal is abnormal in the same area adjacent to soft tissue infection, confidence regarding the diagnosis of osteomyelitis is increased. Terms such as "reactive hyperemia" and "osteitis" should be avoided since they are nebulous, undefined, and unproven terms (**Fig. 5**). An impression characterizing a finding as "osteitis" does not give the clinical team clear guidance regarding treatment options. The term "reactive hyperemia" can give them a false sense of security, suggesting the lack of bone infection, and that less aggressive care is a reasonable option. Refer to a recent white paper from an expert panel of the Society of Skeletal Radiology for more information about the use of terms in musculoskeletal infection.[45]

Patients with diabetes characteristically have other confounding findings on MRI of the foot and ankle that can result in loss of diagnostic confidence. Vasculopathy and neuropathy result in diffuse soft tissue edema and muscle atrophy, with diffusely high T2 signal throughout the soft tissues (see **Fig. 4**). Neuropathic osteoarthropathy can occur anywhere in the foot and ankle but is most common at the midfoot and hindfoot, presenting with joint deformity (involvement at the midfoot and hindfoot results in a "rocker bottom" deformity). Neuropathic joints can show effusions and periarticular

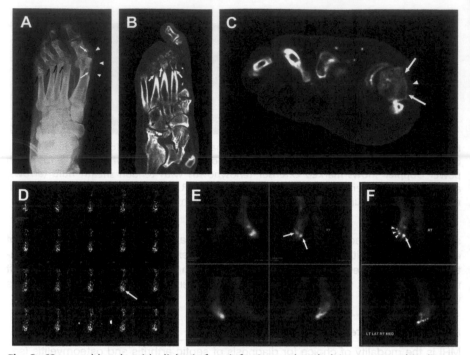

Fig. 3. 62-year-old male with diabetic foot infection and underlying neuropathic disease. (A) AP radiograph of the foot shows neuropathic osteoarthropathy at the second through fifth metatarsophalangeal joints, associated with fractures (*black arrows*) of the distal metatarsal bones. Ulceration (*arrowheads*) is present at the medial margin of the forefoot with erosion at the medial margin of the first metatarsal head and proximal phalanx (*white arrows*) consistent with osteomyelitis. (B) Axial CT image demonstrates the neuropathic fractures of the distal metatarsal bones (*arrows*). (C) Coronal CT image depicts the medial ulceration (*arrowhead*) and erosion of the first metatarsal head (*arrows*). (D) Tc-99m-MDP bone scan early flow images show rapid uptake of radiotracer throughout the forefoot (*arrow*). (E) Blood pool images from Tc-99m-MDP bone scan show coalescence of radiotracer in the region of the metatarsal heads (*arrows*). (F) Delayed images from Tc-99m-MDP bone scan show the concentration of tracer in the region of the first metatarsophalangeal joint (*arrow* - true positive for infection) and the fractured, neuropathic second through fifth metatarsal heads (*arrowheads* – false positive result).

edema or fluid collections, subchondral bone marrow edema, and cystic changes. Decreased sensation can also lead to stress fractures ("neuropathic fractures") which are accompanied by tremendous bone marrow and soft tissue edema. Superimposed noninfectious inflammatory conditions such as gout can also occur in patients with diabetes which can have a similar MR imaging appearance as infection.

As noted above patients with diabetes can develop ulceration over areas of bony prominence. This is seen on MRI as focal disruption of the otherwise continuous skin signal, often with heaped up margins. Underlying cellulitis occurs at the ulcer base, with the replacement of underlying subcutaneous fat signal on T1-weighted images, edema, and enhancement on fluid-sensitive and post-contrast sequences. Sinus tracts can arise from the ulcer and extend to joints, tendon sheaths, or bone. These can be found on MRI as a linear fluid signal with "tram track" enhancement. Soft tissue abscess is a more focal, rounded fluid collection (typically complex) with thick rim enhancement.[9,16,19,27,45,46]

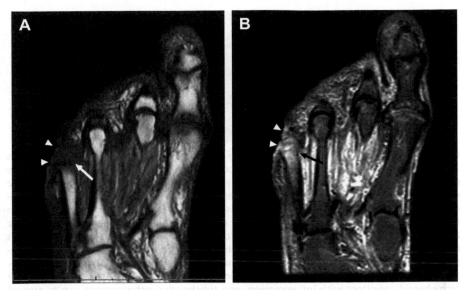

Fig. 4. Recurrent osteomyelitis in a 48-year-old diabetic female with the previous amputation of the third ray and the fifth toe. (*A*, *B*) Axial T1-weighted MR image (*A*) and axial fat-suppressed T2-weighted MR image (*B*) of the forefoot show ulceration (*arrowheads*) over the residual fifth ray. There is a confluent replacement of fat signal and bone marrow edema in the fifth metatarsal head (*arrows*) and distal shaft representing recurrent osteomyelitis. Diffuse soft tissue edema and muscle atrophy is characteristic of advanced diabetes mellitus.

Septic arthritis is seen on MRI as joint effusion, typically with signs of inflammation including pericapsular edema and marginal bone marrow edema at the "bare area" between the cartilage surface and capsule. The fluid is often complex, with thick rim enhancement on post-contrast images (**Fig. 6**).[1,10,16,43,47]

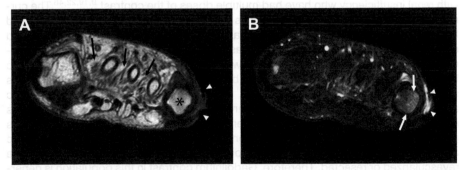

Fig. 5. Early osteomyelitis of the fifth metatarsal head in a 59-year-old male with diabetes mellitus and foot ulceration. (*A*) Sagittal STIR MR image shows complex fluid within the extensor digitorum longus sheath (*arrows*) representing septic tenosynovitis.. Note normal fat signal within the fifth metatarsal head (*asterisk*). (*B*) Coronal T2-weighted fat-suppressed image shows ulceration (*arrowheads*) with underlying soft tissue edema consistent with cellulitis at the ulcer base. Bone marrow edema is present at the lateral margin of the fifth metatarsal head (*arrows*) concerning for early osteomyelitis. Care should be taken to avoid nonspecific or unproven terms such as "reactive hyperemia" or "osteitis" in this scenario.

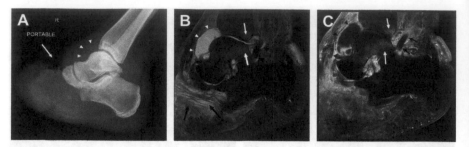

Fig. 6. Septic arthritis and tenosynovitis of the ankle in a 49-year-old female with diabetes and previous amputation with new dorsal ulceration. (*A*) Lateral radiograph of the ankle shows previous amputation at the hindfoot with deep ulceration dorsally (*arrow*). Note effusion in the ankle joint (*arrowheads*). (*B*) Sagittal STIR MR image shows diffuse phlegmonous changes (*black arrows*) in the anterior soft tissues, and a large ankle joint effusion (*white arrowheads*) with subchondral marrow edema (*white arrows*) consistent with septic arthritis and early osteomyelitis. Complex fluid is present along the flexor hallucis longus (FHL) tendon sheath (black *arrowheads*) which communicates with the ankle joint, representing the proximal spread of infection into the lower leg. (*C*) Sagittal T1-weighted fat-suppressed contrast-enhanced MR image shows rim enhancement of the ankle effusion (*black arrowheads*) consistent with inflammation, and subchondral enhancement (*white arrows*) consistent with septic arthritis/early osteomyelitis. Note enhancement/inflammation along the FHL sheath (*black arrows*).

Any structure passing through an area of infection can become secondarily involved. This is particularly true for tendons; if a tendon passes through an area of cellulitis and exhibits fluid or enhancement in the sheath more proximally or distally, there should be an increased concern for septic tenosynovitis (see **Fig. 6**). Tendon sheaths and fascial planes can be conduits for the proximal spread of infection to the ankle and lower leg, and any suspicion should be reported to the surgeon for potential exploration.[9,16,19,27,45,46]

Gadolinium contrast administration has been somewhat controversial in recent years due to the identification of nephrogenic systemic fibrosis (NSF) in patients with renal insufficiency who have had multiple doses of the contrast.[9,19,22,46] The current opinion for its use in pedal infection is as follows: (1) Creatinine clearance should be checked ahead of time, with the risks and benefits discussed with the patient and referring physician; (2) Gadolinium contrast is generally not necessary for the diagnosis of osteomyelitis, since most marrow edema will enhance (except for ischemic bone); and (3) Gadolinium contrast can be useful to assess patients for infectious soft tissue/joint disease (ie, sinus tracts, abscess, septic tenosynovitis, and septic arthritis), and to identify non-enhancing areas representing devitalization (**Fig. 7**). As mentioned above, the extent of involvement is very important information for patients going for surgical debridement/amputation. Identification of devitalized and ischemic areas is also important pre-operative information since those areas will need to be revascularized or resected. Therefore, Gadolinium contrast in this population is generally reserved for patients who are being evaluated for definitive surgery.

Other diagnostic techniques have recently been applied to the diagnosis of pedal infection, including diffusion-weighted imaging (DWI). A recent article by Chhabra and colleagues showed the utility of DWI for identifying abscess without the use of intravenous contrast (**Fig. 8**). PET-MRI fusion imaging is also being applied to pedal infection, and may be useful for the differentiation of osteomyelitis from other conditions such as neuropathic disease (**Fig. 9**).

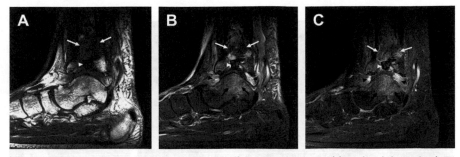

Fig. 7. Chronic osteomyelitis of the distal tibia in a 35-year-old male. (*A*) Sagittal T1-weighted MR image of the ankle shows diffuse replacement of normal marrow signal (*arrows*) consistent with osteomyelitis. A focus of black signal (*arrowhead*) is present near the ankle joint representing a sequestrum. (*B*) Sagittal STIR MR image shows corresponding heterogeneous edema signal within the distal tibia (*white arrows*), with low signal sequestrum (*white arrowhead*). There is a complex fluid signal in the ankle joint (*black arrowheads*) consistent with septic arthritis; there is corresponding marrow edema (*black arrows*) consistent with the spread of infection into the talus. (*C*) Sagittal T1-weighted fat-suppressed contrast-enhanced MR image shows heterogeneous enhancement within the distal tibia (*white arrows*), with a non-enhancing sequestrum (*white arrowhead*). There is diffuse enhancement of the ankle joint effusion (*black arrowheads*) and marrow enhancement (*black arrows*) confirming findings on the pre-contrast images of chronic osteomyelitis of the tibia, focal devitalization, septic arthritis, and spread to the talus.

Nuclear Medicine

Bone scan

Three-phase bone scan can be used for diagnosis of osteomyelitis, using Tc-99m methylene diphosphonate (MDP) which is taken up in areas of bone turnover (see **Fig. 3**). Dynamic flow (angiographic), blood pool, and delayed phases are obtained immediately, 5 minutes, and 3 hours post-tracer injection respectively. Late delayed phase could be obtained 8 and 24 hours posttracer injection. Osteomyelitis shows increased tracer uptake in all phases of the bone scan. Previous studies reported a high sensitivity of bone scintigraphy In osteomyelitis diagnosis; however, pedal disease in patients with diabetes creates particular challenges with macrovascular and microvascular disease leading to false negatives due to lack of uptake, and non-infectious conditions associated with hyperemia (ie, neuropathic osteoathropathy) leading to false positive readings (see **Fig. 3**).[48–51] Arthropathy, trauma, fractures, and malignancy characterized by high osteoblastic activity will all show increased uptake of tracer, lowering specificity.[50,51] Poor anatomical localization of the affected bone is a drawback of nuclear medicine scans in general. Delayed 8 hours and 24 hours are helpful in patient with DM and peripheral vascular disease which may demonstrate delayed bone uptake. Labeled WBC scan can provide increased specificity when correlated with a positive three-phase bone scan. Septic arthritis will show increased tracer uptake on all phases on both sides of the affected joint; however, septic arthritis and noninfectious inflammatory arthritis such as gout can not be differentiated.[51–53]

Bone Biopsy

In many circumstances, musculoskeletal infection is ultimately diagnosed via needle aspiration or bone biopsy. In patients with diabetes with cellulitis and ulceration, an underlying marrow signal abnormality should be considered suspicious for

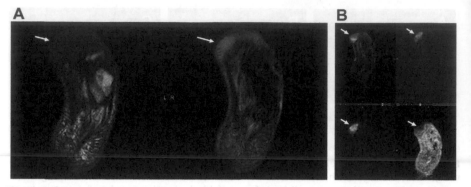

Fig. 8. Soft tissue abscess in a 61-year-old male. Diffusion-weighted imaging. (Figures courtesy Avneesh Chhabra MD FACR, UTSW Medical Center). (*A*) Axial T1-weighted MR image (*left*) and T2-weighted fat-suppressed MR image (*right*) of the forefoot show focal fluid-like signal (*arrows*) in the medial soft tissues. (*B*) Axial MR diffusion-weighted imaging (upper left to lower right, b50, b400, b800 dwi and adc map; adc = 0.79 x10-3 mm²/s) shows restricted diffusion (*arrows*) in the area of abscess.

osteomyelitis, as noted above. It is recommended that this concern should be communicated with the treating physician, who will initiate broad-spectrum antibiotic therapy and institute aggressive wound care, or plan definitive surgery. Follow-up may be performed after non-surgical treatment in 1 to 2 months; many individuals with aggressive conservative care heal their ulcer and the marrow finding resolves. Bone biopsy is generally not recommended because it creates an entryway for infection

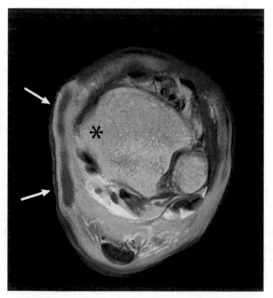

Fig. 9. Ulceration and cellulitis of the medial ankle in a 45-year-old female with diabetes. Axial PET-MRI (co-registration of PET data with T1-weighted MR image) shows increased metabolic activity (*arrows*) over the medial malleolus. No abnormal activity is present in the medial malleolus itself (*asterisk*).

that was not there initially; if the marrow finding did indeed represent "reactive hyper-emia" it is not recommended to create a portal for infection.

On the other hand, a joint effusion with concern for septic arthritis (clinically or by imaging) can and should be aspirated and sent for lab analysis at the first opportunity.

DIFFERENTIAL DIAGNOSIS
Neuropathic Osteoarthropathy

In acute neuropathic (Charcot) osteoarthropathy, the foot shows swelling, erythema, and warmth, which makes clinical differentiation from infection difficult. In chronic neuropathic disease and deformity there may be ulceration with drainage and concern for superimposed infection. On MR imaging, both osteomyelitis and neuropathic disease can show low T1 and high T2 marrow signal, making diagnosis more difficult. The presence of ulcer and/or sinus tract extending to a marrow abnormality, or adjacent soft tissue abscesses is also highly suspicious for infection. Location is important as well; abnormality away from a major joint, that is, at the base of the first or fifth metatarsal, dorsum/terminal tuft of the toes, calcaneus, and malleoli are the more common locations for osteomyelitis. The presence of subchondral cysts and bone debris, joint destruction/subluxation, and midfoot or hindfoot location all favor neuropathic osteoarthropathy.[9,23,24,46,54]

SUMMARY

Radiography is considered the first-line screening exam for clinically suspected osteomyelitis. However, additional evaluation is generally needed since negative radiographs do not exclude osteomyelitis, and positive radiographs require additional investigation for the extent of bone involvement and soft tissue disease. MRI is the definitive diagnostic exam with high sensitivity and specificity combined with excellent anatomic definition. Gadolinium contrast can be useful (if renal function allows) to define the extent of soft tissue disease and to detect areas of ischemia and devitalization for surgical planning. Bone marrow edema on fluid-sensitive images and low signal intensity on T1-weighted images in the presence of secondary MRI findings, including superficial ulcer, sinus tract, and cellulitis with or without abscess are typical findings of osteomyelitis. If there is a contraindication to MRI, three-phase bone scan could be used for diagnosis. Early diagnosis and treatment is essential.

CLINICS CARE POINTS

- Foot and ankle osteomyelitis occurs in patients with diabetes most commonly via contiguous spread from superficial ulcers and sinus tracts.

- MRI is the examination of choice for diagnosis of osteomyelitis and septic arthritis and for the accurate delineation of extent for proper medical or surgical treatment planning.

- Neuropathic osteoarthropathy and neuropathic fracture can clinically simulate osteomyelitis.

DISCLOSURE

The authors have nothing to disclose.

REFERENCES

1. Ledermann HP, Morrison WB, Schweitzer ME. MR image analysis of pedal osteomyelitis: Distribution, patterns of spread, and frequency of associated ulceration and septic arthritis. Radiology 2002;223(3):747–55.
2. Bamberger DM, Daus GP, Gerding DN. Osteomyelitis in the feet of diabetic patients. Long-term results, prognostic factors, and the role of antimicrobial and surgical therapy. Am J Med 1987;83(4):653–60.
3. Wald ER. Risk factors for osteomyelitis. Am J Med 1985;78(6B):206–12.
4. Schaper NC, Nabuurs-Franssen MH, Huijberts MSP. The diabetic foot: a global view. Diabetes Metab Res Rev 2000;16(Suppl 1).
5. Reiber GE, Smith DG, Vileikyte L, et al. Causal pathways for incident lower-extremity ulcers in patients with diabetes from two settings. Diabetes Care 1999;22(1):157–62.
6. Prompers L, Huijberts M, Apelqvist J, et al. High prevalence of ischaemia, infection and serious comorbidity in patients with diabetic foot disease in Europe. Baseline results from the Eurodiale study. Diabetologia 2007;50(1):18–25.
7. Ndosi M, Wright-Hughes A, Brown S, et al. Prognosis of the infected diabetic foot ulcer: a 12-month prospective observational study. Diabet Med 2018;35(1):78–88.
8. Ward JD. The Diabetic Foot: Soft Tissue and Bone Infection. Infect Dis Clin North Am 1990;4(3):409–32.
9. Schweitzer ME, Morrison WB. MR imaging of the diabetic foot. Radiol Clin North Am 2004;42(1):61–71.
10. Ledermann HP, Morrison WB, Schweitzer ME. Pedal abscesses in patients suspected of having pedal osteomyelitis: Analysis with MR imaging. Radiology 2002;224(3):649–55.
11. Faglia E, Clerici G, Caminiti M, et al. Influence of osteomyelitis location in the foot of diabetic patients with transtibial amputation. Foot Ankle Int 2013;34(2):222–7.
12. Winkler E, Schöni M, Krähenbühl N, et al. Foot Osteomyelitis Location and Rates of Primary or Secondary Major Amputations in Patients With Diabetes. Foot Ankle Int 2022;43(7):957–67.
13. Moon MS, Moon JL. Management of Osteomyelitis. J Orthop Surg 2000;8(2).
14. Parsons B, Strauss E. Surgical management of chronic osteomyelitis. Am J Surg 2004;188(1 SUPPL. 1):57–66.
15. Allende JMB, Sánchez MG, Caso AA. Osteomyelitis. Medicine (Spain) 2022;13(52):3041–9.
16. Karchevsky M, Schweitzer ME, Morrison WB, et al. MRI Findings of Septic Arthritis and Associated Osteomyelitis in Adults. Am J Roentgenol 2004;182(1):119–22.
17. Cook EA, Ashcraft JF. Clinical and Laboratory Diagnosis. undefined 2015;43(4):139–41.
18. Shone A, Burnside J, Chipchase S, et al. Probing the validity of the probe-to-bone test in the diagnosis of osteomyelitis of the foot in diabetes [1]. Diabetes Care 2006;29(4):945.
19. Morrison WB, Schweitzer ME, Batte WG, et al. Osteomyelitis of the foot: relative importance of primary and secondary MR imaging signs. Radiology 1998;207(3):625–32.
20. Chihara S, Segreti J. Osteomyelitis. Dis Mon 2010;56(1):6–31.
21. Giurato L, Meloni M, Izzo V, et al. Osteomyelitis in diabetic foot: A comprehensive overview. World J Diabetes 2017;8(4):135.

22. Ledermann HP, Schweitzer ME, Morrison WB. Nonenhancing Tissue on MR Imaging of Pedal Infection. AJR Am J Roentgenol 2012;178(1):215–22.
23. Ledermann HP, Morrison WB. Differential diagnosis of pedal osteomyelitis and diabetic neuroarthropathy: MR Imaging. Semin Muscoskel Radiol 2005;9(3): 272–83.
24. Marcus CD, Ladam-Marcus VJ, Leone J; et al. MR Imaging of Osteomyelitis and Neuropathic Osteoarthropathy in the Feet of Diabetics. Radiographics 1996; 16(6):1337–48.
25. Nardone DA. Probing to Bone in Infected Pedal Ulcers. JAMA 1995;274(11):869.
26. García Morales E, Lázaro-Martínez JL, Aragón-Sánchez FJ, et al. Inter-observer reproducibility of probing to bone in the diagnosis of diabetic foot osteomyelitis. Diabet Med 2011;28(10):1238–40.
27. Sax AJ, Halpern EJ, Zoga AC, et al. Predicting osteomyelitis in patients whose initial MRI demonstrated bone marrow edema without corresponding T1 signal marrow replacement. Skeletal Radiol 2020;49(8):1239–47.
28. Armstrong DG, Lavery LA, Sariaya M, et al. Leukocytosis is a poor indicator of acute osteomyelitis of the foot in diabetes mellitus. J Foot Ankle Surg 1996; 35(4):280–3.
29. Fleischer AE, Didyk AA, Woods JB, et al. Combined clinical and laboratory testing improves diagnostic accuracy for osteomyelitis in the diabetic foot. J Foot Ankle Surg 2009;48(1):39–46.
30. The diagnosis of diabetic foot osteomyelitis: examination findings and laboratory values - PubMed. Available at: https://pubmed.ncbi.nlm.nih.gov/19478702/. Accessed September 27, 2022.
31. Goergens ED, McEvoy A, Watson M, et al. Acute osteomyelitis and septic arthritis in children. J Paediatr Child Health 2005;41(1–2):59–62.
32. Osteomyelitis of the Foot and Ankle. Medical and Surgical Management. Switzerland: Springer International Publishing; 2015. p. 346.
33. Ahmadi ME, Morrison WB, Carrino JA, et al. Neuropathic arthropathy of the foot with and without superimposed osteomyelitis: MR imaging characteristics. Radiology 2006;238(2):622–31.
34. Johnson PW, Collins MS, Wenger DE. Diagnostic utility of T1-weighted MRI characteristics in evaluation of osteomyelitis of the foot. Am J Roentgenol 2009; 192(1):96–100.
35. Gold RH, Hawkins RA, Katz RD. Bacterial osteomyelitis: findings on plain radiography, CT, MR, and scintigraphy. AJR Am J Roentgenol 1991;157(2):365–70.
36. Shults DW, Hunter GC, McIntyre KE, et al. Value of radiographs and bone scans in determining the need for therapy in diabetic patients with foot ulcers. Am J Surg 1989;158(6):525–30.
37. Yuh WTC, Corson JD, Baraniewski HM, et al. Osteomyelitis of the foot in diabetic patients: evaluation with plain film, 99mTc-MDP bone scintigraphy, and MR imaging. AJR Am J Roentgenol 1989;152(4):795–800.
38. Yuh WTC, Corson JD, Baraniewski HM, et al. Osteomyelitis of the foot in diabetic patients: Evaluation with pain film, 99mTc-MDP bone scintigraphy, and MR imaging. Am J Roentgenol 1989;152(4):795–800.
39. Dinh MT, Abad CL, Safdar N. Diagnostic accuracy of the physical examination and imaging tests for osteomyelitis underlying diabetic foot ulcers: Meta-analysis. Clin Infect Dis 2008;47(4):519–27.
40. Newman LG, Waller J, Palestro CJ, et al. Unsuspected osteomyelitis in diabetic foot ulcers. Diagnosis and monitoring by leukocyte scanning with indium in 111 oxyquinoline. JAMA 1991;266(9):1246–51.

41. Lee YJ, Sadigh S, Mankad K, et al. The imaging of osteomyelitis. Quant Imag Med Surg 2016;6(2):184–98.
42. Aliabadi P, Nikpoor N, Alparslan L. Imaging of neuropathic arthropathy. Semin Muscoskel Radiol 2003;7(3):217–25.
43. Chandnani VP, Beltran J, Morris CS, et al. Acute experimental osteomyelitis and abscesses: detection with MR imaging versus CT. Radiology 1990;174(1):233–6.
44. Pineda C, Espinosa R, Pena A. Radiographic Imaging in Osteomyelitis: The Role of Plain Radiography, Computed Tomography, Ultrasonography, Magnetic Resonance Imaging, and Scintigraphy. Semin Plast Surg 2009;23(2):80.
45. Alaia EF, Chhabra A, Simpfendorfer CS, et al. MRI nomenclature for musculoskeletal infection. Skeletal Radiol 2021;50(12):2319–47.
46. McCarthy E, Morrison WB, Zoga AC. MR Imaging of the Diabetic Foot. Magn Reson Imag Clin N Am 2017;25(1):183–94.
47. Offiah AC. Acute osteomyelitis, septic arthritis and discitis: differences between neonates and older children. Eur J Radiol 2006;60(2):221–32.
48. Palestro CJ, Capriolli R, Love C, et al. Rapid diagnosis of pedal osteomyelitis in diabetics with a technetium-99m-labeled monoclonal antigranulocyte antibody. J Foot Ankle Surg 2003;42(1):9–14.
49. Schauwecker DS. The scintigraphic diagnosis of osteomyelitis. Am J Roentgenol 1992;158(1):9–18.
50. Palestro CJ, Love C. Nuclear Medicine and Diabetic Foot Infections. Semin Nucl Med 2009;39(1):52–65.
51. Harvey J, Cohen MM. Technetium-99-labeled leukocytes in diagnosing diabetic osteomyelitis in the foot. J Foot Ankle Surg 1997;36(3):209–14.
52. Love C, Palestro CJ. Nuclear medicine imaging of bone infections. Clin Radiol 2016;71(7):632–46.
53. Noriega-Álvarez E, Domínguez Gadea L, Orduña Diez MP, et al. Role of Nuclear Medicine in the diagnosis of musculoskeletal infection: a review. Rev Española Med Nucl Imagen Mol 2019;38(6):397–407.
54. Berendt AR, Lipsky B. Is this bone infected or not? Differentiating neuro-osteoarthropathy from osteomyelitis in the diabetic foot. Curr Diabetes Rep 2004;4(6):424–9.

Presurgical and Postsurgical MRI Evaluation of Osteochondral Lesions of the Foot and Ankle: A Primer

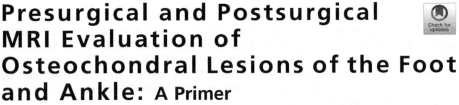

James J. Butler, MB BCh, Taylor Wingo, MD,
John G. Kennedy, MD, MCh, FFSEM, FRCS (Orth)*

KEYWORDS

- Ankle osteochondral lesion • MRI • T2-mapping MRI • dGEMRIC

KEY POINTS

- Osteochondral lesions of the ankle joint are difficult to manage due to the poor regenerative ability of the articular cartilage and thus, are typically managed surgically.
- Plain film radiographs are a useful diagnostic imaging modality but may miss up to 50% of OCLs. CT scans provide an excellent evaluation of the subchondral plate and bone but have a lower sensitivity than MRI at detecting ankle OCLs.
- MRI is the gold standard diagnostic imaging tool for ankle OCLs and is a crucial determinant in patient management.
- Post-operative morphologic MRIs provide a semi-quantitative analysis of the ankle OCL (MOCART scores) but mixed evidence exists regarding the association between MOCART scores and clinical outcomes.
- The gold standard diagnostic imaging tool for ankle OCLs is magnetic resonance imaging, which allows precise evaluation of the articular cartilage and assessment of the surrounding soft tissue structures. Post-operative morphologic MRI assessment via MOCART scores provide semi-quantitative analysis of the repair tissue, but mixed evidence exists regarding its association with post-operative outcomes. Post-operative biochemical MRIs allow assessment of the collagen network of the articular cartilage via T2-mapping and T2* mapping, and assessment of the articular glycosaminoglycan content via delayed gadolinium-enhanced MRI of cartilage (dGEMRIC), T1rho mapping and sodium imaging.

 Video content accompanies this article at http://www.foot.theclinics.com.

Foot and Ankle Division, Department of Orthopaedic Surgery, NYU Langone Health, 171 Delancey Street, 2nd Floor, New York City, NY 10002, USA
* Corresponding author.
E-mail address: john.kennedy@nyulangone.org

Foot Ankle Clin N Am 28 (2023) 603–617
https://doi.org/10.1016/j.fcl.2023.04.010
1083-7515/23/© 2023 Elsevier Inc. All rights reserved.

INTRODUCTION

Osteochondral lesions (OCLs) of the ankle joint represent a defect in the articular cartilage and/or subchondral bone of the talus or tibial plafond.[1] OCLs of the talus (OLT) represents the majority of OCLs at the tibiotalar joint, whereby 1 OLT accounts for 14 to 20 OCLs of the tibial plafond (OLTP).[1] These lesions are often preceded by trauma, and patients typically present with deep ankle pain, ankle swelling, reduced range of motion, and altered gait.[1]

Initial workup includes standard AP and lateral X-rays; however, these do not detect approximately 50% of OCLs.[2,3] More accurate assessment of the ankle cartilage can be obtained via computed tomography (CT) scans, MRI and in recent years, single photon emission computed tomography scans.[4] Although numerous classification systems based on various imaging modalities have been described for ankle OCLs (Tables 1–3),[2,3] they have a poor utility because management is primarily determined by lesion size, containment, cystic appearance, and earlier treatments.[4] MRI is a crucial diagnostic imaging tool that helps guide management. Smaller lesions (<100 mm^2 or <10 mm in diameter) can be treated with arthroscopic debridement, retrograde drilling, and augmentation with biological adjuvants.[4] Larger lesions (>100 mm^2 or >10 mm in diameter), uncontained lesions, cystic lesions, or lesions that have failed earlier operative intervention require more invasive procedures such as autologous osteochondral transfer (AOT).[5]

This review describes the most up-to-date evidence regarding the role of MRI in both preoperative and postoperative assessments of OCLs of the ankle joint. We also address limitations associated with each MRI technique.

PREOPERATIVE MRI FOR ANKLE OCLs—AN OVERVIEW

Early diagnosis of ankle OCLs is essential due to the relentless, progressive nature of this debilitating pathologic condition. Upon presentation to the emergency department following an acute ankle injury, patients initially undergo diagnostic imaging via plain film radiographs. However, radiographic imaging has a poor sensitivity for ankle OCLs because it fails to detect approximately 50% of OCLs.[2,3] Although CT provides excellent assessment of the underlying subchondral plate and bone, they seem to be limited in their assessment of the articular cartilage.[4] MRI seems to be the most optimal single diagnostic imaging tool for ankle OCLs. Verhagen and colleagues demonstrated that MRI had a sensitivity and specificity for OCLs of 96% with a positive predictive value of 89% and a negative predictive value of 99%, underpinning the essential role of MRIs in the assessment of potential ankle OCLs.[5]

To obtain an MRI of the ankle, patients are typically positioned supine in the MRI scanner with the ankle in a neutral position. Patients may also be placed in the prone position with the ankle in maximum plantarflexion so as to limit the number of movement artifacts and to significantly reduce the magic angle effect of the tendons that course around the ankle.[6] We use proton density fat-suppressed sequences in the

Table 1	
Berndt and Harty X-ray classification	
Stage 1	Small area of subchondral compression
Stage 2	Partial fragment detachment
Stage 3	Complete fragment detachment but not displaced
Stage 4	Displaced fragment

Table 2
Ferkel and Sgaglione CT classification

Stage 1	Cystic lesion within dome of talus with an intact roof on all view
Stage 2a	Cystic lesion communication to talar dome surface
Stage 2b	Open articular surface lesion with the overlying nondisplaced fragment
Stage 3	Nondisplaced lesion with lucency
Stage 4	Displaced fragment

sagittal, axial, and coronal planes. We do not use intravenous contrast for our imaging. At our institution, 3 Tesla (3-T) field strength is preferred over 1.5-T field strength given its higher sensitivity for detecting cartilaginous lesions due to its superior signal-to-noise ratio and spatial resolution. A cadaveric study by Barr and colleagues found that corIM fast-spine echo (FSE) 3-T had a higher sensitivity (64% vs 27%) and specificity (99% vs 97%) for detecting cartilage lesions at the ankle compared with corIM FSE 1.5-T.[7] The anatomy of the ankle joint and morphologic characteristics of the articular cartilage pose challenges in obtaining high-quality images. The relatively thin articular cartilage layer and curved surface of the talar dome may lead to partial volume effects, especially in the edge region.[8] To address the partial volume effects, we use higher field strengths that trade higher signal-to-noise ratio for increased spatial resolution.

Advancements in MRI technology have facilitated visualization of the ankle articular cartilage in high resolution. The emergence of three-dimensional (3-D) sequences has provided high-quality spatial resolution and secondary reconstruction possibilities in any spatial direction.[9] A major advantage of 3-D sequences is the use of isotropic voxels without any gap between each individual layer. Three-dimensional sequences tend to limit any partial volume effects precipitated by the curved surface of the talar dome. Furthermore, 3-D MRI sequences have been shown to have higher signal-to-noise ratio[10] or contrast-to-noise ratio[11] in the cartilage in comparison to fluid.

Critical Factors to Report

Lesion location

Raikin and colleagues devised a 3×3 grid system on MRI to evaluate the incidence of talar dome OCLs by both location and morphologic characteristics.[12] They found that 62% of lesions were located in the medial talar dome compared with 34% of lesions located in the lateral talar dome. The most frequently involved zone was the centromedial zone (53%). In addition, they found that medial lesions were deeper and had a larger surface area compared with lateral lesions.

Table 3
Hepple MRI classification

Stage 1	Articular cartilage edema
Stage 2a	Cartilage injury with underlying fracture and surrounding bony edema
Stage 2b	Stage 2a without surrounding bone edema
Stage 3	Detached but nondisplaced fragment
Stage 4	Displaced fragment
Stage 5	Subchondral cyst formation

The location of the lesion is often tied to the mechanism of injury. Lateral injuries are typically posttraumatic (94%).[4] They are shallow, oval-shaped lesions that are created due to shear stress across the talar dome. Medial lesions are most commonly post-traumatic but have a less frequently traumatic etiology compared with lateral lesions (64%). They are typically deeper cup-shaped lesions that occur due to torsional impaction and axial loading. A systematic review conducted by Butler and colleagues evaluated the topographic characteristics of OLTPs.[13] In total, 49.2% of OLTPs occurred on the medial aspect of the tibial plafond and were strongly associated with ankle sprains. In addition, there was a low rate of kissing lesions (17.1%; **Fig. 1**) suggesting that OLTPs stem from chronic, repetitive ankle trauma rather than high-energy impact injuries.

Lesion location has a significant impact on surgical management. Uncontained talar shoulder lesions require more extensive surgical intervention including AOT proced-ure.[14] In addition, when performing an AOT procedure, medial lesions will require a Chevron-type osteotomy of the medial malleolus compared with lateral lesions, which most commonly need a tibial trapezoidal osteotomy.[15] For posterolateral lesions, a tibial trapezoidal osteotomy may not provide adequate access to the lesion, thus, a fibular takedown is warranted.[15]

Lesion size

Lesion size is a critical factor that must be evaluated because it guides treatment stra-tegies. The lesions should be measured in 3 planes—anteroposterior, laterolateral, and depth. The diameter of the lesion is measured at its largest size on both the coronal and sagittal planes of the MRI with the measurement taken from the rim of the cartilage layer

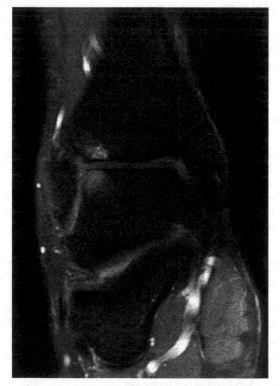

Fig. 1. A 12 × 8 mm talar OCL with associated "kissing" 7 × 8 mm cystic tibial plafond OCL.

to the base of the lesion. Due to the presence of bone marrow edema (BME), MRI can often overestimate the size of the lesion.[16] A retrospective review by Yasui and colleagues demonstrated that MRI overestimated OLT size in the coronal plane in 48.9% of cases and in the sagittal plane in 46.7% of cases compared with arthroscopic examination.[16] To obtain a more accurate assessment of the lesion size, our institution uses the ellipse formula: lesion area = coronal length × sagittal length × 0.79.

Smaller lesions (diameter <10 mm or area <100 mm^2) may be amenable to more conservative surgical techniques such as debridement, anterograde drilling and augmentation with biological adjuvants such as platelet rich plasma or concentrated bone marrow aspirate (CBMA). Ramponi and colleagues found that bone marrow stimulation (BMS) may not be suitable for patients with OLTs greater than 107.4 mm^2 and/or 10.2 mm in diameter.[17] Larger lesions (diameter >10 mm or area >100 mm^2) often require more extensive procedures such as AOT (**Fig. 2**).

Subchondral plate and bone

The subchondral plate and subchondral bone are vital components of the ankle joint. The subchondral bone is an integral structural scaffold, which bears 30% of the compressive load through the joint, in comparison to the 1% to 3% of load absorbed by the articular cartilage.[18] The subchondral bone communicates with the articular cartilage via cross-talk to facilitate a variety of signaling pathways.[17] Important features to report for the subchondral bone are subchondral BME, subchondral cysts, and sclerosis of the subchondral bone.

Subchondral BME is a common finding in patients with ankle OCLs. Asymptomatic, isolated subchondral BME with no significant damage to the articular cartilage may represent an occult cartilage injury that can often be managed nonoperatively, with interval MRIs to assess for the progression of the BME.[19,20] Symptomatic subchondral BME with associated cartilaginous injuries may reflect a progressive and/or unstable lesion that may warrant surgical intervention.

Damage to the articular cartilage may result in fracture of the cartilage and underlying subchondral plate. This facilitates penetration of surrounding fluid through the cartilage, subchondral plate, and into the subchondral bone. This buildup of intraosseous fluid can precipitate osteolysis, devascularization of the bone, and subchondral cyst formation. Both the length and depth of these cysts should be recorded. Cystic lesions are a poor prognostic indicator and often require more aggressive surgical management.

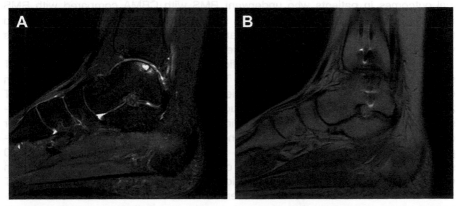

Fig. 2. (*A*) MRI demonstrating an 11 × 13 mm cystic talar OCL. (*B*) MRI 2 months postautologous osteochondral transplantation demonstrating incorporation of the graft into the talus.

Overtime, the intraosseous fluid pressure may reduce in certain patients with the concurrent commencement of bone remodeling. This may result in sclerotic changes to the subchondral bone.

Concomitant pathologic condition

MRI allows for assessment of not only of the native articular cartilage but of the surrounding soft tissue structures. Approximately 80% of patients with OCLs have an associated traumatic cause, the most common of which are ankle sprains.[4] MRI can assess the integrity of the lateral ligament complex and, depending on the degree of damage, concomitant surgical procedures such as a lateral ligament reconstruction can be carried out while simultaneously addressing the OCL. Other concomitant soft tissue pathologic conditions such as peroneal tendon tears, posterior tibial tendon insufficiency, and degenerative abnormalities can also be identified via MRI and an appropriate management plan can be devised.

POSTOPERATIVE MRI ASSESSMENT

At our institution, we obtain postoperative MRIs with T2-mapping for all patients with ankle OCLs regardless of the intervention at 6, 12, 24, and 36 months postop. Postoperative MRI is critical for assessment of not only the degree of healing of the cartilage lesion but also of the subchondral plate, subchondral bone, and surrounding soft tissue structures.

Numerous techniques have been described for postoperative assessment of ankle OCLs. These techniques can be broadly categorized as morphologic MRIs and biochemical MRIs.

Morphologic MRIs

The magnetic resonance observation of cartilage repair tissue (MOCART) score is a list of criteria to quantify MRI results following treatment of OCLs (**Table 4**).[21] It includes 9 distinct variables and provides a reproducible, standardized approach for the morphologic assessment of the repair tissue. This system has found to provide good interobserver reliability, with intraclass correlation coefficients (ICCs) of greater than 0.81 in 8 of the 9 criteria.[21]

The literature demonstrates conflicting evidence regarding the association between MOCART scores and clinical outcomes following surgical management of ankle OCLs. Hannon and colleagues found improved MOCART scores and subjective clinical outcomes in patients who underwent BMS with CBMA compared with BMS alone.[22] Conversely, a recent systematic review by Miglorini and colleagues found no correlation between MOCART scores and subjective clinical outcomes in patients who underwent surgical treatment of ankle and knee OCLs.

During the last number of years, modifications have been made to the MOCART scoring tool to address its deficiencies. Three additional scoring tools have been developed including MOCART 2.0, modified MOCART, and MOCART 3D. MOCART 2.0[23,24] made significant alterations including removing subchondral lamina adhesions, whereas adding other parameters including signal intensity for BME cysts, or osteonecrosis. Casari and colleagues found no correlation between American orthopaedic foot and ankle society (AOFAS) scores and postoperative MOCART 2.0 scores.[24] The modified MOCART score demonstrated inhomogeneous ICCs, with no strong correlation between arthroscopic findings for OLTs and modified MOCART scores.[25] The 3D MOCART score has been shown to correlate with numerous histologic scoring systems but concerns have been raised regarding susceptibility artifacts in the repair tissue.[26]

Table 4
Magnetic resonance observation of cartilage repair tissue

Category	Item	Points
Defect fill	Subchondral bone exposed	0
	Incomplete <50%	5
	Incomplete >50%	10
	Complete	20
	Hypertrophy	15
Cartilage interface	Complete	15
	Demarcating border visible	10
	Defect visible <50%	5
	Defect visible >50%	0
Surface	Surface intact	10
	Surface damaged <50% of depth	5
	Surface damaged >50% of depth	0
Adhesions	Absent	5
	Yes	0
Structure	Homogeneous	5
	Inhomogeneous or cleft formation	0
Signal intensity	Normal	30
	Nearly normal	10
	Abnormal	0
Subchondral lamina	Intact	5
	Not intact	0
	Intact	5
Subchondral bone	Granulation tissue, cyst, sclerosis	0
	Absent	5
Effusion	Yes	0
Total		100

BIOCHEMICAL MRIs

Biochemical MRIs evaluates 2 key components of the articular cartilage, namely the collagen fiber network and the cartilaginous glycosaminoglycan content.[27] These constituents play vital roles in maintaining cartilage homeostasis. In the setting of ankle OCLs, there is disorganization of the collagen fiber network, altered water content, and decreased glycosaminoglycan content.[27] T2-mapping and T2* mapping have been used to assess the collagen network and water content for ankle chondral injuries.[28,29] Delayed gadolinium-enhanced MRI of cartilage (dGEMRIC),[30] T1rho mapping[31] and sodium imaging[32] have been used for the assessment of the glycosaminoglycan content in the ankle joint.

T2-Mapping Evaluation

T2 mapping is a readily available imaging technique that can detect early cartilage degradation before morphologic cartilage degeneration in a multi-echo spin-echo (MESE) sequence.[28] It facilitates examination of the integrity, orientation, and concentration of the collagen fiber network, and the cartilaginous water content without the need for injection of intravenous contrast medium. The organization of the collagen network may reflect the quality of the repair tissue.[28]

At our institution, the senior musculoskeletal radiologist performs T2 mapping using a 16-cm field of view and 512 × 512 matrix (0.3 mm pixel spacing). T2 relaxation values for the repaired cartilage tissue are measured using a linear least squares estimation (FuncTool 3.1; GE Healthcare, Chicago, IL, USA) in a 0.2 mm² region of interest in the deep and superficial articular repair cartilage. T2 relaxation values of the adjacent, healthy cartilage are measured using the same 0.2 mm² region of interest.

T2-mapping MRI correlates with clinical outcomes following surgical intervention of ankle OCLs. A study by Rizzo and colleagues used T2-mapping MRIs with a 1.5 T MRI scanner for patients with OLTs who underwent BMS compared with bone marrow–derived cell transplantation (BMDCT).[28] The BMS cohort had significantly more fibro-cartilage tissue and less hyaline-like tissue compared with the BMDCT cohort, as evidenced by discrepancy in T2 values.[28] In addition, Kubosch and colleagues followed 17 patients with OLTs and found similar T2 relaxation times between the site of the implanted autologous matrix-induced chondrogenesis (AMIC) and the surrounding native cartilage, suggesting that AMIC may produce hyaline-like cartilage.[33] Finally, Ross and colleagues found no significant difference in superficial and deep relaxation times between patients who underwent primary AOT compared with patients who underwent AOT following an earlier failed BMS procedure.[34]

T2-mapping MRIs are a validated, extensively studied, essential component of our postoperative protocol, especially in patients who have undergone AOT procedure. It facilitates detailed analysis of not only the repair tissue but can assess the degree of integration of the donor graft to the recipient cartilage in patients who have undergone AOT procedure (**Fig. 3**).

T2* Mapping

T2* mapping is an alternative biochemical MRI technique that assesses the collagen fiber network and water content of the articular cartilage. T2* mapping is obtained with multigradient recalled echo (GRE) sequences, unlike T2 mapping, which uses

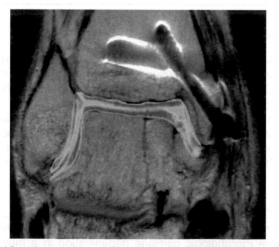

Fig. 3. A 32-year-old patient underwent autologous osteochondral for a medial talar OCL. T2-mapping MRI at 12 months demonstrates good integration of the graft into the recipient talar dome, with restoration of the radius of curvature and color stratification comparable to the native cartilage. *From* Kennedy JG, Murawski CD. The Treatment of Osteochondral Lesions of the Talus with Autologous Osteochondral Transplantation and Bone Marrow Aspirate Concentrate: Surgical Technique. Cartilage. 2011;2(4):327-336. https://doi.org/10.1177/1947603511400726.

MESE sequences. GRE sequences allow for shorter acquisition times, can obtain 3D measurements, and have lower specific absorption rate limits. Although, theoretically, T2 mapping and T2* mapping should yield similar relaxation times for tissues with short relaxation times such as cartilage. Welsch and colleagues found that T2* mapping recorded lower relaxation times for T2* mapping, likely due to the GRE sequence in T2* mapping. However, numerous limitations with T2* mapping exist. First, the interference between the articular cartilage and underlying subchondral bone may yield extremely low T2* values secondary to macroscopic susceptibility effects, creating an illusion of zonal variation that is not present.[28] As a result, zonal variational analysis should not be conducted with T2*-mapping MRIs. Furthermore, the use of postoperative T2* mapping should be avoided in patients with hardware present near the ankle joint due to the high rate of susceptibility artifacts from the metalwork, which greatly reduces the quality of the T2* measurements.

Hu and colleagues evaluated the talar articular cartilage using T2*-mapping MRIs on a 3-T scanner between patients with chronic lateral ankle instability (CLAI) and patients without CLAI.35 The authors demonstrated significantly higher T2* values of the total talar cartilage in the CLAI cohort compared with the healthy cohort. In addition, Schutz and colleagues conducted a study on the articular ankle cartilage of 22 ultralong distance endurance athletes using T2* mapping with a mobile 1.5 T MRI scanner.[36] Although morphologic imaging suggested stable cartilage conditions throughout the event, T2*-mapping MRI demonstrated an increase in T2* values during the initial 2000 km with a subsequent decrease in T2* values for the following 2500 km of the race, illustrating the subtle biochemical changes of the ankle joint that can be detected by T2*-mapping MRIs.

The senior author refrains from using T2* mapping in patients following treatment of their ankle OCLs due to the lack of available clinical evidence supporting its use together with the issues surrounding susceptibility artifacts, particularly in patients who have undergone AOT procedures.

Delayed Gadolinium-Enhanced MRI of Cartilage

DGEMRIC is an MRI technique that was first described in 2001 to evaluate the concentration of cartilaginous glycosaminoglycans via T1 relaxation times. The technique involves intravenous administration of the negatively charged gadolinium diethylene-triamine penta-acetic acid (Gd-DTPA2−), which distributes an inversely proportional manner to the negatively charged glycosaminoglycans in the cartilage.[37] In patients with healthy cartilage, the negatively charged glycosaminoglycans oppose the diffusion of Gd-DTPA2−. In patients with damaged cartilage, more Gd-DTPA2− accumulates in the joint due to the decrease in glycosaminoglycans, leading to a reduction in the T1 relaxation times in a concentration-dependent manner. Typically, the MRI is taken 45 minutes after intravenous administration of the Gd-DTPA2− to allow sufficient penetration of the articular cartilage. To further improve the distribution of the contrast in the articular cartilage, patients must perform ankle ranging exercises.

There have been a limited number of studies examining the use of dGEMRIC for ankle OCLs. Rehnitz and colleagues compared dGEMRIC and T2-mapping MRIs in patients with OLTs who either underwent conservative treatment or microfracture.[30] The authors found that dGEMRIC was superior to T2 mapping at identifying clinical outcomes for patients treated for OLTs but is inferior at discriminating repair tissue from native, hyaline cartilage. Furthermore, Wiewiorski and colleagues used dGEMRIC postoperatively in a cohort of 23 patients with OLTs treated with AMIC, reporting significantly lower GAG levels in the repair tissue compared with the native, healthy cartilage tissue.[38]

At our institution, we limit the use of dGEMRIC to assess postoperative OLTs due to the hindrances of the intravenous contrast administration together with the mandatory time interval before quantitative T1 mapping.

T1-Rho Imaging

T1-rho mapping MRIs are a promising imaging modality that can quantify and assess the cartilaginous GAG content and collagen fiber network of the articular cartilage. T1-rho describes the spin-lattice relaxation time in the rotating frame[39] using SE, FSE, echo planar imaging, spiral imaging, or 3D GE sequences, without the need for intravenous contrast injections.[40] This technique evaluates low-frequency interactions between cartilaginous hydrogen and macromolecules in free water. An in vitro bovine study by Akella and colleagues found that approximately 50% depletion of cartilaginous proteoglycans resulted in significant increases in T1-rho values, demonstrating that T1-rho functions as a proxy for measuring cartilaginous proteoglycan content.[41]

In recent years, numerous clinical studies have been conducted examining the role of T1-rho MRI imaging of the articular ankle cartilage but few clinical studies have been conducted on patients with ankle OCLs. Horiuchi and colleagues used both T1-rho and T2-mapping MRIs to examine the ankle cartilage of ballet dancers.[31] They found that male dancers displayed cartilage with greater thickness and volume compared with the female cohort. Interestingly, the authors found that segmented cartilage on T1-rho imaging demonstrated greater thickness and volume in comparison to T2-mapping. Furthermore, 2 recent studies by Lange and colleagues and Song and colleagues demonstrated increased talar T1-rho values in patients with CLAI suggesting that T1-rho relaxation may be a sensitive marker for CLAI-induced early stage ankle osteoarthritis.[42,43] Finally, Haraguchi and colleagues examined 9 patients who underwent AOT procedure at 2 year follow-up for ankle OCLs using T1-rho 3-T MRIs.[44] The authors found a gradual improvement in proteoglycan content between the donor tissue and native surrounding cartilage via T1-rho values but a discrepancy in T1-rho values still existed at 2-year follow-up suggesting that the cartilage reparation process may be slower than previously thought.

Sodium Imaging

Another method for evaluating the glycosaminoglycans of the articular cartilage is via sodium imaging.[32] The underlying principle of this technique is that negatively charged sites on glycosaminoglycans are equalized by the positively charged sodium molecules.[32] In addition to relaxation times, sodium-corrected signal intensities (cSI) or absolute sodium concentrations can be calculated in the articular cartilage to assess the cartilage glycosaminoglycan content. Although this is a promising MRI technique, there is a litany of drawbacks. First, special multinuclear hardware is required because the concentration of sodium ions is greatly lower than hydrogen ions.[27] In addition, the sensitivity of sodium ions in cartilage is approximately 4000 times lower compared with that of hydrogen ions, resulting in low space-to-noise ratio, which limits spatial resolution of images acquired at 3-T.[27] To achieve a spatial resolution, higher field strengths must be used.

Sodium imaging was first used to evaluate knee articular cartilage and has demonstrated good ICCs and correlation with dGEMRIC.[27] However, a paucity of data exists describing the role of sodium imaging for the ankle joint. Zbyn and colleagues performed sodium MRIs at 7-T on 5 ankle cadaver specimens, 9 asymptomatic healthy volunteers, 6 patients with ankle OCLs treated with microfracture and 6 patients with ankle OCLs treated with matrix-associated autologous chondrocyte transplantation (MACT).[32] The authors demonstrated significantly lower cSI in the healthy cohort compared with the postoperative patients, reflecting lower cartilaginous glycosaminoglycan content. No significant difference in cSI was observed between the microfracture cohort and the MACT cohort suggesting that microfracture and MACT lead to comparable quality of repair tissue. The lack of clinical evidence and extensive limitations with this technique limit its widespread use in the clinical setting.

FUTURE DEVELOPMENTS

Arthroscopic examination is the gold standard method of assessment of OCL size. However, arthroscopy comes with the risk of iatrogenic cartilage injury,[45] soft tissue trauma, risks associated with sedation under general anesthesia and significant costs associated with using the arthroscopic suite in the operating room.

In-office needle arthroscopy (IONA) is an emerging, novel, arthroscopic system that has gained in popularity during the last number of years.[46] IONA uses a 2.2-mm arthroscope and sheath with an optic chip at the tip of arthroscope (400 × 400 pixel image resolution) to visualize, evaluate, and treat the diseased joint.[46] Various surgical instruments such as burrs, graspers, biters, shavers, resectors, scissors, and probes can be used with the IONA technology to treat the specific pathologic condition. IONA procedures are conducted at the beside with the patient fully conscious using wide awake local anesthetic no tourniquet. The minimal soft tissue trauma permits rapid return to daily and sporting activities. IONA has been used to treat various pathologic conditions including anteromedial ankle impingement, peroneal tendon disorders, posterior ankle impingement, anterior talofibular ligament augmentation with suture tape, posterior tibial tendon dysfunction, hallux rigidus, and Achilles tendinosis.

The precise indications for IONA for the treatment of ankle OCLs is yet to be defined, primarily due to its recent reemergence in the last number of years. IONA offers both diagnostic (Video 1) and therapeutic strategies for managing ankle OCLs. In patients with smaller OCLs identified on preprocedure MRIs, IONA can provide an accurate assessment of the lesion size, inspection of the entire ankle joint to identify any concomitant pathologic condition and can be used to directly treat smaller OCLs.

SUMMARY

MRI is a vital diagnostic tool that guides management of ankle OCLs. MRI not only facilitates extensive evaluation of the OCL but also permits assessment of the underlying subchondral bone and surrounding soft tissue structures. Postoperative assessment via T2-mapping MRI allows for a biochemical analysis of the collagen fiber network and cartilaginous water content of the repair tissue, and can evaluate the integration of the donor graft into the recipient talar cartilage. Promising biochemical MRI techniques include T2*-mapping, dGEMRIC, T1-rho mapping, and sodium imaging; however, further research is warranted to determine their role in the management of ankle OCLs. Although the MOCART scoring tool facilitates a semiquantitative analysis of the repair tissue, there is conflicting clinical evidence supporting its use. IONA provides both accurate assessment of the size of the OCL and potential soft tissue pathology, and treatment of the lesion but its exact role is yet to be determined.

CLINICS CARE POINTS

- There is mixed evidence regarding the efficacy of the MOCART score for postoperative assessment of ankle OCL repair tissue.

- T2-mapping MRIs is a validated technique for biochemical assessment of the repair articular cartilage.
- The main drawback of dGEMRIC is the requirement of intravenous contrast administration together with the mandatory time interval before quantitative T1 mapping.
- Limited evidence exists for other biochemical techniques including T2* mapping, T1-rho mapping and sodium imaging.
- IONA provides accurate assessment of the size of the OCL and potential soft tissue pathology, and treatment of the lesion OCL.

DISCLOSURE

The authors report the following potential conflicts of interest or sources of funding: J.G. Kennedy is a consultant to Arteriocyte Industries (Isto *Biologics) and Arthrex Inc, and receives support from Ohnell Family Foundation, United States and Mr and Mrs Michael J. Levitt. J.G. Kennedy reports as a board or committee member for the American Orthopaedic Foot and Ankle Society, European Society of Sports Traumatology, Knee Surgery and Arthroscopy, Ankle and Foot Associates, and International Society for Cartilage Repair of the Ankle.

ACKNOWLEDGEMENTS

We would like to thank Dr. Mohammad T. Azam and Dr. Nathan W. Jia for their expertise and assistance throughout all aspects of our study and for their help in writing the manuscript.

SUPPLEMENTARY DATA

Supplementary data related to this article can be found online at https://doi.org/10.1016/j.fcl.2023.04.010.

REFERENCES

1. Elias I, Raikin SM, Schweitzer ME, et al. Osteochondral lesions of the distal tibial plafond: localization and morphologic characteristics with an anatomical grid. Foot Ankle Int 2009;30(6):524–9.
2. Loomer R, Fisher C, Lloyd-Smith R, et al. Osteochondral lesions of the talus. Am J Sports Med 1993;21(1):13–9.
3. Hepple S, Winson IG, Glew D. Osteochondral lesions of the talus: a revised classification. Foot Ankle Int 1999;20(12):789–93.
4. Looze CA, Capo J, Ryan MK, et al. Evaluation and Management of Osteochondral Lesions of the Talus. Cartilage 2017;8(1):19–30.
5. Verhagen RaW, Maas M, Dijkgraaf MGW, et al. Prospective study on diagnostic strategies in osteochondral lesions of the talus. Is MRI superior to helical CT? J Bone Joint Surg Br 2005;87(1):41–6.
6. Mengiardi B, Pfirrmann CWA, Schöttle PB, et al. Magic angle effect in MR imaging of ankle tendons: influence of foot positioning on prevalence and site in asymptomatic subjects and cadaveric tendons. Eur Radiol 2006;16(10):2197–206.
7. Barr C, Bauer JS, Malfair D, et al. MR imaging of the ankle at 3 Tesla and 1.5 Tesla: protocol optimization and application to cartilage, ligament and tendon pathology in cadaver specimens. Eur Radiol 2007;17(6):1518–28.

8. Millington SA, Li B, Tang J, et al. Quantitative and topographical evaluation of ankle articular cartilage using high resolution MRI. J Orthop Res 2007;25(2):143–51.

9. Weber MA, Wünnemann F, Jungmann PM, et al. Modern Cartilage Imaging of the Ankle. Röfo 2017;189(10):945–56.

10. Stevens KJ, Busse RF, Han E, et al. Ankle: isotropic MR imaging with 3D-FSE-cube–initial experience in healthy volunteers. Radiology 2008;249(3):1026–33.

11. Notohamiprodjo M, Kuschel B, Horng A, et al. 3D-MRI of the ankle with optimized 3D-SPACE. Invest Radiol 2012;47(4):231–9.

12. Elias I, Zoga AC, Morrison WB, et al. Osteochondral lesions of the talus: localization and morphologic data from 424 patients using a novel anatomical grid scheme. Foot Ankle Int 2007;28(2):154–61.

13. Butler JJ, Mercer NP, Hurley ET, et al. Osteochondral Lesions of the Tibial Plafond: A Systematic Review. Orthop J Sports Med 2021;9(11). 23259671211029210.

14. Hurley ET, Murawski CD, Paul J, et al. Osteochondral Autograft: Proceedings of the International Consensus Meeting on Cartilage Repair of the Ankle. Foot Ankle Int 2018;39(1_suppl):28S–34S.

15. Kennedy JG, Murawski CD. The Treatment of Osteochondral Lesions of the Talus with Autologous Osteochondral Transplantation and Bone Marrow Aspirate Concentrate: Surgical Technique. Cartilage 2011;2(4):327–36.

16. Yasui Y, Hannon CP, Fraser EJ, et al. Lesion Size Measured on MRI Does Not Accurately Reflect Arthroscopic Measurement in Talar Osteochondral Lesions. Orthop J Sports Med 2019;7(2). 2325967118825261.

17. Ramponi L, Yasui Y, Murawski CD, et al. Lesion Size Is a Predictor of Clinical Outcomes After Bone Marrow Stimulation for Osteochondral Lesions of the Talus: A Systematic Review. Am J Sports Med 2017;45(7):1698–705.

18. Shimozono Y, Hurley ET, Yasui Y, et al. The Presence and Degree of Bone Marrow Edema Influence Midterm Clinical Outcomes After Microfracture for Osteochondral Lesions of the Talus. Am J Sports Med 2018;46(10):2503–8.

19. The Treatment of Osteochondral Lesions of the Talus with Autologous Osteochondral Transplantation and Bone Marrow Aspirate Concentrate: Surgical Technique - PubMed. Available at: https://pubmed.ncbi.nlm.nih.gov/26069591/. Accessed November 21, 2022.

20. Marlovits S, Striessnig G, Resinger CT, et al. Definition of pertinent parameters for the evaluation of articular cartilage repair tissue with high-resolution magnetic resonance imaging. Eur J Radiol 2004;52(3):310–9.

21. Marlovits S, Singer P, Zeller P, et al. Magnetic resonance observation of cartilage repair tissue (MOCART) for the evaluation of autologous chondrocyte transplantation: determination of interobserver variability and correlation to clinical outcome after 2 years. Eur J Radiol 2006;57(1):16–23.

22. Hannon CP, Ross KA, Murawski CD, et al. Arthroscopic Bone Marrow Stimulation and Concentrated Bone Marrow Aspirate for Osteochondral Lesions of the Talus: A Case-Control Study of Functional and Magnetic Resonance Observation of Cartilage Repair Tissue Outcomes. Arthroscopy 2016;32(2):339–47.

23. Schreiner MM, Raudner M, Marlovits S, et al. The MOCART (Magnetic Resonance Observation of Cartilage Repair Tissue) 2.0 Knee Score and Atlas. Cartilage 2021;13(1_suppl):571S–87S.

24. Casari FA, Germann C, Weigelt L, et al. The Role of Magnetic Resonance Imaging in Autologous Matrix-Induced Chondrogenesis for Osteochondral Lesions of the Talus: Analyzing MOCART 1 and 2.0. Cartilage 2021;13(1_suppl):639S–45S.

25. Lee KT, Lee YK, Young KW, et al. Factors influencing result of autologous chondrocyte implantation in osteochondral lesion of the talus using second look arthroscopy. Scand J Med Sci Sports 2012;22(4):510–5.

26. Goebel L, Zurakowski D, Müller A, et al. 2D and 3D MOCART scoring systems assessed by 9.4 T high-field MRI correlate with elementary and complex histological scoring systems in a translational model of osteochondral repair. Osteoarthritis Cartilage 2014;22(10):1386–95.

27. Schreiner MM, Mlynarik V, Zbýň Š, et al. New Technology in Imaging Cartilage of the Ankle. Cartilage 2017;8(1):31–41.

28. Rizzo G, Cristoforetti A, Marinetti A, et al. Quantitative MRI T2 Mapping is Able to Assess Tissue Quality After Reparative and Regenerative Treatments of Osteochondral Lesions of the Talus. J Magn Reson Imaging 2021;54(5):1572–82.

29. Welsch GH, Mamisch TC, Hughes T, et al. In vivo biochemical 7.0 Tesla magnetic resonance: preliminary results of dGEMRIC, zonal T2, and T2* mapping of articular cartilage. Invest Radiol 2008;43(9):619–26.

30. Rehnitz C, Kuni B, Wuennemann F, et al. Delayed gadolinium-enhanced MRI of cartilage (dGEMRIC) and T2 mapping of talar osteochondral lesions: Indicators of clinical outcomes. J Magn Reson Imaging 2017;46(6):1601–10.

31. Horiuchi S, Yu HJ, Luk A, et al. T1rho and T2 mapping of ankle cartilage of female and male ballet dancers. Acta Radiol 2020;61(10):1365–76.

32. Zbýň S, Stelzeneder D, Welsch GH, et al. Evaluation of native hyaline cartilage and repair tissue after two cartilage repair surgery techniques with 23Na MR imaging at 7 T: initial experience. Osteoarthritis Cartilage 2012;20(8):837–45.

33. Kubosch EJ, Erdle B, Izadpanah K, et al. Clinical outcome and T2 assessment following autologous matrix-induced chondrogenesis in osteochondral lesions of the talus. Int Orthop 2016;40(1):65–71.

34. Ross AW, Murawski CD, Fraser EJ, et al. Autologous Osteochondral Transplantation for Osteochondral Lesions of the Talus: Does Previous Bone Marrow Stimulation Negatively Affect Clinical Outcome? Arthroscopy 2016;32(7):1377–83.

35. Hu Y, Zhang Y, Li Q, et al. Magnetic Resonance Imaging T2* Mapping of the Talar Dome and Subtalar Joint Cartilage 3 Years After Anterior Talofibular Ligament Repair or Reconstruction in Chronic Lateral Ankle Instability. Am J Sports Med 2021;49(3):737–46.

36. Schütz UHW, Ellermann J, Schoss D, et al. Biochemical cartilage alteration and unexpected signal recovery in T2* mapping observed in ankle joints with mobile MRI during a transcontinental multistage footrace over 4486 km. Osteoarthritis Cartilage 2014;22(11):1840–50.

37. Maroudas A, Muir H, Wingham J. The correlation of fixed negative charge with glycosaminoglycan content of human articular cartilage. Biochim Biophys Acta 1969;177(3):492–500.

38. Wiewiorski M, Miska M, Kretzschmar M, et al. Delayed gadolinium-enhanced MRI of cartilage of the ankle joint: results after autologous matrix-induced chondrogenesis (AMIC)-aided reconstruction of osteochondral lesions of the talus. Clin Radiol 2013;68(10):1031–8.

39. Sepponen RE, Pohjonen JA, Sipponen JT, et al. A method for T1 rho imaging. J Comput Assist Tomogr 1985;9(6):1007–11.

40. Witschey WRT, Borthakur A, Elliott MA, et al. T1rho-prepared balanced gradient echo for rapid 3D T1rho MRI. J Magn Reson Imaging 2008;28(3):744–54.

41. Akella SV, Regatte RR, Gougoutas AJ, et al. Proteoglycan-induced changes in T1rho-relaxation of articular cartilage at 4T. Magn Reson Med 2001;46(3):419–23.

42. Lange T, Sturm L, Jungmann PM, et al. Biomechanical Effects of Chronic Ankle Instability on the Talar Cartilage Matrix: The Value of T1ρ Relaxation Mapping Without and With Mechanical Loading. J Magn Reson Imaging 2022. https://doi.org/10.1002/jmri.28267.

43. Song K, Pietrosimone B, Tennant JN, et al. Talar and Subtalar T1ρ Relaxation Times in Limbs with and without Chronic Ankle Instability. Cartilage 2021; 13(1_suppl):1402S–10S.

44. Haraguchi N, Ota K, Nishida N, et al. T1ρ mapping of articular cartilage grafts after autologous osteochondral transplantation for osteochondral lesions of the talus: A longitudinal evaluation. J Magn Reson Imaging 2018;48(2):398–403.

45. Harris JD, Brand JC, Rossi MJ, et al. Iatrogenic Arthroscopic Cartilage Injury: Arthroscrapes Result From Iatrogenesis Imperfecta. Arthroscopy 2020;36(8):2041–2.

46. Colasanti CA, Mercer NP, Garcia JV, et al. In-Office Needle Arthroscopy for the Treatment of Anterior Ankle Impingement Yields High Patient Satisfaction With High Rates of Return to Work and Sport. Arthroscopy 2022;38(4):1302–11.

Weight-Bearing Computed Tomography of the Foot and Ankle—What to Measure?

Jaeyoung Kim, MD[a], Scott Ellis, MD[a], John A. Carrino, MD, MPH[b],*

KEYWORDS

- Weight-bearing • CT • Ankle arthritis • Syndesmosis
- Progressive collapsing foot deformity • Hallux valgus • Lisfranc

KEY POINTS

- Weight-bearing computed tomography (WBCT) provides the visualization of foot and ankle deformities in 3 dimensions (3D) and during loaded conditions.
- With 3D spatial analysis of WBCT images, subtle ligamentous injuries of the foot and ankle may be detected earlier.
- The clinical significance of WBCT findings must be determined.

INTRODUCTION

Ten years have passed since the use of weight-bearing computed tomography (WBCT) in foot and ankle surgery began. Since its implementation, WBCT has greatly enhanced our knowledge of foot and ankle pathologic condition that was not readily visualized with conventional approaches or in an unloaded state. We now have a powerful tool for evaluating and treating foot and ankle patients that overcomes the inaccuracies and biases of conventional methods, such as bone superimposition, x-ray beam projection angle, and magnification problems.[1–3]

Understanding what is now being assessed and evaluated in the foot and ankle field using WBCT would be beneficial for analyzing its past and future applications. Earlier research evaluated whether WBCT produces measurements of the same value as conventional weight-bearing radiographs, including Meary's angle and talonavicular coverage angle (TNC), in progressive collapsing foot deformity (PCFD).[4] In addition, attempts have been made to define the normal WBCT range of these parameters to determine whether WBCT measurements may be used to diagnose diseases and

[a] Foot and Ankle Service, Hospital for Special Surgery, 532 East 72nd Street, New York, NY, USA;
[b] Department of Radiology, Hospital for Special Surgery, 535 East 70th Street, New York, NY, USA
* Corresponding author.
E-mail address: carrinoj@hss.edu

Foot Ankle Clin N Am 28 (2023) 619–640
https://doi.org/10.1016/j.fcl.2023.04.004
1083-7515/23/© 2023 Elsevier Inc. All rights reserved.

foot.theclinics.com

assess postoperative improvement.[5,6] Then, metrics that cannot be measured using standard methods were specified, such as the inclination of the subtalar joint surface in weight-bearing condition, subluxation of the talocalcaneal joint, and axial plane rotation of the bones within or across the ankle and subtalar joints.[7–13] Recently, digitally reconstructed radiographs (DRR) have been created and implemented,[14] revealing the potential for WBCT to one day replace conventional weight-bearing radiographs (**Fig. 1**), thereby reducing radiation risk and expense and maximizing patient convenience. Foot and ankle pathologic conditions can now be examined in greater detail due to the numerous possibilities afforded by three-dimensional (3D) image processing from WBCT images. The combination of distance mapping, joint coverage mapping, joint volume measurements, and biometric analysis exemplifies the future direction and field use of WBCT.[15–19]

This article aims to provide an overview of what is measured in WBCT images of the foot and ankle by introducing common WBCT applications and parameters examined in the field, including ankle arthritis, syndesmosis injuries, PCFD, hallux valgus (HV) deformity, and Lisfranc injuries.

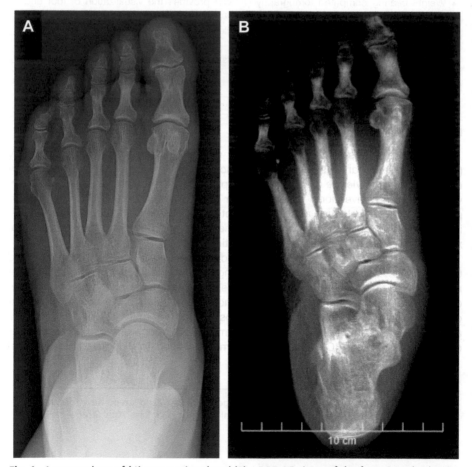

Fig. 1. A comparison of (*A*) conventional and (*B*) a DRR AP views of the foot. Standard radiographic parameters that have previously been assessed using conventional radiography can be measured using a DRR.

ANKLE ARTHRITIS
Assessing the Tibiotalar Joint

With the conventional approach, ankle arthritis has been classified based on the coronal (varus or valgus) or sagittal (anterior or posterior) alignment of the joint, without knowledge of the axial plane orientation. Access to the axial plane alignment of bones within the ankle and subtalar joint may be one of the most significant advantages of adopting WBCT to evaluate ankle arthritis, and this is likely to have a substantial impact on our current practice.

Two studies have measured abnormal talar rotation in the axial plane in varus ankle arthritis.[8,20] In a WBCT investigation of patients with varus ankle arthritis, Kim and colleagues measured the talus rotation ratio to examine abnormal internal rotation of the talus and found that patients with varus ankle arthritis had a higher talus rotation ratio than the control group.[8] Moreover, the talus rotation ratio showed a higher incidence in patients with severe varus ankle osteoarthritis when compared with the moderate group, indicating that the talus is abnormally internally rotated in varus ankle arthritis. This implies that ankle arthritis must be understood in 3D planes, meaning that the varus ankle arthritis observed on the plain anteroposterior (AP) radiograph is a combination of deformities from 2 additional planes, including rotation of the talus in the axial plane (**Fig. 2**). Song and colleagues confirmed, using simulated WBCT, that the talus was abnormally internally rotated in mild-to-severe varus ankle arthritis, as Kim and colleagues described.[20] In addition, they demonstrated that a supramalleolar osteotomy decreases the talar rotation ratio compared with the preoperative value, showing that it corrects the abnormal internal rotation of the talus in the axial plane.

Occasionally, WBCT findings may differ from our understanding of ankle arthritis based on conventional radiography (**Fig. 3**). In a WBCT assessment of medial gutter arthritis, Kim and colleagues examined the ratio of medial gutter width to tibial plafond-talar dome space in coronal images of the anterior, middle, and posterior ankle (ratio <0.5: medial gutter narrowing).[21] Importantly, the anterior part of the ankle joint demonstrated valgus talar tilt rather than varus, contradicting our existing belief that medial gutter arthritis is a feature of a subtype of varus ankle arthritis (Takakura 3a, **Fig. 4**).[22] This implies that the surgical treatment of ankle arthritis, particularly from a joint preservation standpoint, would change significantly following the application of WBCT to assess ankle arthritis.

Hindfoot Alignment and Subtalar Joint Compensation

Assessing the hindfoot alignment and the behavior of the subtalar joint is a crucial aspect of ankle arthritis treatment. It has been reported that the projection angle of the beam and the orientation of the foot at the time of the hindfoot alignment view is taken have a substantial effect on the results,[3] making WBCT particularly useful for evaluating hindfoot alignment. Krahenbühl and colleagues evaluated the subtalar vertical angle (SVA) in coronal images in WBCT images in order to compare subtalar joint orientation between varus, valgus ankle arthritis, and healthy controls.[23] Subtalar joint orientation was more varus in patients with varus ankle arthritis and more valgus in patients with valgus ankle arthritis, suggesting that subtalar joint orientation may be a risk factor for developing ankle arthritis.

Compensation of the subtalar joint is another area of interest for surgeons treating ankle arthritis; yet two-dimensional (2D) radiographs limit their ability to elucidate it (accurate assessment has been impeded by superposition caused by the midfoot). With the WBCT, subtalar orientation and hindfoot alignment can be identified more precisely. Krahenbühl and colleagues measured the SVA to evaluate subtalar joint

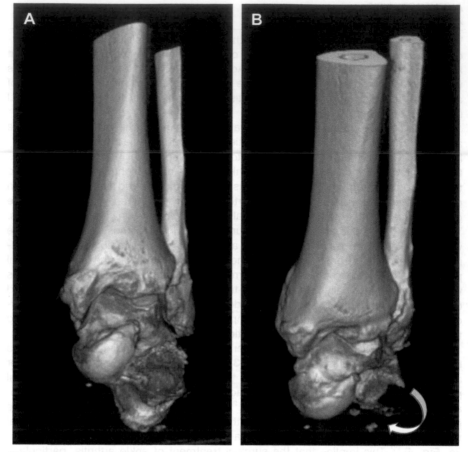

Fig. 2. Three-dimensional weight-bearing computed tomography images of a patient with varus ankle arthritis exhibiting varus tilt of the talus (*A*) and internal rotation of the talus within the mortise (*B*). The *arrow* in figure (*B*) indicates varus tilt and simultaneous internal rotation of the talus.

orientation in reference to the ground, subtalar inclination angle (SIA) to evaluate infra-malleolar compensation for supramalleolar abnormalities, and inftal-subtal angle to evaluate talar configuration.[24] They found that that varus ankle arthritis was associated with increased SIA compared with control patients, suggesting compensation, whereas valgus ankle arthritis was not associated with compensation. Importantly, when comparing different stages of ankle osteoarthritis, no significant differences in subtalar joint alignment were observed, which contradicted the findings of an earlier study on subtalar joint compensation using plain radiography.[25] Using WBCT images, Kang and colleagues determined the SIA and calcaneal inclination angle (CIA) to evaluate coronal plane subtalar compensation in varus ankle arthritis.[10] They found that subtalar compensation in the coronal plane was decreased in advanced varus ankle arthritis (Takakura 3b and 4) and concluded that talar tilt angles greater than 9.5° have a significant likelihood of a noncompensated heel. In addition, they proposed that the coronal plane calcaneal axis at the medial border of the calcaneus (CIA) more correctly represents the coronal orientation of the calcaneus than the SIA.

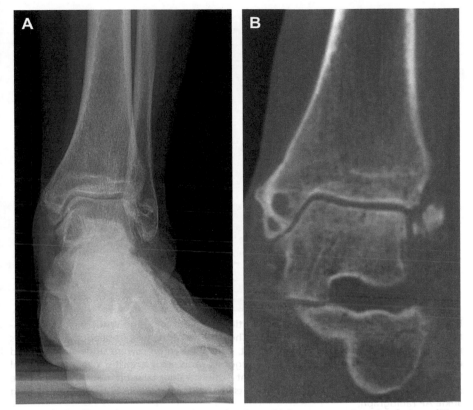

Fig. 3. WBCT allows for a more precise evaluation of joint space under a loaded condition. Weight-bearing ankle AP views do not clearly demonstrate narrowing of the medial gutter (*A*); however, WBCT coronal images (*B*) demonstrate medial gutter narrowing and cyst formation in the tibia, indicating that the severity of ankle arthritis is more advanced than what is seen on plain radiographs.

Burssens and colleagues described changes of subtalar joint alignment after supramalleolar osteotomy.[26] They created 3D bone models from WBCT images and identified the principal axes of the tibia, talus, and calcaneus and the angle between those bones was measured before and after supramalleolar osteotomy. The study demonstrated the talocalcaneal alignment changes in the sagittal and axial plane, not the coronal plane after SMO, and this indicates that WBCT can be used to elucidate subtalar joint behavior in ankle arthritis, which was impeded in 2D approach.

Despite the aforementioned research, it remains unclear whether subtalar joint compensation actually exists or whether malalignment of the hindfoot is the cause of the tibiotalar deformity. The authors think that either WBCT analysis of ankle arthritis in conjunction with lower limb alignment or the use of WBCT that extends to the hip joint will better reveal subtalar joint behavior in ankle arthritis and provide an answer to the question.

Surgical Planning in Total Ankle Arthroplasty

Literature describing the use of WBCT in total ankle arthroplasty (TAA) is also increasing. Computed tomography (CT)-derived patient-specific instrumentation (PSI) alignment guides enable more accurate bone cuts in TAA, which is one of the

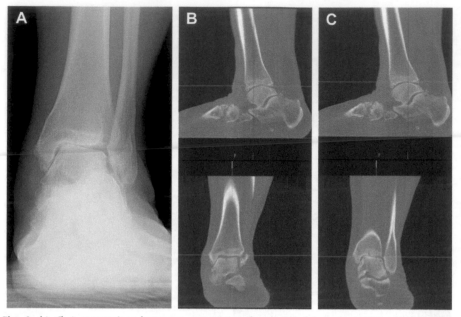

Fig. 4. (A–C) A comparison between conventional radiographic and WBCT images in a patient with medial gutter ankle arthritis. (A) The AP view of the weight-bearing ankle shows medial gutter narrowing and varus talar tilt, which, based on current understanding and conventional radiographic interpretation, suggests varus ankle arthritis. WBCT scans reveal that the anterior aspect of the tibiotalar joint exhibits valgus talar tilt, not varus, while the posterior aspect of the tibiotalar joint exhibits varus tilt, comparable to the weight-bearing ankle AP radiograph.

most prominent clinical applications of the WBCT in TAA.[27,28] Currently, this is performed by PSI reports generated based on the mechanical axis or anatomic axis and has shown to provide appropriate implant size and satisfactory tibial and talar component alignment postoperatively (**Fig. 5**). The cutting guides are produced based on the patient's specific anatomy, which has the potential to improve ankle alignment and prosthesis insertion reproducibility. Now that WBCT can be performed up to the level of the knee or higher, it can be utilized to determine, among other factors, the anatomic and mechanical axis of the tibia, allowing the surgeon to place an implant with precise alignment.

Preoperative WBCT is also helpful for the evaluation of procedures that are performed in conjunction with TAA, including calcaneal osteotomies, ligament reconstruction, and adjacent joint arthrodesis. de Cesar Netto and colleagues investigated preoperative WBCT generated foot and ankle offset (FAO) and found that preoperative FAO can predict the number of bony realignment procedures necessary for TAA implantation to obtain a plantigrade foot.[29] Compared with patients with varus malalignment, patients with valgus malalignment required a greater number of bony realignment procedures.

Authors think that the application of WBCT in TAA will significantly improve the early detection of cyst formation or lucency if it can be incorporated into follow-up imaging (**Fig. 6**). WBCT can reveal whether there is a correlation between the weight-bearing alignment following TAA and the formation and location of cysts.[30] This will also explain more about the causes of nonrevision reoperation, which is still reported at

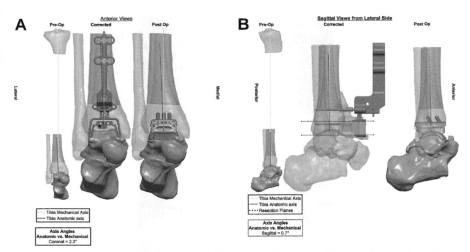

Fig. 5. The perioperative weight-bearing computed tomography can be used to design patient-specific instruments with customized cutting guides. The patient-specific report offers the coronal (*A*) and sagittal (*B*) analysis, enabling the surgeon to make preoperative modifications to the implant size and position.

a relatively high rate after TAA.[31,32] For instance, malpositioning of the component relative to the malleolus in the axial plane would be clearly depicted by WBCT scans, which would explain the cause of pain and ultimately aid in determining the optimal axial plane position of the implant.

What to Measure in Ankle Arthritis?

- Axial rotation of the talus (Talar rotation ratio)
- Medial joint space narrowing (ratio of medial gutter width to tibial plafond-talar dome space)
- Subtalar joint and hindfoot alignment
- Surgical planning in TAA (patient specific instrumentation)

SYNDESMOSIS INJURY

Injuries that disrupt the syndesmosis continue to be difficult to identify using conventional radiography,[33] particularly if the injury is subtle, because the measurements are substantially influenced by the beam projection angle to the ankle joint. Nonweight-bearing CT scans have been used to diagnose syndesmotic injuries[34] but their inherent inability to examine the syndesmosis under load or stress limits their utility. WBCT scans have been used to assess motion and explore biomechanics in the distal tibiofibular syndesmosis due to the imaging capabilities under load and rotational stress. Using WBCT scans, Lepojarvi and colleagues assessed syndesmosis motion under weight-bearing conditions in healthy control patients.[35] They measured sagittal translation of the fibula, anterior or posterior widths of the distal tibiofibular syndesmosis, tibiofibular clear space, and rotation of the fibula. In 88% of subjects, the fibula was anterior to the tibial incisura when the ankle was neutrally loaded. When the ankle was rotated, the incisura underwent physiologic motion as the fibula moves, on average, 1.5 mm anterior-posterior and 3° in external rotation. Burssens and colleagues compared the WBCT scan measurements of syndesmotic injury patients (high ankle sprain, n = 12) with those of contralateral uninjured ankle. The lateral malleolus in the incisura shifted 1.6 mm in the mediolateral direction and 0.9 mm in the AP

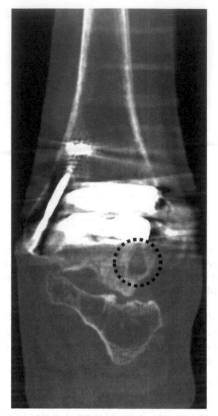

Fig. 6. A postoperative weight-bearing computed tomography coronal image of a patient who developed a cyst (*dotted circle*) following TAA.

direction in patients with syndesmotic injuries.[36] In addition, a 4.7° increase in external rotation was seen in the injured side.

In contrast, Hamard and colleagues found that WBCT scans were less effective than standard nonweight-bearing multiplanar CT scans at differentiating pathologic syndesmotic injury after measuring 10 metrics in both modalities.[37] The findings of this study indicated that conventional nonweight-bearing multiplanar CT scans were more reliable at detecting syndesmotic injury. They attributed this observation to the physiologic widening of the distal tibiofibular syndesmosis under load-bearing conditions.

The aforementioned studies relied on linear measurements in plain radiographs or single-plane CT scans, in which the distance or angle between the fibula and tibia varies based on the measurement level and is therefore vulnerable to bias. The introduction of recent research utilizing syndesmotic area or volumetric assessment has proven higher accuracy in detecting syndesmosis injury (**Figs. 7** and **8**).[15,16] Bhimani and colleagues evaluated the area of the syndesmosis in axial serial images and determined the volume of the syndesmosis in patients with syndesmotic instability and the control group (**Fig. 9**).[16] On the injured side, the 3D volumetric measurement of the syndesmosis joint was significantly greater than on the uninjured side, whereas in the control group, there was no difference between sides. Moreover, they found that 3D volumetric measurements are more sensitive than 2D measurements for identifying syndesmosis instability. They also determined the optimal level at which to measure the volume of the

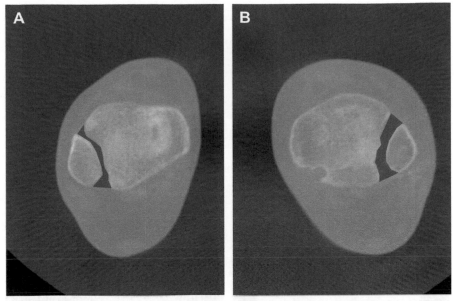

Fig. 7. Bilateral axial weight-bearing computed tomography scans reveal an enlarged syndesmosis area (colored in red) and irregularity of the distal tibiofibular joint surface on the injured side (B) compared with the contralateral uninjured side (A).

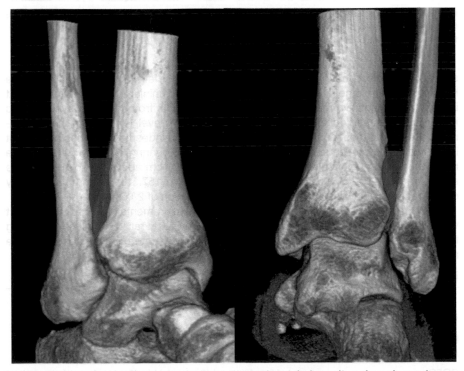

Fig. 8. After measuring the syndesmosis area in each axial plane slice, the volumetric measurement can be constructed and measured (red-colored area).

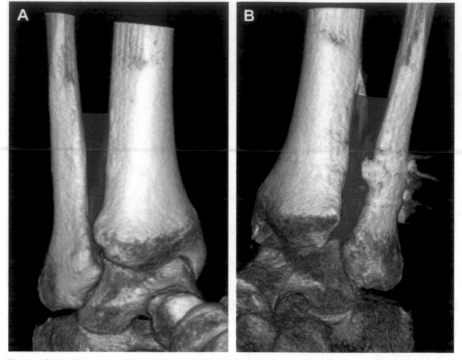

Fig. 9. Three-dimensionally reconstructed ankle images of the uninjured contralateral side (*A*) and malreduced syndesmosis (*B*), demonstrating a wider space (red-colored area) between the tibia and fibula.

syndesmosis, discovering that from the tibial plafond to a level 5 cm proximally had the highest relative volumetric ratio between the injured and uninjured sides, indicating that it is the most sensitive method for distinguishing stable from unstable syndesmotic injury. Raheman and colleagues discovered in a recent level 1 study that the syndesmotic area is the most accurate metric for assessing syndesmotic injuries because it increased in the presence of instability during weight-bearing.[38] They found that the mean area of the tibiofibular syndesmosis measured 1 cm above the joint line in the axial plane was 112.5 ± 6.7 mm², which increased to 157.5 ± 6.7 mm² after injury compared with uninjured ankles by a standard deviation of 29.5 mm².

Due to relatively large intersubject variation in measurements and less intrasubject variation, WBCT diagnosis of syndesmosis has previously relied on bilateral imaging for comparison. More data in the future would allow us to determine the absolute value and type of measurement required to detect syndesmosis injury using WBCT.

What to Measure in Syndesmosis Injuries?

- Syndesmosis area
- Syndesmosis volume

PROGRESSIVE COLLAPSING FOOT DEFORMITY
Foot and Ankle Offset

PCFD encompasses a spectrum of forefoot, midfoot, and hindfoot deformities, each of which requires a 3D assessment to determine the most appropriate treatment.[39] In addition, understanding in 3 dimensions is essential for comprehending the impact of specific procedures on a particular bone, its adjacent joints, and the foot tripod as a whole. FAO is probably one of the comprehensive approaches to understanding the deformity and the consequences of surgical treatment. It is shown as a percentage of the distance between the orthogonal projection of the center of the ankle (talus) and the center of the foot, divided by the AP foot length (**Fig. 10**).[18] It can be measured semi-automatically using a dedicated software where 3 weight-bearing points that correspond to the foot tripod and the center of the ankle are manually marked by an observer. FAO corresponded with 2D measurements of hindfoot alignment and forefoot abduction and varus, enabling a general assessment of the PCFD deformity.[40] Day and colleagues evaluated the FAO before and after PCFD reconstruction and found a significant decrease following surgical treatments, indicating that PCFD correction aids in reducing the biomechanical imbalance between the ankle, foot, and hindfoot.[41]

Subtalar Joint Anatomy and Alignment

As described in an earlier study utilizing a simulated WBCT by Ananthakrisnan and colleagues, talocalcaneal (subtalar) joint subluxation is regarded as a primary

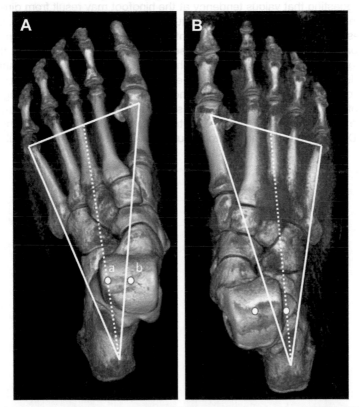

Fig. 10. Three-dimensionally reconstructed foot images of patients with PCFD demonstrating the calculation method for FAO. The solid lines represent the orthogonal projection of the foot tripod onto the foot, whereas the dashed line represents the length of the foot. The FAO is the percentage of the distance between the orthogonal projection of the highest and most central point of the talus (*B*) and the center of the foot (*A*) divided by the foot length (*dashed line*). The patient (*B*) with more advanced PCFD showed a greater FAO than PCFD that was relatively mild (*A*).

pathomechanism in PCFD.[42] They constructed a 3D model of the talocalcaneal articulation and found that there is a marked subluxation of the talocalcaneal joint in patients with PCFD, with only 68% of the posterior facet of the calcaneus in contact with the talus, compared with 92% in control patients. This was later supported by a study by de Cesar Netto and colleagues, which described the uncoverage percentage and incongruence angle of the middle facet of the subtalar joint.[12] They compared patients with PCFD and controls and reported that patients in the case group had higher values of uncoverage and incongruence than those in the control group (**Fig. 11**).

Other studies also focused on elucidating whether there are differences in the anatomy of the talus and calcaneus at the subtalar joint that eventually lead to collapsing of the foot. Probasco and colleagues evaluated the inclination of the subtalar joint's posterior facet between patients with PCFD and controls.[43] They measured inftal-suptal angle (between the superior and inferior margins of the talus), inftal-hor angle (between the inferior margin of the talus and the horizontal plane of the floor), and the inftal-supcal angle (between the inferior margin of the talus and the superior margin of the calcaneus). They found that the inftal-hor and inftal-suptal angles were significantly greater in patients with PCFD, whereas the inftal-supcal angle did not differ significantly, suggesting that valgus tendency at the hindfoot may result from direct valgus angulation of the bones and not from valgus obliquity at the joint surfaces. Cody and colleagues compared the inftal-hor and inftal-suptal angles with the common radiographic parameters used for PCFD assessment.[7] They reported that the inftal-suptal angle was positively correlated with the TNC, Meary's angle, calcaneal pitch, medial column height, and hindfoot alignment measurements, with Meary's angle having the strongest correlation. In addition, they found that the inftal-suptal angle greater than 17° of valgus can be used to distinguish patients with PCFD from control patients due to the higher prevalence of inftal-suptal angles greater than 17° among patients with PCFD compared with the control group. Although these studies on subtalar joint

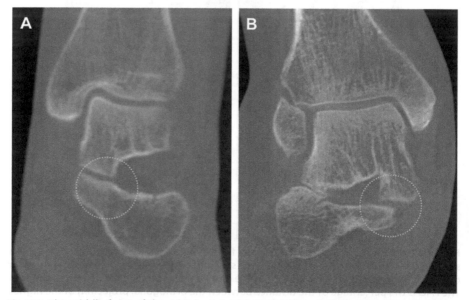

Fig. 11. The middle facet of the subtalar joint (*dotted yellow circle*) in a healthy control patient (*A*) and a PCFD (*B*). Greater subluxation of the middle facet of the subtalar joint is observed in patients with PCFD.

anatomy indicated susceptibility of patients with PCFD to developing the deformity, they did not account for the rotational profile of the talus and calcaneus when evaluating angles in WBCT slices. Therefore, future studies with a 3D bone model are required to determine whether the aforementioned angles are truly different from controls. Moreover, greater valgus angulation of the posterior facet in patients with PCFD and their surgical outcomes with anterior or posterior calcaneal osteotomies must be studied to determine whether valgus obliquity of the subtalar joint is indicative of subtalar fusion to prevent further subluxation at the subtalar joint even after calcaneal osteotomies.

Lateral Impingement

Lateral impingement either at the sinus tarsi or at calcaneofibular (also known as subfibular) area is thought to be an extra-articular consequence of talocalcaneal subluxation (**Fig. 12**). These findings have been associated with patient symptoms as well as the degree of deformity or peritalar ligament failure.[44–47] Malicky and colleagues used simulated WBCT images from patients with PCFD and assessed for lateral impingements.[46] They found that sinus tarsi impingement was observed in 92% of the CT scans and calcaneofibular impingement in 66%, which differed markedly from control patients, who had rates of 5% and 0%, respectively. Jeng and colleagues also assessed sinus tarsi and calcaneofibular impingements using WBCT scans.[47] For the lateral talocalcaneal distance, the measurement of the shortest distance between the tip of the lateral process of the talus and the superior margin of the calcaneus was performed in the sagittal plane. For the calcaneofibular distance, the shortest distance to the lateral margin of the posterior facet of the calcaneus was measured in the coronal image, visualizing the most inferior end of the fibula. However, Kim and colleagues measured the talocalcaneal distance at the sinus tarsi and calcaneofibular

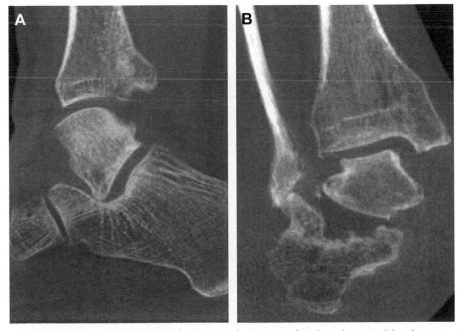

Fig. 12. Weight-bearing computed tomography images showing sinus tarsi impingement (A) and calcaneofibular impingement (B).

distance in WBCT images and assessed their correlations to common radiographic parameters to sought radiographic cutoff value predicting lateral impingements verified in WBCT.[45] They found that TNC was most associated with the talocalcaneal distance at the sinus tarsi and hindfoot moment arm (HMA) was most associated with the calcaneofibular distance. Moreover, a TNC of 41.2° had a 100% positive predictive value for predicting sinus tarsi impingement, whereas an HMA threshold of 38.1 mm had a 100% positive predictive value. This study has an important clinical implication because the majority of foot and ankle centers still do not have access to WBCT, which provides findings crucial to the new PCFD staging system as well as establishment of the surgical plan.

Distance Mapping Technique

Despite using WBCT images, measurements for determining subluxation of the joint have been performed in 1D or 2D, which can result in a large degree of variability between observers, particularly when deciding which slice to measure. In addition, the number of joints in the foot and ankle, as well as their complex 3D arrangement, makes 2D imaging interpretation challenging and imprecise. Distance mapping examines the relative positions between joint surfaces in 3 dimensions.[17,48] It offers quantitative visualization of the joint surface distance distribution via color-coded maps shown on each articular bone, as well as quantification and comparison of joint surface interactions (**Fig. 13**). Changes in surface-to-surface distance in the ankle, subtalar, and midfoot joints were observed, elucidating how the articular spaces undergo morphologic changes in PCFD versus control individuals.[49]

This technology is currently available through the postprocessing of WBCT pictures by engineers; however, a dedicated software or future integration into a picture archiving and communication system will facilitate its everyday use in a clinic.

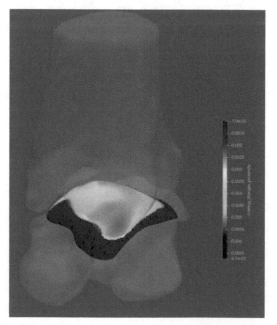

Fig. 13. An example of the distance mapping technique. Color-coded distance maps depict the intra-articular distances between the surfaces of adjacent bones.

What to Measure in Progressive Collapsing Foot Deformity?

- FAO
- Incongruence angle of the middle facet of the subtalar joint
- Inclination of the posterior facet of the subtalar joint
- Sinus tarsi or calcaneofibular bony impingement
- Talocalcaneal distance at the sinus tarsi or calcaneofibular distance
- Distance map (ankle, subtalar, talonavicular, and midfoot joints)

HALLUX VALGUS DEFORMITY
Measuring Common Radiographic Parameters for Evaluating Hallux Valgus

One of the earliest studies utilizing WBCT in HV deformity by Collan and colleagues compared the common radiographic parameters of conventional weight-bearing radiographs to those of WBCT.[50] In their investigation, the correlation between hallux valgus angle (HVA) and intermetatarsal angle (IMA) from 3D CT and conventional 2D plain radiographs was strong, leading the authors to conclude that WBCT can be used in isolation to evaluate patients with HV deformity. Coughlin and colleagues assessed the intraobserver and interobserver consistencies and reliability of angular measurements with WBCT in HV deformity.[51] The authors conclude that although the study verifies the reliability of IMA and HVA measurements, the reliability of the distal metatarsal articular angle and metatarsophalangeal joint (MTPJ) congruency is uncertain, primarily due to the difficulty of identifying medial and lateral articular surfaces. More recently, de Carvalho and colleagues examined manual and semiautomatic 3D measures using a specialized software in HV and control patients and found that semiautomatic measurements are comparable to manual measurements.[52] In addition, the software distinguished between pathologic and nonpathologic conditions when semiautomatic measurements were performed. These studies suggest that WBCT has the potential to replace the current approach of conventional radiography. Additionally, WBCT allows us to evaluate the HV pathomechanism in 3 dimensions, as described below.

Pronation of the First Metatarsal and Sesamoid Position

Studies using plain radiographs have suggested that the first metatarsal pronates in HV but concluded that the pronation of the metatarsus is difficult to evaluate in plain radiographs.[53] With WBCT, we understood the importance of the coronal plane deformity in HV. Collan and colleagues evaluated the rotational profile of the first metatarsal in HV and found a nonsignificant increase in the pronation of the first metatarsal in patients with HV compared with controls, whereas the pronation of the proximal phalanx was significantly greater in patients with HV than in controls.[50] This study suggested that WBCT scans could be used to assess the coronal component of the HV deformity **(Fig. 14)**.

Pronation of the first metatarsal was identified in the following study. Using simulated WBCT images, Kim and colleagues demonstrated an increase in pronation of the first ray in patients with HV relative to control patients when the alpha angle was measured.[54] This was the first study to report first metatarsal rotation in HV and in their cohort, 87.3% of HV cases demonstrated excessive first metatarsal rotation. Three-dimensional modeling was also used in measuring first metatarsal rotation. Using a 3D model of the first metatarsal and measuring the pronation of the first ray using the second metatarsal as a reference, Campbell and colleagues found a 9.9° increase in first metatarsal pronation compared with normal control patients.[55]

Studies also have observed changes in pronation following HV correction. Scheele and colleagues compared preoperative to postoperative pronation angles from the

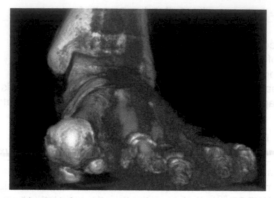

Fig. 14. In a patient with HV deformity, a 3D rendering image reveals pronation of the first metatarsal and minimal subluxation of the sesamoids.

metatarsal head and sesamoids and found that the pronation of the first metatarsal and the sesamoids were significantly reduced by the modified Lapidus procedure.[56] Interestingly, they noticed elevation of the second metatarsal head following surgery, which could be explained by the considerable plantarization of the lateral sesamoid caused by recentering the sesamoids under the head of the first metatarsal (**Fig. 15**). Conti and colleagues examined the link between changes in pronation following the modified Lapidus operation and Patient-Reported Outcomes Measurement Information System (PROMIS) scores.[9] Patients with decreased first metatarsal pronation demonstrated a substantially higher improvement in PROMIS physical function compared with those with no change or increased first metatarsal pronation. In the group with decreased first metatarsal pronation, recurrence rates were considerably lower than in the group with no change or increased first metatarsal pronation. In addition, the group with a moderate pronation change (2°–8° decrease) that left the first metatarsal slightly undercorrected had a better PROMIS outcome than those with a lesser or greater degree change. This indicates that when treating HV with the modified Lapidus method, care must be taken not to overcorrect the first metatarsal pronation.

Future research is necessary to understand the clinical implications of first ray pronation, and surgical correction targeting this deformity is necessary. Additional research is also required to identify the locations of rotational deformities. Despite multiple studies demonstrating the pronation of the first metatarsal in HV, there is weak evidence that shows a link between radiographic parameters and the pronation detected via WBCT.[55] As will be detailed in the following section, HV deformity involves a rotational component and midfoot instability in addition to the first metatarsal

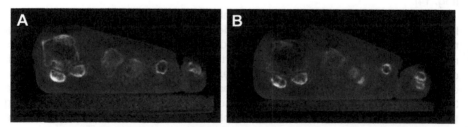

Fig. 15. Changes in the alignment of the first metatarsal head and sesamoids in the coronal plane from preoperative (*A*) to postoperative (*B*) conditions after a modified Lapidus procedure for HV deformity.

deformity. As reported by Ota and colleagues, pronation detected with WBCT scans can also be caused by the intrinsic rotation of the first metatarsal head resulting from torsion.[57] Finally, clinical outcome studies evaluating the relationship between patient-reported outcomes and various surgical methods for HV correction are required.

Three-Dimensional Midfoot Hypermobility

In a study that evaluated patients with HV compared with healthy volunteers using simulated WBCT scan, Kimura and colleagues found that instability of the first ray in HV occurs not only at the tarsometatarsal (TMT) joint but also at the adjacent joints that constitutes the first ray.[58] Moreover, this hypermobility occurs in 3D planes; for example, patients with HV have greater inversion and adduction of the first TMT relative to the medial cuneiform, not only dorsiflexion. Their results showed that in patients with HV compared with controls, there was significantly greater dorsiflexion at the talonavicular joint; significantly greater eversion and abduction at the medial cuneonavicular joint; significantly greater dorsiflexion, inversion, and adduction at the first tarsometatarsal joint; and finally, significantly greater eversion and abduction at the first MTPJ. In a separate study, they also found instability at the intercuneiform joint (between medial and middle) in patients with HV compared with healthy controls, using the same WBCT protocol used for the prior study.[59] They concluded that HV deformity is also associated with hypermobility of the joint between the medial and middle cuneiforms, hypothesizing that this joint should be potentially stabilized in patients with severe first ray hypermobility.

Geng and colleagues inspected mobility of the first metatarsal-cuneiform joint in HV and controls during weight-bearing using 3D CT.[60] During body weight-bearing conditions, the first metatarsal-cuneiform joint in HV feet dorsiflexed, supinated, and internally rotated to a greater degree than controls. Furthermore, the joint in HV feet widened significantly compared with the controls and tended to translate more in the dorsal-plantar direction. This shows some of the physiologic and pathologic movement at this joint and suggests multidirectional hypermobility at the joint in HV.

What to Measure in Hallux Valgus Deformity?

- Pronation of the first metatarsal bone (alpha angle) and the medial column
- Sesamoid subluxation

LISFRANC INJURY

The use of WBCT in Lisfranc injuries has been reported in more recent publications compared with other foot and ankle diseases. Although increasing, there is currently a limited number of publications that describe the utility of WBCT in Lisfranc injury. Compared with fracture/dislocation of the Lisfranc joint, subtle injury/instability of the Lisfranc joint caused by low-energy trauma may be difficult to identify with conventional weight-bearing radiographs because of their relatively low sensitivity.[61] MRI or conventional CT can detect ligament rupture and midfoot joint space widening, respectively; however, their ability to detect the physiologic alignment of the midfoot joints is limited by the unloaded condition during the examination.

Use of WBCT is reported, with a particular emphasis on diagnosing subtle Lisfranc injuries. WBCT is less affected by the projection angle on the Lisfranc joint because Lisfranc joints require an average craniocaudal x-ray beam angulation[62] but it is difficult to adapt to a variation in arch height between individuals. Studies have shown that the WBCT can be used to diagnose Lisfranc ligament injuries that are subtle.[61,63] In a study involving 24 cadaveric specimens, the distance between the medial cuneiform

(C1) and second metatarsal base (M2), which represents the origin and insertion of the Lisfranc ligament, was measured after sequential isolated sectioning of individual aspects of the Lisfranc ligament complex followed by ligaments surrounding the Lisfranc region under 3 different loading conditions.[64] The study found that sectioning of the Lisfranc ligament complex alone was insufficient to depict more than a 2 mm widening of the C1-M2 space compared with the intact condition, which is the current gold standard for diagnosing Lisfranc injury with standard radiographs. They concluded that a relative widening of greater than 1.5 mm under partial weight-bearing (40 kg) on axial WBCT imaging can clinically indicate a complete Lisfranc injury. To have a greater than 2 mm widening, which is the diagnostic threshold in standard radiographs; however, some degree of adjacent ligament injury is required. This also suggests that a subset of Lisfranc injuries involving damage to only a portion of the Lisfranc ligament complex may go undiagnosed with simple radiographs and a 2-mm radiographic cutoff in a clinical setting.

Another clinical study showed the value of WBCT 1, 2, and 3D measurements for assessing Lisfranc injuries.[63] Comparing 14 patients with surgically confirmed Lisfranc instability to 36 control patients using WBCT and measuring the distances, alignment, and volume of the Lisfranc joint, they found that 3D had a higher sensitivity for detecting Lisfranc injury.[63] Notably, they found that coronal 3D measurements were more sensitive than axial because the dislocation occurs both laterally and superiorly. This finding demonstrates the true value of WBCT in comparison to conventional methods, as well as the necessity and value of transforming the obtained images into a 3D analysis. Despite these findings, the clinical utility of WBCT in the setting of acute injury is questionable. Obtaining a WBCT in a fully weight-bearing state may be difficult in patients with Lisfranc injuries; therefore, a cutoff value in nonweight-bearing radiographs and CT scans or a ligament injury on MRI must exist to avoid missing the diagnosis at this stage.

WHAT TO MEASURE IN LISFRANC INJURIES?

- Medial cuneiform-second metatarsal base distance
- Lisfranc joint area
- Lisfranc joint volume

SUMMARY

WBCT has significantly increased our understanding of common foot and ankle diseases; nonetheless, its contribution to clinical decision-making remains unclear. From the clinical data and information collected, we expect to have a 3D comprehension of the disease and its prognosis, as well as postoperative changes in WBCT parameters and their clinical significance. However, WBCT's global use is currently limited, and 3D analysis requires the use of specialized software or professionals. Access to the WBCT machine, as well as a processing technique and software solutions, and a concerted effort to correlate radiography findings with WBCT findings are required to address foot and ankle disease in a large playground.

CLINICS CARE POINTS

- Weight-bearing computed tomography (WBCT) facilitates a more comprehensive comprehension of foot and ankle diseases.

- Post-processing WBCT images into three-dimensional horizons, along with biometric analysis, further enhances the understanding of foot and ankle diseases.

CONFLICT OF INTEREST

S. Ellis: Consultant for Vilex, Nextremity/Medartis, Stryker, and Paragon 28. American Orthopedic Foot and Ankle Society (AOFAS) board of directors. J. A. Carrino: Consultant: Pfizer, AstraZenca, Regeneron, Globus, Covera, Image Analysis Group. Editorial Board: Radiology, Arthritis and Rheumatology, Osteoarthritis Imaging.

REFERENCES

1. Lintz F, de Cesar Netto C, Barg A, et al. Weight-bearing cone beam CT scans in the foot and ankle. EFORT open reviews 2018;3(5):278–86.
2. Baverel L, Brilhault J, Odri G, et al. Influence of lower limb rotation on hindfoot alignment using a conventional two-dimensional radiographic technique. Foot Ankle Surg 2017;23(1):44–9.
3. Barg A, Amendola RL, Henninger HB, et al. Influence of ankle position and radiographic projection angle on measurement of supramalleolar alignment on the anteroposterior and hindfoot alignment views. Foot Ankle Int 2015;36(11):1352–61.
4. Haleem AM, Pavlov H, Bogner E, et al. Comparison of deformity with respect to the talus in patients with posterior tibial tendon dysfunction and controls using multiplanar weight-bearing imaging or conventional radiography. JBJS 2014;96(8):e63.
5. Steadman J, Bakshi N, Arena C, et al. Normative distribution of first metatarsal axial rotation. Foot Ankle Int 2021;42(8):1040–8.
6. Najefi A-A, Zaveri A, Alsafi MK, et al. The assessment of first metatarsal rotation in the normal adult population using weightbearing computed tomography. Foot Ankle Int 2021;42(10):1223–30.
7. Cody EA, Williamson ER, Burket JC, et al. Correlation of talar anatomy and subtalar joint alignment on weightbearing computed tomography with radiographic flatfoot parameters. Foot Ankle Int 2016;37(8):874–81.
8. Kim J-B, Yi Y, Kim J-Y, et al. Weight-bearing computed tomography findings in varus ankle osteoarthritis: abnormal internal rotation of the talus in the axial plane. Skeletal Radiol 2017;46(8):1071–80.
9. Conti MS, Willett JF, Garfinkel JH, et al. Effect of the modified Lapidus procedure on pronation of the first ray in hallux valgus. Foot Ankle Int 2020;41(2):125–32.
10. Kang HW, Kim D-Y, Park GY, et al. Coronal plane Calcaneal-Talar Orientation in Varus Ankle Osteoarthritis. Foot Ankle Int 2022;43(7):928–36.
11. de Cesar Netto C, Silva T, Li S, et al. Assessment of posterior and middle facet subluxation of the subtalar joint in progressive flatfoot deformity. Foot Ankle Int 2020;41(10):1190–7.
12. de Cesar Netto C, Godoy-Santos AL, Saito GH, et al. Subluxation of the middle facet of the subtalar joint as a marker of peritalar subluxation in adult acquired flatfoot deformity: a case-control study. JBJS 2019;101(20):1838–44.
13. Kim J, Rajan L, Henry J, et al. Axial plane rotation of the talus in progressive collapsing foot deformity: a weightbearing computed tomography analysis. Foot Ankle Int 2023;44(4):281–90.
14. Fuller RM, Kim J, An TW, et al. Assessment of Flatfoot Deformity Using Digitally Reconstructed Radiographs: Reliability and Comparison to Conventional Radiographs. Foot Ankle Int 2022;43(7):983–93.

15. Ashkani Esfahani S, Bhimani R, Lubberts B, et al. Volume measurements on weightbearing computed tomography can detect subtle syndesmotic instability. J Orthop Res 2022;40(2):460–7.

16. Bhimani R, Ashkani-Esfahani S, Lubberts B, et al. Utility of volumetric measurement via weight-bearing computed tomography scan to diagnose syndesmotic instability. Foot Ankle Int 2020;41(7):859–65.

17. Dibbern KN, Li S, Vivtcharenko V, et al. Three-dimensional distance and coverage maps in the assessment of peritalar subluxation in progressive collapsing foot deformity. Foot Ankle Int 2021;42(6):757–67.

18. Lintz F, Welck M, Bernasconi A, et al. 3D biometrics for hindfoot alignment using weightbearing CT. Foot Ankle Int 2017;38(6):684–9.

19. Zhang JZ, Lintz F, Bernasconi A, et al. 3D biometrics for hindfoot alignment using weightbearing computed tomography. Foot Ankle Int 2019;40(6):720–6.

20. Song JH, Kang C, Kim TG, et al. Perioperative axial loading computed tomography findings in varus ankle osteoarthritis: Effect of supramalleolar osteotomy on abnormal internal rotation of the talus. Foot Ankle Surg 2021;27(2):217–23.

21. Kim J-B, Park CH, Ahn J-Y, et al. Characteristics of medial gutter arthritis on weightbearing CT and plain radiograph. Skeletal Radiol 2021;50(8):1575–83.

22. Tanaka Y, Takakura Y, Hayashi K, et al. Low tibial osteotomy for varus-type osteoarthritis of the ankle. The Journal of bone and joint surgery British 2006;88(7):909–13.

23. Krähenbühl N, Tschuck M, Bolliger L, et al. Orientation of the subtalar joint: measurement and reliability using weightbearing CT scans. Foot Ankle Int 2016;37(1):109–14.

24. Krähenbühl N, Siegler L, Deforth M, et al. Subtalar joint alignment in ankle osteoarthritis. Foot Ankle Surg 2019;25(2):143–9.

25. Hayashi K, Tanaka Y, Kumai T, et al. Correlation of compensatory alignment of the subtalar joint to the progression of primary osteoarthritis of the ankle. Foot Ankle Int 2008;29(4):400–6.

26. Burssens A, Susdorf R, Krähenbühl N, et al. Supramalleolar Osteotomy for Ankle Varus Deformity Alters Subtalar Joint Alignment. Foot Ankle Int 2022;43(9):1194–203.

27. Zeitlin J, Henry J, Ellis S. Preoperative Guidance With Weight-Bearing Computed Tomography and Patient-Specific Instrumentation in Foot and Ankle Surgery. HSS J 2021;17(3):326–32.

28. Thompson MJ, Consul D, Umbel BD, et al. Accuracy of Weightbearing CT Scans for Patient-Specific Instrumentation in Total Ankle Arthroplasty. Foot & Ankle Orthopaedics. 2021;6(4). 24730114211061493.

29. de Cesar Netto C, Day J, Godoy-Santos AL, et al. The use of three-dimensional biometric Foot and Ankle Offset to predict additional realignment procedures in total ankle replacement. Foot Ankle Surg 2022;28(7):1029–34.

30. Lintz F, Mast J, Bernasconi A, et al. 3D, weightbearing topographical study of periprosthetic cysts and alignment in total ankle replacement. Foot Ankle Int 2020;41(1):1–9.

31. Day J, Kim J, O'Malley MJ, et al. Radiographic and clinical outcomes of the Salto Talaris total ankle arthroplasty. Foot Ankle Int 2020;41(12):1519–28.

32. Kim J, Rajan L, Fuller R, et al. Mid-term functional outcomes following reoperation after total ankle arthroplasty: A retrospective cohort study. Foot Ankle Surg 2022;28(8):1463–7.

33. Beumer A, Van Hemert W, Niesing R, et al. Radiographic measurement of the distal tibiofibular syndesmosis has limited use. Clin Orthop Relat Res 2004;423: 227–34.

34. Ebraheim NA, Lu J, Yang H, et al. Radiographic and CT evaluation of tibiofibular syndesmotic diastasis: a cadaver study. Foot Ankle Int 1997;18(11):693–8.

35. Lepojärvi S, Niinimäki J, Pakarinen H, et al. Rotational dynamics of the normal distal tibiofibular joint with weight-bearing computed tomography. Foot Ankle Int 2016;37(6):627–35.

36. Burssens A, Vermue H, Barg A, et al. Templating of Syndesmotic Ankle Lesions by Use of 3D Analysis in Weightbearing and Nonweightbearing CT. Foot Ankle Int 2018;39(12):1487–96.

37. Hamard M, Neroladaki A, Bagetakos I, et al. Accuracy of cone-beam computed tomography for syndesmosis injury diagnosis compared to conventional computed tomography. Foot Ankle Surg 2020;26(3):265–72.

38. Raheman FJ, Rojoa DM, Hallet C, et al. Can Weightbearing Cone-beam CT Reliably Differentiate Between Stable and Unstable Syndesmotic Ankle Injuries? A Systematic Review and Meta-analysis. Clin Orthop Relat Res 2022;480(8): 1547–62.

39. Myerson MS, Thordarson DB, Johnson JE, et al. Classification and Nomenclature: Progressive Collapsing Foot Deformity. Foot Ankle Int 2020;41(10):1271–6.

40. de Cesar Netto C, Bang K, Mansur NS, et al. Multiplanar Semiautomatic Assessment of Foot and Ankle Offset in Adult Acquired Flatfoot Deformity. Foot Ankle Int 2020;41(7):839–48.

41. Day J, de Cesar Netto C, Nishikawa DRC, et al. Three-Dimensional Biometric Weightbearing CT Evaluation of the Operative Treatment of Adult-Acquired Flatfoot Deformity. Foot Ankle Int 2020;41(8):930–6.

42. Ananthakrisnan D, Ching R, Tencer A, et al. Subluxation of the talocalcaneal joint in adults who have symptomatic flatfoot. J Bone Joint Surg Am 1999;81(8): 1147–54.

43. Probasco W, Haleem AM, Yu J, et al. Assessment of coronal plane subtalar joint alignment in peritalar subluxation via weight-bearing multiplanar imaging. Foot Ankle Int 2015;36(3):302–9.

44. de Cesar Netto C, Saito GH, Roney A, et al. Combined weightbearing CT and MRI assessment of flexible progressive collapsing foot deformity. Foot Ankle Surg 2021;27(8):884–91.

45. Kim J, Rajan L, Fuller R, et al. Radiographic Cutoff Values for Predicting Lateral Bony Impingement in Progressive Collapsing Foot Deformity. Foot Ankle Int 2022;43(9):1219–26.

46. Malicky ES, Crary JL, Houghton MJ, et al. Talocalcaneal and subfibular impingement in symptomatic flatfoot in adults. J Bone Joint Surg Am 2002;84(11):2005–9.

47. Jeng CL, Rutherford T, Hull MG, et al. Assessment of Bony Subfibular Impingement in Flatfoot Patients Using Weight-Bearing CT Scans. Foot Ankle Int 2019; 40(2):152–8.

48. Siegler S, Konow T, Belvedere C, et al. Analysis of surface-to-surface distance mapping during three-dimensional motion at the ankle and subtalar joints. J Biomech 2018;76:204–11.

49. Bernasconi A, De Cesar Netto C, Siegler S, et al. Weightbearing CT assessment of foot and ankle joints in Pes Planovalgus using distance mapping. Foot Ankle Surg 2022;28(6):775–84.

50. Collan L, Kankare JA, Mattila K. The biomechanics of the first metatarsal bone in hallux valgus: a preliminary study utilizing a weight bearing extremity CT. Foot Ankle Surg 2013;19(3):155–61.
51. Coughlin MJ, Freund E, Roger A, et al. The reliability of angular measurements in hallux valgus deformities. Foot Ankle Int 2001;22(5):369–79.
52. de Carvalho KAM, Walt JS, Ehret A, et al. Comparison between Weightbearing-CT semiautomatic and manual measurements in Hallux Valgus. Foot Ankle Surg 2022;28(4):518–25.
53. Maldin RA. Axial rotation of the first metatarsal as a factor in hallux valgus. J Am Podiatry Assoc 1972;62(3):85–93.
54. Kim Y, Kim JS, Young KW, et al. A New Measure of Tibial Sesamoid Position in Hallux Valgus in Relation to the Coronal Rotation of the First Metatarsal in CT Scans. Foot Ankle Int 2015;36(8):944–52.
55. Campbell B, Miller MC, Williams L, et al. Pilot Study of a 3-Dimensional Method for Analysis of Pronation of the First Metatarsal of Hallux Valgus Patients. Foot Ankle Int 2018;39(12):1449–56.
56. Scheele CB, Christel ST, Fröhlich I, et al. A cone beam CT based 3D-assessment of bony forefoot geometry after modified Lapidus arthrodesis. Foot Ankle Surg 2020;26(8):883–9.
57. Ota T, Nagura T, Kokubo T, et al. Etiological factors in hallux valgus, a three-dimensional analysis of the first metatarsal. J Foot Ankle Res 2017;10:43.
58. Kimura T, Kubota M, Taguchi T, et al. Evaluation of First-Ray Mobility in Patients with Hallux Valgus Using Weight-Bearing CT and a 3-D Analysis System: A Comparison with Normal Feet. J Bone Joint Surg Am 2017;99(3):247–55.
59. Kimura T, Kubota M, Suzuki N, et al. Comparison of Intercuneiform 1-2 Joint Mobility Between Hallux Valgus and Normal Feet Using Weightbearing Computed Tomography and 3-Dimensional Analysis. Foot Ankle Int 2018;39(3):355–60.
60. Geng X, Wang C, Ma X, et al. Mobility of the first metatarsal-cuneiform joint in patients with and without hallux valgus: in vivo three-dimensional analysis using computerized tomography scan. J Orthop Surg Res 2015;10:140.
61. Kennelly H, Klaassen K, Heitman D, et al. Utility of weight-bearing radiographs compared to computed tomography scan for the diagnosis of subtle Lisfranc injuries in the emergency setting. Emerg Med Australas 2019;31(5):741–4.
62. Rankine JJ, Nicholas CM, Wells G, et al. The diagnostic accuracy of radiographs in Lisfranc injury and the potential value of a craniocaudal projection. AJR Am J Roentgenol 2012;198(4):W365–9.
63. Bhimani R, Sornsakrin P, Ashkani-Esfahani S, et al. Using area and volume measurement via weightbearing CT to detect Lisfranc instability. J Orthop Res 2021;39(11):2497–505.
64. Sripanich Y, Weinberg M, Krähenbühl N, et al. Change in the First Cuneiform-Second Metatarsal Distance After Simulated Ligamentous Lisfranc Injury Evaluated by Weightbearing CT Scans. Foot Ankle Int 2020;41(11):1432–41.

Image-Guided Foot and Ankle Injections

Ryan C. Kruse, MD[a],*, Brennan Boettcher, DO[b]

KEYWORDS

- Ultrasound • Injection • Foot • Ankle

KEY POINTS

- The foot and ankle is a complex anatomic region.
- Image-guided procedures should be considered over palpation-guided procedures.
- Ultrasound is a valuable tool for both soft tissue and intra-articular image-guided procedures.
- Fluoroscopy may be considered for intra-articular injections.

INTRODUCTION

The foot and ankle is a complex anatomic region that is prone to various pathologic conditions. These include intra-articular conditions, as well as acute and chronic injuries to extra-articular soft tissues. Most conditions in this region can be treated without surgical intervention, and minimally invasive options such as injection-based therapies should be considered first line as part of a comprehensive nonoperative treatment program.

Traditionally, procedures were performed based on palpation or anatomic landmarks. As fluoroscopy and ultrasound (US) have become more readily available, image-guided injections have demonstrated several benefits, including increased accuracy, improved therapeutic effect, and better clinical outcomes.[1] US demonstrates the advantage of allowing visualization of the needle within the target structure, which is necessary for injections around nerves. Fluoroscopy is very accurate for joint injections, but confers the negative of ionizing radiation, and frequently the need for contrast material.

With US-guided procedures in the foot and ankle, there are a few key points to keep in mind. Most structures in this region are small and relatively superficial. As a result, a

---

[a] Department of Orthopedics and Rehabilitation, University of Iowa Sports Medicine, 2701 Prairie Meadow Drive, Iowa City, IA 52246, USA; [b] Division of Sports Medicine, Department of Orthopedic Surgery, 200 First Street SW, Rochester, MN 55905, USA
* Corresponding author.
E-mail address: ryan-kruse@uiowa.edu

Foot Ankle Clin N Am 28 (2023) 641–665
https://doi.org/10.1016/j.fcl.2023.04.005
1083-7515/23/© 2023 Elsevier Inc. All rights reserved.

foot.theclinics.com

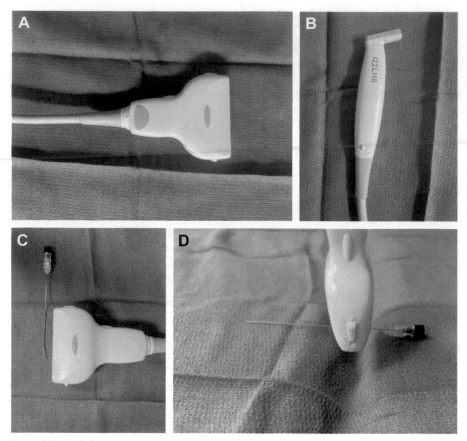

Fig. 1. (*A*). High-frequency, linear array transducer. (*B*). Hockey stick transducer. (*C*). In-plane injection approach. (*D*). Out-of-plane injection approach.

small footprint, high-frequency linear array transducer should be used (**Fig. 1**A). If available, a hockey stick transducer may be considered (**Fig. 1**B). Additionally, although in-plane (needle parallel to the transducer) injections are preferred due to improved needle visualization, out-of-plane (needle perpendicular to the transducer) injections are commonly used due to small joint spaces (**Fig. 1**C, D).

Injectate choice will vary based on the pathologic condition and injection goals. For therapeutic injections, corticosteroids are commonly used due to low cost and limited postprocedural restrictions. However, their safety has recently been called more into question.[2,3] Many clinicians offer alternative injection options, such as orthobiologics (OBX), which do not carry the same risks and may provide more durable pain relief.[4] Finally, anesthetic only injections are often used to confirm or refute a particular structure as a pain generator.

In this article, we describe the procedural techniques and considerations for common US-guided intra-articular, perineural, and soft tissue injections in the foot and ankle. The focus of this article is on US-guided techniques due to the authors' procedural practices; however, fluoroscopic guidance can be considered for most intra-articular injections in this region.

INTRA-ARTICULAR INJECTIONS

Intra-articular injections comprise the vast majority of foot and ankle injections. A thorough understanding of the complex anatomy in this region is critical to ensure procedural accuracy. Radiographs are essential for the evaluation of bony anatomy and the presence of anomalies such as accessory ossicles, which may result in confusion when planning the procedural approach, and potentially incorrect injection targets.

Tibiotalar Joint

The tibiotalar joint is a diarthrodial joint formed by the distal tibia, distal fibula, and talus. It functions as a hinge joint, allowing for dorsiflexion and plantarflexion of the ankle. It is stabilized by 3 ligamentous groups; anterior talofibular ligament (ATFL), the tibiofibular syndesmosis (which includes the anterior inferior tibiofibular ligament, posterior tibiofibular ligament, and the interosseous membrane), and the deltoid ligament complex.

Normal sonoanatomy

Laterally, the hyperechoic bony cortices of the distal fibula and talus are seen. The hyperechoic fibrillar structure spanning these 2 structures is the ATFL. Anteriorly, a longitudinal view of the joint demonstrates the hyperechoic talus with a thin anechoic line overlying the talus, representing the talar cartilage. In a transverse view, the hyperechoic cortices of the distal tibia and talus are in view. Medially, again seen are the distal tibia and talus with the hyperechoic deltoid ligament spanning this region.

Lateral, out-of-plane
Patient positioning
- Lateral decubitus, with pillow or bolster underneath ankle to promote ankle inversion.

Approach
- Transducer oriented over ATFL. The needle is advanced lateral to medial, deep to the ATFL (**Fig. 2**A).

Needle
- Gauge: 25 to 27g.
- Length: 1.25 to 2.5In.

Injectate volume
- 2 to 4 mL.

Procedural considerations
- Avoid injecting into ATFL.
- "Walk down" technique can be helpful to avoid iatrogenic injury.

Medial, out-of-plane
Patient positioning
- Lateral decubitus, with pillow or bolster underneath ankle to promote ankle eversion.

Approach
- Transducer at the medial ankle joint. The needle is advanced medial to lateral, deep to the deltoid ligament (**Fig. 2**B).

Needle
- Gauge: 25 to 27g.
- Length: 1.25 to 2.5in.

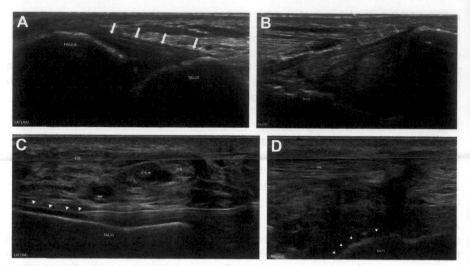

Fig. 2. Tibiotalar joint injection approaches. (*A*) Lateral, Out-of-plane. (*B*) Medial, Out-of-plane. (*C*) Anterior, In-plane. (*D*) Anterior, Out-of-plane. Closed arrowheads, talar cartilage; Closed arrows, ATFL; DP, dorsalis pedis artery; EDL, extensor digitorum longus tendon; EHL, extensor hallucis longus tendon; EHLm, extensor hallucis longus muscle; Open arrows, deltoid ligament.

Injectate volume
- 2 to 4 mL.

Procedural considerations
- Avoid nearby tibial nerve and branches.

Anterior, out-of-plane
Patient positioning
- Supine.

Approach
- Transducer over the anterior ankle joint in an anatomical sagittal plane. The needle can be advanced medial to lateral or lateral to medial (**Fig. 2**C).

Needle
- Gauge: 25 to 27g.
- Length: 1.25 to 2.5in.

Injectate volume
- 2 to 4 mL.

Procedural considerations
- Avoid nearby anterior ankle tendons, dorsalis pedis artery, and deep fibular nerve (DFN).

Anterior, in-plane
Patient positioning
- Supine.

Approach
- Transducer over the talus in an anatomic axial plane. The needle can be advanced medial to lateral or lateral to medial, and should be guided directly superficial to the talar cartilage (**Fig. 2**D).

Needle
- Gauge: 25 to 27g.
- Length: 1.25 to 2.5in.

Injectate volume
- 2 to 4 mL.

Procedural considerations
- The position of the DFN and dorsalis pedis artery needs to be considered.
- Injectate should be seen coursing medially and laterally. If injectate is seen localizing at the injection site, the needle tip is likely not intra-articular.

Subtalar Joint

The subtalar joint comprises posteriorly the talus and calcaneus (forming the posterior facet) and anteriorly the talus, calcaneus, and navicular (forming the middle and anterior facets).[5] These regions are connected by an interosseous tunnel called the sinus tarsi. Within the sinus tarsi is a complex network of ligamentous structures, small vasculature, and sensory nerve fibers.[6] The subtalar joint allows for multiplanar motion; however, the primary function of the joint is to allow inversion and eversion.

Normal sonoanatomy
The anterolateral subtalar joint can be found by identifying the hyperechoic fibular tendons and following them distally past the lateral malleolus. As they course around the lateral malleolus, the fibrillar calcaneofibular ligament (CFL) is seen underneath the tendons. Deep to the CFL, the subtalar joint is visualized as a cleft between the bony surfaces of the talus and calcaneus.

The posterolateral joint is visualized just lateral to the Achilles tendon. The hyperechoic cortices of the posterior tibial, talus, and calcaneus can be seen (and therefore the posterior tibiotalar and subtalar joints). Medially, the posteromedial joint line can be visualized by first finding the hyperechoic cortices of the medial malleolus and talus. The transducer is then translated anteriorly, and the joint space is found immediately anterior to the sustentaculum tali, deep to the flexor digitorum longus (FDL) and posterior tibialis (PT) tendons. Finally, the sinus tarsi can be readily identified at the anterolateral ankle by finding the hyperechoic cortices of the talus and calcaneus, with the transducer is a sagittal oblique orientation.

Anterolateral, out-of-plane
Patient positioning
- Lateral decubitus, with pillow or bolster underneath ankle to promote ankle inversion.

Approach
- Transducer at the anterolateral subtalar joint, parallel to the calcaneofibular ligament. The needle is advanced anterolateral to posteromedial (**Fig. 3**A).

Needle
- Gauge: 25 to 30g.
- Length: 1.25 to 2in.

Injectate volume
- 1 to 2 mL.

Procedural considerations
- Avoid injecting into fibular tendons or nearby sural nerve.

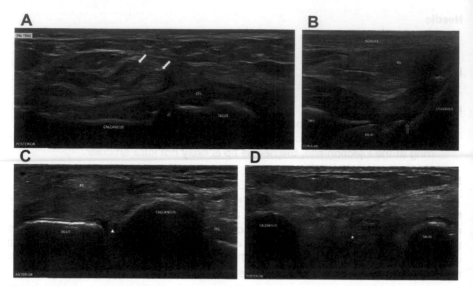

Fig. 3. Subtalar joint injection approaches. (*A*) Anterolateral, Out-of-plane. (*B*) Posterolateral, In-plane. (*C*) Posteromedial, Out-of-plane. (*D*). Sinus tarsi injection, Out-of-plane. Asterisk, Sinus tarsi; CFL, calcaneofibular ligament; Closed arrowhead, posteromedial subtalar joint; Closed arrows, fibular tendons; FHL, flexor hallucis longus tendon; Kfp, Kager's fat pad; Open arrow, posterolateral subtalar joint; PT, posterior tibialis tendon.

Posterolateral, in-plane
Patient positioning
- Prone with ankle in dorsiflexion.

Approach
- Transducer oriented in an anatomic sagittal plane, directly lateral to the Achilles tendon, angled slightly medially. The needle is advanced posterolateral to anteromedial (**Fig. 3**B).

Needle
- Gauge: 25 to 30g.
- Length: 1.25 to 2in.

Injectate volume
- 1 to 2 mL.

Procedural considerations
- This is a very steep approach and visualization can be challenging. Care should be taken to visualize the needle tip at all times.
- The nearby sural nerve should be identified and avoided.

Posteromedial, out-of-plane
Patient positioning
- Lateral decubitus, with pillow or bolster underneath ankle to promote ankle eversion.

Approach
- Transducer is oriented over the sustentaculum tali and the talus, with the spring ligament spanning the 2 bony cortices. The needle is advanced medial to lateral (**Fig. 3**C).

Needle
- Gauge: 25 to 30g.
- Length: 1.25 to 2in.

Injectate volume
- 1 to 2 mL.

Procedural considerations
- The tibial neurovasculature is nearby and should be identified.

Sinus tarsi
Patient positioning
- Lateral decubitus, with pillow or bolster underneath ankle to promote ankle inversion.

Approach
- Transducer is oriented in an anatomic coronal oblique plane, spanning the anterior process of the calcaneus and the talar neck. The needle is advanced in a posteromedial direction (**Fig. 3**D).

Needle
- Gauge: 25 to 30g.
- Length: 1.25 to 2in.

Injectate volume
- 1 to 2 mL

Procedural considerations
- This injection approach can also be used in cases of soft tissue/sinus tarsi impingement.

Talonavicular Joint

The talonavicular joint is functionally and anatomically connected to 2 separate joint complexes.[7] It contributes to the subtalar joint complex as part of the talocalcaneonavicular joint, and also articulates with the calcaneocuboid joint to form the transverse tarsal (Chopart's) joint. The joint primarily allows inversion and eversion.

Normal sonoanatomy
The talonavicular joint is identified by following the PT tendon distally to its insertion on the navicular. The transducer is then rotated in a clockwise manner, and the hyperechoic cortex of the talus should come into view.

Out-of-plane
Patient positioning
- Lateral decubitus, with pillow or bolster underneath ankle to promote ankle eversion.

Approach
- Transducer is oriented in an anatomic sagittal oblique plane. The needle is advanced medial to lateral (**Fig. 4**).
- Alternatively, an in-plane, proximal to distal approach may be used.

Needle
- Gauge: 27 to 30g.
- Length: 0.75 to 1.5in.

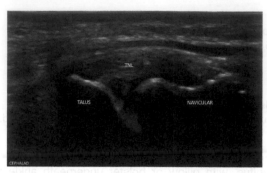

Fig. 4. Talonavicular joint injection approach. TNL, dorsal talonavicular ligament.

Injectate volume
- 0.5 to 1 mL.

Procedural considerations
- Be mindful of an os naviculare because a synchondrosis between it and the navicular could be confused for the talonavicular joint.

Calcaneocuboid Joint

The calcaneocuboid joint, along with the talonavicular joint, forms the transverse tarsal joint.[8] The calcaneocuboid joint is a modified saddle joint, with minimal motion except slight translation during inversion and eversion. The joint is stabilized plantarly by the short and long plantar ligaments, medially by the medial calcaneocuboid ligament, and dorsally by the dorsal calcaneocuboid ligament.

Normal sonoanatomy
In an anatomic sagittal plane, the hyperechoic bony cortices of the calcaneus and cuboid are seen, with the hyperechoic dorsal calcaneocuboid ligament spanning the 2 structures.

Out-of-plane
Patient positioning
- Lateral decubitus, with pillow or bolster underneath ankle to promote ankle inversion.
- Alternatively, patient may lay supine.

Approach
- Transducer oriented in an anatomic sagittal plane, with the needle advanced lateral to medial (**Fig. 5**).
- Alternatively, an in-plane, proximal to distal approach may be used.

Needle
- Gauge: 27 to 30g.
- Length: 0.75 to 1.5in.

Injectate volume
- 0.5 to 1 mL.

Procedural considerations
- The nearby fibular tendons should be identified and avoided.

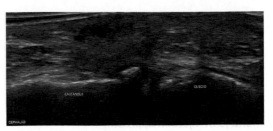

Fig. 5. Calcaneocuboid joint injection approach.

Naviculocuneiform Joint

The naviculocuneiform joint is formed by the articulations between the navicular and the 3 cuneiform bones.[9] Motion is minimal across the joint. The joint is primarily stabilized by both dorsal and plantar ligaments, with the plantar ligaments being further supported by small slips from the PT tendon.

Normal sonoanatomy

The hyperechoic bony cortices of the navicular and each cuneiform bone are seen, typically with a small joint space.

Out-of-plane
Patient positioning
- Lateral decubitus, with pillow or bolster underneath ankle to promote ankle eversion.

Approach
- Out-of-plane, medial to lateral (**Fig. 6**).

Needle
- Gauge: 27 to 30g.
- Length: 0.75 to 1.5in.

Injectate volume
- 0.5 to 1 mL.

Procedural considerations
- A far lateral approach should be avoided due to the nearby superficial and deep fibular nerves.

Tarsometatarsal Joints

The tarsometatarsal (TMT) joints are arthrodial joints, formed by the articulations between the proximal metatarsals and the cuneiforms and cuboid. Although each TMT joint is considered a separate entity, there is a normal communication between the second and third TMT joints.[10] The joints are stabilized by dorsal, plantar, and interosseous ligaments, the most important of which is the Lisfranc ligament, which connects the medial cuneiform to the base of the second metatarsal.

Normal sonoanatomy

In a transverse plane, the metatarsals, cuneiforms, and cuboid all seem as hyperechoic, relatively flat structures. Hyperechoic, fibrillar extensor tendons may be seen in long axis dorsal to the joints.

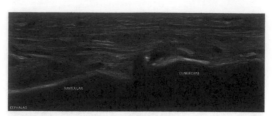

Fig. 6. Naviculocuneiform joint injection approach.

Out-of-plane
Patient positioning
- Supine, knee flexed, foot flat on bed.

Approach
- Anatomic sagittal orientation over dorsal foot. The needle is advanced medial to lateral or lateral to medial (**Fig. 7**).

Needle
- Gauge: 27 to 30g.
- Length: 0.75 to 1.5in.

Injectate volume
- 0.5 to 1 mL.

Procedural considerations
- Avoid overlying neurovasculature, including dorsal pedis artery and superficial/ deep fibular nerves.
- To identify which TMT joint is visualized, it can be helpful to trace the metatarsals in an axial plane to the TMT joint and rotate the transducer.

Metatarsophalangeal Joints

The metatarsophalangeal (MTP) joints are formed by the articulations of the metatarsal heads and proximal phalanges. They are condyloid joints, which allow for flexion, extension, abduction, and adduction. The joints are stabilized by collateral ligaments, plantar ligaments, deep transverse metatarsal ligaments, and plantar plate.

Normal sonoanatomy
From a dorsal view, the metatarsal head has a characteristic rounded, hyperechoic appearance. The hyperechoic dorsal joint capsule is easily visualized, with the hyperechoic, fibrillar extensor tendons seen in long axis dorsal to the joints.

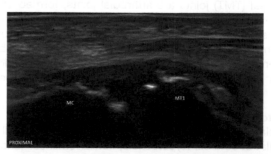

Fig. 7. TMT joint injection approach. MC, medial cuneiform; MT1, first metatarsal.

Out-of-plane
Patient positioning
- Supine, knee flexed, foot flat on bed.

Approach
- Anatomic sagittal orientation over dorsal foot, with a transverse view of joint. The needle is advanced medial to lateral or lateral to medial (**Fig. 8**).

Needle
- Gauge: 27 to 30g.
- Length: 0.75 to 1.5in.

Injectate volume
- 0.25 to 0.5 mL.

Procedural considerations
- Small volume injectate preferred to avoid overdistension of the joint.

Interphalangeal Joints

The interphalangeal joints are small joints formed by the articulations of the proximal and middle phalanges as well as the middle and distal phalanges. They are hinge joints, allowing for flexion and extension. Stabilization is provided by plantar and collateral ligaments.

Normal sonoanatomy
Bony margins seem as hyperechoic, well-corticated structures, with a small joint space between. Hyperechoic, fibrillar extensor tendons are seen dorsal to the joint.

Out-of-plane
Patient positioning
- Supine, knee flexed, foot flat on bed.

Approach
- Anatomic sagittal orientation over dorsal foot, with a transverse view of joint. The needle is advanced medial to lateral or lateral to medial (**Fig. 9**).

Needle
- Gauge: 27 to 30g.
- Length: 0.5 to 1.5in.

Injectate volume
- 0.5 to 1 mL.

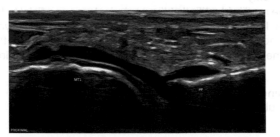

Fig. 8. MTP joint injection approach. MT1, first metatarsal; PP, proximal phalanx.

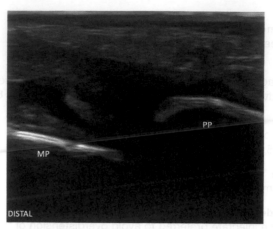

Fig. 9. Interphalangeal joint injection approach. PP, proximal phalanx; MP, middle phalanx.

Procedural considerations
- Identify and avoid nearby interdigital nerves.
- Consider rotating the transducer into an in-plane view to confirm depth of the needle to avoid intracapsular injection.

PERINEURAL INJECTIONS

Nerve pathology about the foot and ankle is common and can have primary or secondary causes. When performing perineural injections, there are a few key points to consider. Injecting slowly with local anesthetic while advancing the needle toward the neve can help prevent penetrating the nerve because it will start to push away from the needle tip when the needle enters the perineural space. It is also important to ensure circumferential, perineural spread of injectate to limit the chance of a false-negative response, especially when injecting for diagnostic purposes. Finally, the authors recommend the use of a nonparticulate steroid to reduce the chance of a thromboischemic injury to the nerves.

Sural Nerve

The sural nerve is a sensory nerve that provides sensation to the posterolateral aspect of the distal one-third of the leg as well as the lateral foot and ankle. It is formed by the confluence of the lateral and medial sural cutaneous nerves. Distally, the nerve terminates as the lateral sural cutaneous nerve.

Normal sonoanatomy
The nerve can be readily identified at the posterior leg, superficial to the distal gastrocnemius muscles. It seems as a multifascicular, hyperechoic, honeycomb structure. It courses directly adjacent to the anechoic lesser saphenous vein. At the ankle, it can be seen lateral to the Achilles tendon and posterior to the fibular tendons.

Fascial exit
Patient positioning
- Lateral decubitus or prone.

Approach
- In-plane (**Fig. 10**A).

Needle
- Gauge: 25 to 30g.
- Length: 0.75 to 2in.

Injectate volume
- 1 to 2 mL.

Procedural considerations
- Avoid intravascular injection of the lesser saphenous vein.

Foot/ankle
Patient positioning
- Lateral decubitus, pillow or bolster under ankle to promote inversion.

Approach
- In-plane (**Fig. 10**B).

Needle
- Gauge: 25 to 30g.
- Length: 0.75 to 2in.

Injectate volume
- 1 to 2 mL.

Procedural considerations
- Avoid intravascular injection of the lesser saphenous vein.

Superficial Fibular Nerve

The superficial fibular nerve (SFN) is 1 of 2 branches of common fibular nerve (CFN), originating just distal to the fibular head. It is a mixed nerve. It supplies sensation to most of the lateral leg and dorsum of the foot (with the exception of the first web space), as well as motor innervation to the lateral compartment musculature. Distally, it bifurcates into 2 terminal sensory branches—the medial and intermediate dorsal cutaneous nerves.

The most common site of nerve compression is at the distal one-third of the leg as it pierces the crural fascia. Posttraumatic compression can be seen at the foot and ankle after sprains, fractures, or surgical intervention.

Normal sonoanatomy
The nerve seems as a small, hyperechoic, honeycomb structure coursing between the fibularis longus (FL) and brevis muscle bellies. At the distal one-third of the leg, it is

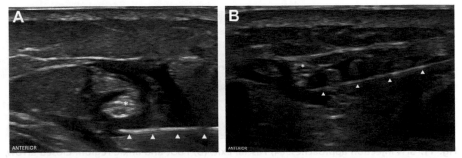

Fig. 10. Sural nerve injection approaches. (*A*) Fascial exit. (*B*) Foot and ankle region. Closed arrowheads, needle; Asterisk, sural nerve.

seen piercing the crural fascia because it becomes cutaneous before it bifurcates further distally.

Fascial exit
Patient positioning
- Lateral decubitus.

Approach
- In-plane, posterior to anterior or anterior to posterior (**Fig. 11**A).

Needle
- Gauge: 25 to 30g.
- Length: 0.75 to 2in.

Injectate volume
- 1 to 2 mL.

Procedural considerations
- If injecting for diagnostic purposes, important to ensure injectate spreads just proximal to fascial exit as well.

Foot/ankle
Patient positioning
- Lateral decubitus, pillow or bolster under ankle to promote inversion.
- Alternatively, supine.

Approach
- In-plane (**Fig. 11**B).

Needle
- Gauge: 25 to 30g.
- Length: 0.75 to 2in.

Injectate volume
- 1 to 2 mL.

Procedural considerations
- Follow terminal branches distally to confirm identification of nerve.

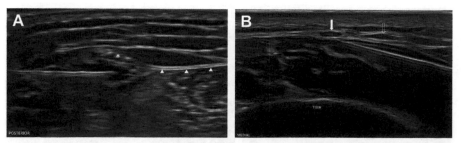

Fig. 11. SFN injection approaches. (*A*) Fascial exit. (*B*) Foot and ankle region. Closed arrow, medial dorsal cutaneous nerve; Open arrow, intermediate dorsal cutaneous nerve; Asterisk, SFN; Closed arrowheads, crural fascia.

Deep Fibular Nerve

The DFN is a mixed nerve and is 1 of 2 terminal branches of the CFN. At the CFN bifurcation, the nerve enters the anterior compartment of the leg and travels distally adjacent to the anterior tibial artery. Within the leg, the nerve provides motor innervation to the anterior compartment musculature. At the level of the tibiotalar joint, the nerve bifurcates into medial and lateral terminal branches. The medial terminal branch is a sensory nerve, which provides sensation to the first web space. The lateral terminal branch is a mixed nerve, providing motor innervation to the extensor digitorum brevis and extensor hallucis brevis muscles and sensory innervation to the second to fourth TMT and MTP joints.

There DFN can become entrapped deep to the inferior extensor retinaculum, otherwise known as "anterior tarsal tunnel syndrome." Additionally, the medial sensory branch can be compressed from tight-fitting shoe wear, dorsal osteophytes secondary to osteoarthritis (OA), or as it courses deep to the extensor digitorum brevis muscle/tendon unit.

Normal sonoanatomy

The nerve is a small, hyperechoic, honeycomb structure. After piercing the extensor digitorum longus muscle, it can be challenging to visualize because it is located deep within the anterior compartment. At the distal leg, it can be seen within the anterior tarsal tunnel before it bifurcates at the tibiotalar joint. Distally, the medial terminal branch is seen immediately adjacent to the dorsalis pedis artery.

Anterior Ankle/Anterior Tarsal Tunnel
Patient positioning
- Supine.

Approach
- In-plane, lateral to medial (**Fig. 12A**).

Needle
- Gauge: 25 to 30g.
- Length: 0.75 to 2in.

Injectate volume
- 1 to 2 mL.

Procedural considerations
- A lateral to medial approach is preferred as the dorsalis pedis artery most often lies medial to the nerve.

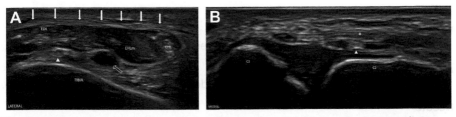

Fig. 12. DFN injection approaches. (*A*) Anterior tarsal tunnel. (*B*) Deep to extensor digitorum brevis tendon. Asterisk, extensor digitorum brevis tendon; C1, first cuneiform; C2, second cuneiform; Closed arrow, inferior extensor retinaculum; Closed arrowhead, DFN; EDL, extensor digitorum longus tendon; EHL, extensor hallucis longus tendon; EHLm, extensor hallucis longus muscle; Open arrow, anterior tibial artery.

Medial branch deep to extensor digitorum brevis tendon
Patient positioning
- Supine.

Approach
- In-plane, lateral to medial (**Fig. 12B**).

Needle
- Gauge: 25 to 30g.
- Length: 0.75 to 2in.

Injectate volume
- 1 to 2 mL.

Procedural considerations
- Ensure careful needle placement to avoid intravascular injection of the dorsalis pedis artery.

Tibial Nerve

The tibial nerve is a mixed nerve and is 1 of 2 terminal branches of the sciatic nerve. It provides sensory innervation to the posterior heel and most of the plantar foot. It provides motor supply to the deep and superficial posterior compartment musculature as well as the foot intrinsic muscles. The nerve courses deep within the posterior leg before entering the tarsal tunnel at the medial ankle. Here, the nerve most typically trifurcates into the medial calcaneal, medial plantar, and lateral plantar nerves; however, the branching pattern is highly variable. The medial calcaneal nerve is a sensory nerve, while the medial and lateral plantar nerves are mixed nerves.

Within the foot and ankle, the most common site of compression is the tarsal tunnel. The medial plantar nerve can be compressed because it courses between the abductor hallucis muscle and the navicular. Additionally, the inferior calcaneal nerve can become compressed because it courses between the abductor hallucis and quadratus plantar muscles.[11] Finally, the common digital plantar nerves can be chronically compressed, which may give rise to focal nerve enlargement, also known as a "Morton neuroma."

Normal sonoanatomy
The nerve seems as a large, hyperechoic, fascicular structure that can be easily identified within the distal leg. As it enters the tarsal tunnel, it is often posterior to the anechoic posterior tibial vasculature. The characteristic hyperechoic, fibrillar architecture of the flexor hallucis longus (FHL) tendon is seen deep to the tibial nerve.

Tarsal tunnel
Patient positioning
- Prone, foot hanging off the edge of the bed.

Approach
- In-plane, posterolateral to anteromedial, deep to the Achilles tendon (**Fig. 13A**).

Needle
- Gauge: 25 to 30g.
- Length: 0.75 to 2in.

Injectate volume
- 1 to 3 mL.

Procedural considerations
- Avoid the nearby posterior tibial vasculature.
- Ensure differentiation of the tibial nerve from the FHL tendon because these can have a similar echotexture.

Medial plantar nerve
Patient positioning
- Prone or lateral decubitus.

Approach
- In-plane (**Fig. 13**B).

Needle
- Gauge: 25 to 30g.
- Length: 0.75 to 2in.

Injectate volume
- 1 to 2 mL.

Procedural considerations
- Avoid nearby flexor tendons.

Inferior calcaneal nerve
Patient positioning
- Prone or lateral decubitus.

Approach
- In-plane (**Fig. 13**C).

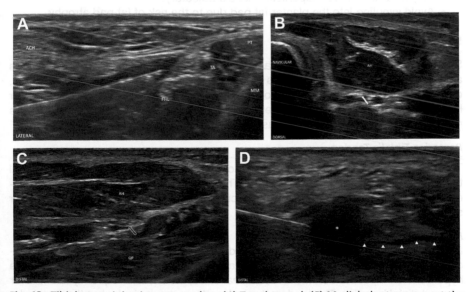

Fig. 13. Tibial nerve injection approaches. (*A*) Tarsal tunnel. (*B*) Medial plantar nerve at the abductor hallucis/navicular interval. (*C*) Inferior calcaneal nerve at the abductor hallucis/quadratus plantae interval. (*D*) Common digital plantar nerve. Closed arrow, medial plantar nerve; Open arrow, inferior calcaneal nerve; Closed arrowheads, common digital plantar nerve; Asterisk, common digital plantar nerve neuroma; ACH, Achilles tendon; AH, abductor hallucis muscle; FHL, flexor hallucis longus tendon; MM, medial malleolus; PT, posterior tibialis tendon; QP, quadratus plantae muscle; TA, posterior tibial artery.

Needle
- Gauge: 25 to 30g.
- Length: 0.75 to 2in.

Injectate volume
- 1 to 2 mL.

Procedural considerations
- Circumferential spread should be seen as the nerve is separated from the surrounding tissues.

Common digital plantar nerve (Morton neuroma)
Patient positioning
- Supine.

Approach
- In-plane, plantar approach, distal to proximal (**Fig. 13**D)
- Alternatively, in-plane, dorsal approach, proximal to distal

Needle
- Gauge: 25 to 30g.
- Length: 0.75 to 2in.

Injectate volume
- 1 to 2 mL.

Procedural considerations
- The nerve is located plantar to the intermetatarsal bursa, so a plantar approach may provide a more "superficial" needle trajectory.
- Avoid injecting into the plantar fat pad due to the risk of fat pad atrophy.

SOFT TISSUE INJECTIONS

Soft tissue injections in the foot and ankle region are primarily limited to peritendinous and intratendinous targets, as well as the plantar fascia (PF). As mentioned previously, corticosteroid should be reserved for peritendinous/perifascial injections and never injected directly into these structures. If an intratendinous/intrafascial procedure is required, a noncorticosteroid such as an OBX should be considered.

Posterior Tibialis Tendon

The PT originates from the deep posterior compartment and passes through the tarsal tunnel, posterior to the medial malleolus. The tendon turns anterior and plantar, ultimately inserting on tuberosity of the navicular, the plantar cuneiforms, and plantar second-fourth metatarsal bases.

Normal sonoanatomy
In the posterior lower leg, the PT is visualized deep and lateral to the FDL muscle, adjacent to the posterolateral border of the tibia and the interosseous membrane. As the hyperechoic PT passes below the medial malleolus, the tendon frequently fans out for a broad distal insertion. The tendon always inserts on the navicular but the remainder of the insertion sites is highly variable.[12]

Patient positioning
- Lateral decubitus, with pillow or bolster underneath ankle to promote ankle eversion.

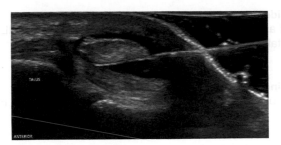

Fig. 14. PT tendon sheath injection approach.

Approach
- In-plane. The target is between the tendon sheath and PT tendon (**Fig. 14**).

Needle
- Gauge: 25 to 30g.
- Length: 1 to 2in.

Injectate volume
- 1 to 3 mL.

Procedural considerations
- Care should be taken to avoid the medial calcaneal nerve, which passes superficial to the PT and flexor retinaculum.

Flexor Hallucis Longus Tendon

The FHL sits anterior to the soleus and posterior to the PT muscle in the lower leg. The tendon passes posteromedial to the groove for the FHL in the talus, and subsequently the groove for the FHL in the calcaneus. The tendon courses deep to the FDL tendon at the Master Knot of Henry before continuing to its insertion at the great toe.

Normal sonoanatomy
In the distal posterior leg, the FHL seems as a hypoechoic muscle with a hyperechoic tendon forming in the posteromedial muscle belly. As it approaches the talus, the hyperechoic ovoid tendon sits within a crescentic groove in the talus, subsequently passing adjacent to the calcaneus in a slightly shallower groove. At these locations, the tibial or medial and lateral plantar nerves are visualized adjacent to the tendon and may seem similar in echotexture to the tendon.

At ankle
Patient positioning
- Prone, with the ankle at the edge of the bed and in a neutral position.

Approach
- In-plane, posterolateral to anteromedial, deep to the Achilles tendon (**Fig. 15A**).

Needle
- Gauge: 25 to 27g.
- Length: 1.5 to 2in.

Injectate volume
- 1 to 2 mL.

Procedural considerations
- The medial and lateral plantar nerves pass posterior to the FHL tendon and care should be taken to avoid these nerves.

Foot region
Patient positioning
- Lateral decubitus, with pillow or bolster underneath ankle to promote ankle eversion.

Approach
- In-plane, medial to lateral.
- The target is adjacent to the FHL tendon at the level of the FHL/FDL intersection (**Fig. 15B**).

Needle
- Gauge: 25 to 27.
- Length: 1.25 to 2in.

Injectate volume
- 1 to 3 mL.

Procedural considerations
- Identify and avoid the medial plantar nerve, which sits adjacent to the FDL/FHL intersection in the foot.

Fibularis longus and fibularis brevis tendons
The FL muscle originates from the fibular head and lateral border of the fibula, as well as the intramuscular septum. Distally, it inserts on the plantar medial cuneiform and base of the first metatarsal. The fibularis brevis tendon originates from the lateral aspect of the fibula and adjacent intramuscular septum. It courses between the lateral malleolus and FL before inserting on the fifth metatarsal.

Normal sonoanatomy
At the level of the midfibula, the typical hypoechoic muscular architecture and a notable superficial hyperechoic FL tendon can be seen. At the lateral malleolus, 2 hyperechoic ovoid tendons are seen, which wrap along the posterior/inferior lateral malleolus, superficial to the CFL and deep to the fibular retinaculum. In the inframalleolar region, they are separated by an osseous prominence on the calcaneus called the fibular tubercle, before they diverge to their distal insertions.

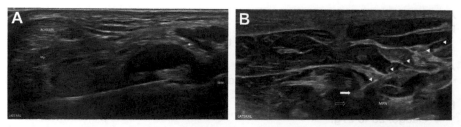

Fig. 15. FHL tendon sheath injection approaches. (*A*) Ankle, deep to Achilles tendon. (*B*) Foot region, Master Knot of Henry. Closed arrow, FDL tendon; Open arrow, FHL tendon; Closed arrowheads, needle; Asterisk, tibial nerve; Kfp, Kager's fat pad; MM, medial malleolus; MPN, medial plantar nerve.

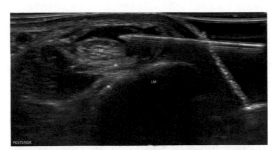

Fig. 16. Fibular tendon sheath injection approach. Br, fibularis brevis tendon; Lg, fibularis longus tendon; LM, lateral malleolus.

Patient positioning
- Lateral decubitus, with pillow or bolster underneath ankle to promote ankle eversion.

Approach
- In-plane, anterior to posterior or posterior to anterior (**Fig. 16**).

Needle
- Gauge: 25 to 30.
- Length: 1 to 2in.

Injectate volume
- 1 to 3 mL.

Procedural considerations
- A gel standoff can help with needle entry location.

Anterior Ankle Tendons

In the lower leg, the anterior tibialis (AT), extensor hallucis longus (EHL), and extensor digitorum longus (EDL) originate from the lateral tibia and interosseous membrane; medial fibula and interosseous membrane; and lateral tibia, medial fibula, and interosseous membranes, respectively. In most individuals, a separate muscle, the fibularis tertius, is seen lateral to the EDL, inserting on the fifth metatarsal. The AT inserts on the inferomedial cuneiform and base of the first metatarsal. The EHL inserts dorsally on the base of the first toe distal phalanx. The EDL tendon diverges into separate tendinous slips in the anterior ankle, inserting on the dorsal aspect of the distal phalanges of toes 2 to 5.

Normal sonoanatomy
The AT and EDL are identified proximally in the anterior compartment as hypoechoic muscle bellies. Approximately halfway down the lower leg, the EHL muscle arises. As the tendons approach the superior extensor retinaculum, they hypoechoic muscles give way to hyperechoic, ovoid tendons, with the AT slightly larger than the EHL. The EDL begins to form into separate tendinous slips as it approaches the tibiotalar joint.

Patient positioning
- Supine, with the ankle comfortably plantarflexed.

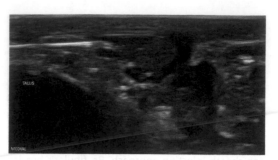

Fig. 17. AT tendon sheath injection approach.

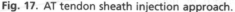

Approach
- In-plane, medial to lateral or lateral to medial for peritendinous injections (**Fig. 17**).
- Mixed in-plane/out-of-plane, distal to proximal for intratendinous injections.

Needle
- Gauge: 22 to 25.
- Length: 0.5 to 1.5in.

Injectate volume
- 1 to 3 mL.

Procedural considerations
- The positions of the SFN and DFN branches should be identified, as the SFN crosses the EHL and EDL, whereas the DFN courses deep to the EHL.

Plantar Fascia

The PF is a thick fascial band arising from the calcaneus, with terminal slips to the toes distally. It is composed of central and lateral cords and a much smaller medial band.

Normal sonoanatomy
The PF seems as a fibrillar, hyperechoic structure, which typically measures less than 4 mm thick at its origin.[13] The distal bands become thin and fan out, making the distal PF sometimes difficult to follow.

Patient positioning
- Prone, with the ankle comfortably plantarflexed.
- Alternatively, lateral decubitus, in neutral ankle position with the medial ankle facing the ceiling.

Approach
- In-plane, medial to lateral for the superficial target (**Fig. 18**A).
- Mixed in-plane/out-of-plane for the deep PF or intrafascial injections (**Fig. 18**B).

Needle
- Gauge: 22 to 27.
- Length: 1.25 to 2in.

Injectate volume
- 1 to 3 mL.

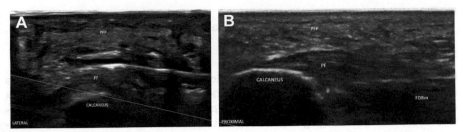

Fig. 18. PF injection approaches. (*A*) In-plane, superficial perifascial. (*B*). Out-of-plane, intra-fascial or deep perifascial. FDBm, flexor digitorum brevis muscle; PF, plantar fascia; PFP, plantar fat pad.

Procedural considerations
- A superficial PF injection target with corticosteroid faces the risk of atrophy of the plantar fat pad.

Retrocalcaneal Bursa

The retrocalcaneal bursa is a synovial lined space, bordered by the calcaneus, Kager's fat pad, and Achilles tendon.

Normal sonoanatomy
The retrocalcaneal bursa is a potential space and is not well visualized sonographically in the absence of bursal fluid. With dynamic motion, the differential motion among Kager's fat pad, the Achilles, and the calcaneus can identify this space. In the normal state, a small rim of anechoic fluid can be seen.

Patient positioning
- Prone, or side-lying.

Approach
- In-plane, medial to lateral or lateral to medial (**Fig. 19**).

Needle
- Gauge: 25 to 27.
- Length: 1.25 to 1.5in.

Injectate volume
- 0.5 to 2 mL

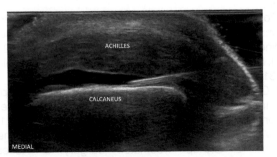

Fig. 19. Retrocalcaneal bursa injection approach.

Pearls/pitfalls
- The position of the tibial, medial calcaneal, and sural nerves must be considered.

SUMMARY

Foot and ankle pathologic condition is ubiquitous, and injection-based treatments are an effective, low risk, treatment option. A thorough understanding of the complex anatomy in this region is critical to ensure procedural accuracy. Due to the high-resolution, real-time imaging capabilities of US, it should be considered as a first-line imaging modality for procedural guidance, whereas fluoroscopy can also be considered for intra-articular injections.

CLINICS CARE POINTS

- Image-guided injections are more accurate and result in better clinical outcomes compared to palpation-guided injections.
- Although in-plane injections are preferred to out-of-plane due to easier needle tracking, an out-of-plane technique is often required due to the small joint spaces in the foot and ankle.
- Nonparticulate corticosteroids should be considered for perineural injections in order to reduce the risk of thromboembolic injury.
- Corticosteroids should never be injected directly into a tendon due to the risk of tendon rupture.

DISCLOSURES

The authors declare no conflicts of interest and do not have any financial disclosures relevant to this study.

REFERENCES

1. Jelsing E, Finnoff J. Efficacy of Ultrasound-Guided Corticosteroid Injections. Current Physical Medicine and Rehabilitation Reports 2016;4:132–7.
2. Kompel AJ, Roemer FW, Murakami AM, et al. Intra-articular corticosteroid injections in the hip and knee: perhaps not as safe as we thought? Radiology 2019; 293(3):656–63.
3. Bucci J, Chen X, LaValley M, et al. Progression of knee osteoarthritis with use of intraarticular glucocorticoids versus hyaluronic acid. Arthritis Rheumatol 2022; 74(2):223–6.
4. Vernese L, Pourcho A, Henning TP. Ultrasound-Guided Orthobiologics of the Foot and Ankle. In: El Miedany Y, editor. Musculoskeletal ultrasound-guided regenerative medicine. Cham: Springer International Publishing; 2022. p. 195–220.
5. Bartoníček J, Rammelt S, Naňka O. Anatomy of the Subtalar Joint. Foot Ankle Clin 2018;23(3):315–40.
6. Lektrakul N, Chung CB, Lai Y-m, et al. Tarsal Sinus: Arthrographic, MR Imaging, MR Arthrographic, and Pathologic Findings in Cadavers and Retrospective Study Data in Patients with Sinus Tarsi Syndrome. Radiology 2001;219(3):802–10.
7. Seringe R, Wicart P. The talonavicular and subtalar joints: The "calcaneopedal unit" concept. J Orthop Traumatol: Surgery & Research 2013;99(6, Supplement):S345–55.

8. Sammarco VJ. The talonavicular and calcaneocuboid joints: anatomy, biomechanics, and clinical management of the transverse tarsal joint. Foot Ankle Clin 2004;9(1):127–45.
9. Renner K, McAlister JE, Galli MM, et al. Anatomic Description of the Naviculocuneiform Articulation. J Foot Ankle Surg 2017;56(1):19–21.
10. Hansford BG, Mills MK, Stilwill SE, et al. Naviculocuneiform and Second and Third Tarsometatarsal Articulations: Underappreciated Normal Anatomy and How It May Affect Fluoroscopy-Guided Injections. Am J Roentgenol 2019; 212(4):874–82.
11. Presley JC, Maida E, Pawlina W, et al. Sonographic visualization of the first branch of the lateral plantar nerve (baxter nerve): technique and validation using perineural injections in a cadaveric model. J Ultrasound Med 2013;32(9): 1643–52.
12. Willegger M, Seyidova N, Schuh R, et al. The tibialis posterior tendon footprint: an anatomical dissection study. J Foot Ankle Res 2020;13(1):25.
13. Ahul K, Ozer D, Sakizlioglu SS, et al. Detection of normal plantar fascia thickness in adults via the ultrasonographic method. J Am Podiatr Med Assoc 2015; 105(1):8–13.

The Emerging Role of Automation, Measurement Standardization, and Artificial Intelligence in Foot and Ankle Imaging: An Update

Samir Ghandour, MD[a], Soheil Ashkani-Esfahani, MD[a,b,*,1],
John Y. Kwon, MD[a,b,1]

KEYWORDS

- Artificial intelligence • Computer-assisted image analysis • Deep learning
- Weight-bearing CT • Portable ultrasound

KEY POINTS

- New imaging technologies, though improved in quality, safety, accessibility, and software aspects, need to also consider the costs, accessibility for underprivileged areas, and include dynamic views in different planes particularly in foot and ankle.
- Standardization and calibration of the measurements and position of the patients while obtaining the images should be considered in developing imaging protocols.
- Educating the clinicians and imaging technicians can reduce the amount of bias and variances among the images making it easier to develop standardized databases for developing registry systems.
- Anapplication of artificial intelligence techniques needs large and granular data sets screened and annotated by expert and validated by externally.

INTRODUCTION

Advancements in medical imaging have escalated far beyond our imagination, especially during the past 2 decades with the development of various imaging techniques and modalities including MRI with different sequences, ultrasound (US) devices with

[a] Department of Orthopaedic Surgery, Foot & Ankle Research and Innovation Lab (FARIL), Massachusetts General Hospital, Harvard Medical School, FARIL Center, 158 Boston Post Road, Weston, MA 02493, USA; [b] Department of Orthopaedic Surgery, Foot and Ankle Center, Massachusetts General Hospital, Harvard Medical School, 52 2nd Avenue, Waltham, MA 02451, USA
[1] Co-senior authors, equal contribution.
* Corresponding author. Yawkey 3, 55 Fruit Street, Boston, MA 02114.
E-mail address: sashkaniesfahani@mgh.harvard.edu

Foot Ankle Clin N Am 28 (2023) 667–680
https://doi.org/10.1016/j.fcl.2023.04.006
1083-7515/23/© 2023 Elsevier Inc. All rights reserved.

Abbreviations	
ROC	Receiver Operating Characteristic
PCC	Pearson correlation coefficient

more accuracy and accessibility, PET with high sensitivity and precision, weight-bearing computed tomography (WBCT) with vivid three-dimensional (3D) views of the bilateral extremities, and many more technologies and modalities that improved orthopedic care mainly in the process of diagnosis and decision-making.[1] The detailed imaging of the structures of the foot and ankle is fundamental to understand the pathologies of various issues that arise in this region. Amid the exponential advances in clinical imaging, the hardware and software aspects of clinical imaging, there are still several rarely explored or even unexplored techniques that clinicians, especially in orthopedic surgery, need to surf and unveil.

In recent years, imaging in foot and ankle orthopedics has improved significantly, especially with the introduction of WBCT and portable handheld US that enables providers to examine the patient under physiologic load.[2] Imaging in weight-bearing conditions enables viewing the joints in their dynamic anatomic position shows the relationships among the structures and the distances better and helps clinicians in detecting pathologies and abnormalities with greater accuracy.[2] However, a concern among clinicians regarding interpretation techniques for these imaging methods is whether they should use the previous methods of measurement and diagnosis or new consensus, new methods of measurement, and new interpretation techniques for these advanced imaging technologies. Automation and computer-assisted image interpretation and measurements have been thought to be a great way of improving accuracy while saving time and effort among orthopedic providers, specifically in foot and ankle.[2,3] Other than numerous achievements in applying computer-assisted technologies and automated measurement methods in orthopedic practice, breakthroughs in the world of artificial intelligence (AI), machine learning (ML), and deep learning as a more recent achievement of AI technology are influencing and transforming the practice of imaging and image interpretation majorly.[4,5] AI has generally offered a broad range of applications to various fields in medical science, and orthopedics is on the ever-expanding list. Not only it assists in the meticulous evaluation of radiological images but also supports the training of surgical residents and can even perform excellent machine-assisted decision-making and treatment of orthopedic patients.[6] Moreover, with the new technologies come new needs for developing diagnostic methods, consensus and cut-off values for measurements, and educating providers to incorporate these methods in their practice to improve the quality of health care. Given the new imaging technologies introduced to foot and ankle orthopedic practice, including WBCT and the portable US, the aim of this study is to highlight the applications, achievements, methods of diagnosis, challenges, and unmet needs in incorporating AI and computer-assisted decision-making in foot and ankle imaging. The authors explore literature reporting the use of automated measurement and interpretation, the methods of standardization of the measurements, the use of AI and ML, and methods of computer-assisted decision-making in foot and ankle imaging.

METHODS

The literature acquisition and selection were conducted in accordance with PRISMA guidelines. A thorough search was conducted using PubMed/Medline and PubMed

Central databases using keywords, as summarized in **Table 1**. The authors also performed cross-referencing of the primarily searched studies to collect further related articles as a secondary search. The inclusion criteria used for selection of the studies were (1) original articles (clinical trials, retrospectives, prospective studies, case-control studies, cohort studies); (2) reporting the applications and the use of new imaging technologies incorporating AI, computer-assisted solutions, and methods of standardization in foot and ankle as described in **Table 1**; (3) appropriate population of adult patients, data analysis, and statistical methods; and (4) published in the past 5 years. Studies that did not have an appropriate population or data analysis methods, systematic and literature reviews, case reports, editorials, and book chapters were excluded. Duplicates were also assessed and removed. The outcome of the literature search was assessed by two expert orthopedic clinical researchers first by their titles and abstracts, and those who were found to be appropriate were then screened by the full text and were included in this review if they met the inclusion/exclusion criteria. The included studies were then classified based on the imaging modality that was used, including CT scan, x-ray, and US, and the results are discussed under their related subheadings. To keep the record of the literature included, a spreadsheet was created that included the name of the first author, publication year, title, study population, imaging modality used in the study, new technologies that were reported in the study, and outcome summary. The authors divided the studies based on the imaging modalities they used in their methodologies to the following subheadings for further discussion: (1) Radiography in Foot and Ankle, (2) CT scan in Foot and Ankle, (3) US in Foot and Ankle, and (4) Other imaging modalities. The authors discussed the advances of each of these modalities subsequently under these subheadings.

Table 1
The search strategy was used to obtain the literature from PubMed/Medline and PubMed Central databases

Terms	Variations (Separated by OR)
Foot/ankle	Foot, foot joints, foot injuries, foot diseases, foot bones, ankle, ankle joint, ankle injuries, ankle fractures
[AND]	
Artificial intelligence/computer-assisted interpretations/standardization	Artificial intelligence, machine intelligence, computational intelligence, machine learning, supervised-machine learning, unsupervised machine learning, automation, pattern recognition, automated, automatic data processing, radiographic image interpretation, computer-assisted image processing, computer-assisted image interpretation, computer-assisted, diagnosis, computer-assisted decision-making, computer-assisted standardization, standards, reference, consensus, clinical alarms
[AND]	
Imaging techniques	Cone-beam computed tomography, computed tomography, x-ray, diagnostic imaging, ultrasonography, diagnostic ultrasound

MeSH keywords were used in this search strategy, and different variations of each term were entered in the search algorithm.

DISCUSSION
Radiography in Foot and Ankle

Although radiography and x-ray imaging have assisted foot and ankle health care providers for a long time, efforts to improve the quality of images, the accuracy, and speed of interpretation are still ongoing. The importance of imaging under physiologic weight-bearing has been emphasized for a long time by various investigators.[7,8] Many researchers have tried to introduce new measurement methods for the diagnosis of foot and ankle pathologies using weight-bearing radiographs as that condition exposes the different bones, joints, ligaments, and muscles of the lower extremity to physiologic stressors, allowing health care providers to better characterize and evaluate their pathologies.[7,9] A study on the influence of percentage weight-bearing on foot radiographs found that when body weight percentage was increased, the talonavicular coverage angle and talocalcaneal angle increased while the cuboid height to ground decreased significantly; however, there were no differences in hallux valgus angle (HVA), 1 to 2 intermetatarsal angle (IMA), forefoot width, LisFranc distance, and talo-first metatarsal angle. Shelton and colleagues postulate that these figures reveal a flattening of the medial arch, increasing hindfoot, valgus, and midfoot external rotation and abduction when body weight percentage applied to a foot is increased.[10] Miller and colleagues assessed the accuracy of weight-bearing radiographs on ankle and foot, hypothesizing that patients only place 50% of their body weight on the affected foot during imaging. However, the findings illustrated significant variability in the actual weight patients applied, raising questions about reliability when it comes to assessment of weight-bearing radiographs, and providing future ground work for research on the accuracy of this imaging method and the need for calibration.[11] Consequently, in a review of 31 studies on various measurement methods in weight-bearing radiography of foot and ankle, the need for standardization and calibration and the necessity of defining reference values for anatomic measurement have been emphasized on and given as recommendation for future research in this field.[12]

It is assumed that using computer-assisted measurements, automated measurements, and AI in conducting measurements and interpreting radiographs can not only improve the accuracy and speed of diagnosis but also improve the reproducibility of the techniques and interobserver agreement. Measurement automation can also help providers analyze larger data sets in a shorter amount of time and base the new reference values for each measurement on a larger and more reliable data set. Using computer-assisted methods and AI, Lauder and colleagues led a pilot study attempting to develop a software capable of fully automating radiographic measurements associated with foot collapse, including Meary's angle, Cuboid height, and Calcaneal tilt. The investigators proposed that the discussed measurements can be produced automatically and without human input in less than a minute[6] compared with an average of 667 seconds required to take the same measurements manually.[13] With the values of 2.4 and 3.6 for the calcaneal tilt and cuboid height, respectively, the variance between the experts was found to be insignificant as well as the percentage of variance that the experts contributed (10%) for all measurements. The intraclass correlation estimates are between 0.78 and 0.86. The investigators found no discernible difference between the manual geometric measurements and the derived geometric measurements computed, suggesting that the fully automatic system provides an unbiased estimate for these measurements and is in agreement with the observers with a strong correlation between the manual and the automatically derived measurements (PCC = 0.71, PCC = 0.84, and PCC = 0.82 for calcaneal tilt, cuboid height, and Meary's angle, respectively).[6] According to the software developers, this software plays an important role in diagnosing mild Charcot neuroarthropathy cases early and monitoring the progression of moderate Charcot neuroarthropathy cases. Pei and colleagues found a high feasibility and reliability modality for the automated measurement of the hip-knee-ankle (HKA) axis using deep-learning x-rays; The automatically calculated HKA using the suggested technique (176.41° ± 12.08°) was statistically close to the ground truth with no significant deviation. Also, the technique's intraclass correlation coefficient (ICC) is 0.99 ($P < .001$). The average angle of deviation between prediction and reality is 0.49°. This approach suggests a high degree of reliability and feasibility in clinical settings.[14] New research has also set about to create an automated modality to determine the calcaneal-fifth metatarsal angle on weight-bearing lateral foot radiographs. In this regard, Koo and colleagues found that their recommended method automatically measuring Meary's angle and calcaneal pitch can potentially and competently support doctors in the measurement of arch angles on weight-bearing lateral foot radiographs for the evaluation of pes planus. The calculated ICC for the algorithm and human-determined Meary's angle and calcaneal pitch measurements was 0.89 (95% CI 0.82–0.94) and 0.992 (95% CI 0.98–0.99), respectively. Regarding interobserver agreement, ICC with algorithms for Meary's angle and calcaneal pitch showed a statistically significant increase ($P < .001$) compared with ICC without algorithms. Combining all of the reader data reveals that the Meary angle ICC without algorithms was 0.815 (95% CI 0.78–0.85) and ICC with algorithms was 0.896 28 (95% CI 0.87–0.92), significantly higher ($P < .0001$) with algorithm use than without. Regarding calcaneal pitch, the ICC resulting from the combination of all three readers without algorithms was 0.963 (CI: 0.95–0.97) and ICC with algorithms was 0.97 (0.97–0.98), significantly higher ($P = .002$) with algorithm use than without.[15]

With advances in AI and particularly deep learning, foot and ankle investigators have also tried to implement these technologies into their practice. Kitamura and colleagues set out to create and train de novo an ankle fracture detection ML ensemble model using both one and three radiographic views from a total of 596 normal and abnormal ankle cases that were collected and processed, comparing their ensemble model's accuracy to preexisting pretrained models that used larger data sets (using up to ~256,000 wrist, hand, and ankle radiographs) and required manual feature engineering. The investigators found that their ensemble models reached an up to 81% accuracy, 80% sensitivity, 88% specificity, 85% positive predictive value (PPV), and 81% negative predictive value (NPV) when three-view radiographs were used, higher than when the ensemble models used one-view radiographs and in line with the accuracy of other models using a much higher number of cases and implementing manual feature extraction.[16] In an evaluation of the performance of two different (Inception V3 and Resnet-50) deep convolutional neural networks (DCNN), using radiographs obtained from 1050 patients with ankle fractures and 1050 healthy controls, in detecting ankle fractures, Ashkani-Esfahani and colleagues discovered that the DCNNs displayed a better performance using three-view images compared with single-view images, achieving 99% sensitivity, 99% specificity, 99% PPV, 99% NPV, 99% F-score, 99% area under the ROC curve (AUC) with the Inception V3 model.[17] The aforementioned studies highlight not only the power of AI in ankle detection but also the importance of using multiple views to train the associated models. In assessing a new AI-based automatic measurement tool for the IMA in hallux valgus (HV) from Digitally Reconstructed Radiographs (DRRs) under weight-bearing, Day and colleagues found that the software is capable of reliably discriminating patients with HV from controls, discovering that there were significant intermethod correlations between the DRR IMA and the auto two-dimensional (2D) (HV, r = 0.61; control, r = 0.60; all P < .001) and auto 3D (HV, r = 0.63; control, r = 0.52; all P < .001) measurements, respectively, reaching near 100% intermethod reproducibility within the software. The automated measurements also improved measurement speeds compared with manual measurements, as those measurements took 23.6 ± 2.31 seconds and 14.5 ± 1.18 seconds, respectively.[18] Ashkani-Esfahani and colleagues have also demonstrated a great performance of deep learning methods and DCNNs in detecting subtle Lisfranc instabilities on radiographs. They used a population of 640 patients with Lisfranc malalignments and showed that the DCNN trained on this database can detect Lisfranc malalignment with 94.8% sensitivity, 96.9% specificity, 98.6% accuracy, 95.8% F-score, and 99.4% AUC. Their model outperformed the clinicians by reducing the rate of misdiagnosis by 10%.[19] Despite the promising potential of computer-assisted image analysis and AI-based methods, one of the main concerns in developing these solutions is the size, validity, and reliability of the data sets given to the machine. These data have to be screened, annotated, and labeled by expert clinicians. The larger the data sets are, the more accurate the solution can become. Moreover, most of these models have to be externally validated and the granularity of the data sets plays a significant role in the success of these models in external validation on various populations.

Computed Tomography of Foot and Ankle

Although CT scan has been the gold standard for detecting bone traumas and fractures with a high accuracy and sensitivity, adding weight-bearing component to it and developing WBCT has promoted the quality and accuracy of diagnosis to a great extent, particularly for subtle injuries and joint instabilities.[4,20] Lawlor and colleagues investigated the use of WBCT, compared with gravity stress radiographs and gravity stress CT, for the detection of ankle instability after supination external rotation (SER) ankle fractures. In this cadaver study on ten specimens, six with stable and four with unstable ankles, they used medial clear space (MCS) ≥ 0.5 mm as a threshold for instability. Before inducing the fracture, imaging on the specimens was done to serve as the control group. Despite the small sample size, the investigators found that MCS measurements between stable and unstable SER were significantly different in the WBCT experimental group (P = .02) while among other groups. Only the controls that underwent gravity stress radiographs showed a significant difference between stable and unstable ankles (P = .04). WBCT performance in detecting instability of the ankle after SER fracture was shown to be better compared with gravity stress radiographs and non-weight-bearing CT scan.[21] Willey and colleagues, in a study on 20 patients with intra-articular tibial pilon fractures, reported that a significant loss of joint space (21% average) can be seen 6 months after the injury on bilateral WBCT images when comparing the injured and uninjured ankles.[22] They tried to develop a simple, standardized, and reliable method to quantify tibiotalar joint space narrowing after tibial pilon fracture on WBCT. Analysis showed that the middle-lateral and middle-central regions of the ankle joint had the greatest decrease in space with an ICC of 88%, and the test–retest reproducibility of 80%. Reviewing these reports on various aspects of ankle fracture assessment shows that WBCT has added a great value to the diagnostic and decision-making processes, whereas research and development still needs to go on to reveal further application of this new modality.

Using WBCT to assess ankle syndesmotic instability, Malhotra and colleagues in their efforts to shed light on the difference weight-bearing causes in the anatomy of the syndesmosis on imaging, compared WBCT with conventional CTs and reported that weight-bearing results in lateral and posterior translation and external rotation of the fibula in relation to the incisura.[2] In a cadaver study by Krähenbühl and colleagues, it was shown that torque application helps to diagnose incomplete syndesmotic injuries on WBCT. The tibiofibular overlap was reported to be a good measure for identifying incomplete syndesmotic injuries, whereas the MCS and tibiofibular clear space could indicate more complete injuries.[23] Patel and colleagues used bilateral WBCT to determine reference values for syndesmotic instability diagnosis and also to see if there is any difference between males and females.[24] They suggested 5.3 mm as the upper limit of lateral translation in uninjured ankles as the threshold for detecting syndesmotic injury. Other measurements including anteroposterior translation (ranged 0.31–2.59 and −1.48–3.44 mm, respectively) and the difference between right and left ankles were not considerable. Increasing age was correlated in their results with a reduction in lateral translation. Hagemeijer and colleagues investigated the usefulness of area measurement at the level of 1 cm proximal to the tibial plafond for detecting instability. They showed that all the values including area, anterior, middle, and posterior differences, and sagittal translation differed significantly between the healthy and unhealthy ankles of the patients who had unilateral syndesmotic instability confirmed intraoperatively ($P < .001$).[25] In another study by Elghazy and colleagues, WBCT was used to assess the quality of reduction comparing suture buttons with screw fixation of the syndesmosis. Their study showed insufficient reduction of the syndesmosis in both groups based on the area of the syndesmosis measurement in WBCT, whereas the surgeon seemed satisfied with the reduction after the surgery.[26] Later, in a study by Bhimani and colleagues, 3D volume measurement of syndesmosis was proposed using bilateral WBCT images. They reported that 3D volume measurement of the syndesmosis up to 5 cm proximal to the tibial plafond has a higher accuracy and reliability compared with area and distance measurements suggested in previous studies.[27] The same group in another study assessing the ability of WBCT to diagnose syndesmotic instability among patients with unilateral Weber B ankle fractures (with a symmetric MCS) found that it can be effective and successful. When detecting instability, 3D volume measurements are more sensitive than conventional distance measurements; they should be taken up to a height of 5 cm above the tibial plafond. The research ascertained that the 3D volume measurements used in WBCT have higher sensitivity than traditional distance measurements but must be measured to a height of 5 cm above the tibial plafond. According to ROC curve analysis, the distal tibiofibular articulation's 3D volume assessed on WBCT from the plafond to a height of 5 cm proximally had an AUC of 0.96 (95% confidence interval: 0.85–1.0), indicating a highly effective diagnostic test.[28] Ashkani-Esfahani and colleagues agree that measurement must be taken up to 5 cm proximal to the plafond, concluding that 3D volume measurements on weight-bearing CT are also capable of diagnosing syndesmotic instability, especially for subtle injured ankle cases that are hard to detect, using conventional diagnostic methods with 95.8% sensitivity and 83.3% specificity. The research proved this by successfully superimposing the 3D model of the injured side on the uninjured contralateral side, which gave them the ability to visualize the pattern of changes in different planes.[17] Guss and colleagues introduced a new standardized method of measurement and bilateral comparison using percentage of changes instead of direct measurement and the use of cutoff values. They introduced a new cutoff value (25.4%) for percentage of changes in the measurement of syndesmotic 3D volume. In the next steps, these researchers tried to automate the process of volume measurement on WBCT images of the syndesmosis and reported 99% inter-rater agreement using the computer-assisted measurement compared with 75% among clinicians.[29] The time consumed for each 3D volume measurement by the automated method was 2.9 $\pm$ 0.3 seconds compared with

268.4 ± 56.4 seconds among the clinicians showing a significant amount of time saved using automated methods. Borjali and colleagues later used DCNNs to improve the accuracy of syndesmotic instability diagnosis using bilateral WBCT images. In their efforts to develop an accurate model with a higher F1-score, they introduced a combination of DCNN and long-short-term memory DCNN that outperformed the clinicians by an accuracy of 93%, F1-score of 91%, sensitivity of 100%, and specificity of 90%. However, their sample size ($n = 144$) was a limitation to their great performance and the need for training these models on larger sample sizes still remains.[30]

Other applications of WBCT for foot pathologies that were investigated in the past years also include assessing the Lisfranc joint for instability, particularly in subtle cases with isolated ligament injuries. In this regard, research by Sripanich and colleagues proposed that coronal WBCT imaging, used through a protocol that localizes the interosseous Lisfranc ligament (ILL), is a potential new clinical method for the measurement of C1–C2 distance in Lisfranc joints that is simple and reproducible. After analyzing the reproducibility and reliability of two different methods (parameter I vs parameter II) and two different planes (coronal vs axial) to localize the ILL, the investigators found C1–M2 distance measurement as the most reliable parameter on coronal images which showed R values of 0.81 for interobserver and 0.84 for intraobserver reliability.[31] Bhimani and colleagues confirmed that the WBCT scan could successfully discern between stable and unstable Lisfranc injuries and postulated that this method's success has high clinical implications for diagnosing Lisfranc instability. All WBCT readings (Lisfranc joint medial cuneiform-base of second metatarsal area, C1–C2 intercuneiform area, C1–M2 distance, C1–C2 distance, M1–M2 distance, first tarsometatarsal [TMT1] angular alignment, second tarsometatarsal [TMT2] angular alignment, TMT1 dorsal step off distance, and TMT2 dorsal step off distance along with the volume of the Lisfranc joint in the coronal and axial plane) were higher on the injured side than the contralateral uninjured side in patients with unilateral Lisfranc instability ($P = .001–.008$). Compared with 2D and 1D Lisfranc joint assessments, volumetric measurements in the coronal and axial planes demonstrated higher sensitivity (92.3% and 91.6%, respectively) and specificity (97.7% and 96.5%, respectively); this suggests that they are the most accurate in identifying Lisfranc instability.[32] Our recent experience with the use of deep learning to improve the accuracy of Lisfranc instability diagnosis on WBCT has shown the potential of developing a model with an accuracy, F1-score, sensitivity, and specificity of over 90%; however, the results highly rely on the sample size and our aim is to increase the sample size to produce a more valid and reliable method for publication and use in practice as a decision assistant. Applications of WBCT were also investigated in other foot conditions. Sangoi and colleagues created a novel approach using computer-assisted 3D axis calculation on foot WBCT that allowed for more accurate assessment of foot alignment or deformity when compared with 2D manual measurements, showing ICC greater than 0.996 for all measurements. Significant variations in calcaneal pitch and Meary's angle were seen in the sagittal plane in Charcot-Marie-Tooth (CMT) cavovarus foot. In comparison to manual 2D measurements, the automated 3D values measured, respectively, 2.42° and 7.29° more. The automated 3D group's talar-first metatarsal angle was on average 10.61° lower (ie, less adducted foot) than the manual 2D groups in the axial plane of CMT cavovarus feet. This technique is proposed to play a role in accurately assessing and evaluating the cavovarus foot, which may inform further treatment algorithms.[33] Bernasconi and colleagues found that, with the exception of the forefoot arch angle, 2D measures between CMT pes cavus and idiopathic pes cavus were not significantly different ($P = .04$). Also, CMT pes cavus had a more severe hindfoot varus malalignment than idiopathic pes cavus, according to 3D measures of the foot and ankle offset, calcaneal offset, and hindfoot alignment angle (P = .03, .04, and 0.02, respectively).[34] De Cesar Netto and colleagues found not only that using 3D WBCT to characterize the valgus hindfoot alignment in patients with adult acquired flatfoot deformity was more reliable and repeatable, but also that the acquired measurements using this method were significantly different as well from clinical evaluation of hindfoot alignment. This proposed method showed overall substantial to almost perfect intra-(range: 0.87–0.97) and interobserver agreements (range: 0.51–0.88) for all 3D WBCT measurements, enabling clinicians to standardize hindfoot alignment measurements in these patients and therefore improve their long-term care and follow-up.[35] However, no comparison of this method's measurements with a ground truth was performed. More distal to the hindfoot while working on HV, in a study comparing WBCT semiautomatic and manual measurements of HVA and IMA, De Carvalho and colleagues found that the semiautomatic measurements were reproducible as well as capable of differentiating pathologic from non-pathologic conditions when measuring the HVA and IMA (P < .05).[36] As the reliability and applications of these tools on WBCT expands, automatic measurements will not only improve treating physician efficiency but also lead to greater strides to measurement standardization and repeatability.

In attempts to improve the quality of CT imaging, introduction of a hybrid imaging modality in nuclear medicine called single-photon emission CT (SPECT-CT) has led to solutions correcting for signal attenuation in the images via SPECT while still maintaining the 3D imaging capabilities of CT scan. SPECT-CT offers a higher spatial resolution as well as a greater sensitivity and accuracy compared with conventional CT, particularly for evaluation of degenerative changes, inflammatory conditions, benign, and malignant lesions.[37] Claassen and colleagues found that SPECT-CT had not only higher inter-rater and intra-rater diagnostic reliability (kappa values for inter-rater reliability were higher for SPECT-CT at 0.68 and MRI + SPECT-CT at 0.71 compared with 0.38 for MRI alone [P < .05]) but also a great impact on final treatment decisions for various complex foot and ankle pathologies. They proposed that the main indications for SPECT-CT over MRI alone are bony pathologies with diagnostic uncertainty, especially in compacted structures such as the joints of the midfoot, occult coalitio, stress fractures, verification or exclusion of nonfusion, periprosthetic disorders after total ankle replacement, and osteochondral lesions in cases of combined pathologies.[38] Toward further modifying CT imaging to improve the quality while lowering the radiation risks, Alagic and colleagues set out to assess the clinical usefulness of ultra-low-dose CT (ULD-CT) as an alternative to DRRs in the evaluation of acute ankle fractures, among others. In 203 extremities, DRR and ULD-CT detected 73 and 109 fractures, respectively (P < .001). They found that ULD-CT detects significantly more fractures than DRR and provides additional clinically relevant data at a comparable radiation dose when compared with DRR (DRR 0.59 $\pm$ 0.33 μSv, 95% CI 0.47–0.59 vs ULD-CT 0.53 $\pm$ 0.43 μSv, 95% CI 0.54–0.64). The investigators also found that ULD-CT provides faster examination and reporting times, accelerating the delivery of care to these acute patients (ULD-CT 7.6 $\pm$ 2.5 minute, 95% CI 7.1–8.1 vs DRR 9.8 $\pm$ 4.7 minute, 95% CI 8.8–10.7; P = .002).[39] Although most of these modalities are promising, investigators have insisted on the need for standardization of the measurement methods and diagnostic protocols as well as calibrations with the aim of increasing the validity, reliability, and reproducibility of these diagnostic imaging technique.

Ultrasonography and Other Imaging Techniques in Foot and Ankle

US has always been a favorable imaging tool as it provides a good to perfect accuracy in detecting several pathologies, especially soft tissue and ligament injuries, and is used for various therapeutic injections and diagnostic aspirations, whereas it has no risk of radiation or other adverse effects on the patient. Recent developments in the realm of US imaging were more focused on the accessibility and accuracy of imaging.[40,41] Researchers and clinicians have conducted several studies on the use of portable handheld US in detecting foot and ankle pathologies.[40] Saengsin and colleagues in a cadaver study compared the measurement of MCS on SER ankle fractures on fluoroscopy versus a portable handheld US device.[42] The US values showed a moderate to strong positive correlation with fluoroscopy (P values <0.001). Inter-rater (US: 0.97, 95%CI: 0.96–0.98) and intra-rater reliability (US: 0.95, 95%CI: 0.94–0.96) were excellent. Saengsin and colleagues also introduced MCS optimal cutoff point to distinguish SER ankle injury stage IVb from other injury stages ranged from 10.4 to 13.8 during the gravity stress test, 4.2 to 7.9 during weight-bearing, and 10.6 to 17.9 during the external rotation stress test with a sensitivity of 60% to 100%, specificity of 84% to 100%, and AUC of 80% to 100%.[42] They suggested portable handheld US with stress examination as a radiation-free, noninvasive, accessible, and low-cost tool to detect medial ankle instability. The same group of researchers also showed the usefulness of portable US for the assessment of syndesmotic instability in cadaver models with good to excellent interobserver and intraobserver reliability.[43] Saengsin and his team also used the portable US for assessment of lateral ankle instability compared with fluoroscopy and showed excellent interobserver and intraobserver agreement using both methods (P < .05). They showed that US could assist the clinicians in measuring the anterior drawer and talar tilt tests first performed with all lateral ligaments intact and then with sequential transection of the anterior talofibular ligament, calcaneofibular, and posterior talofibular ligament.[44]

Ultrasonography and WBCT were not the only imaging modalities that were subject to hardware and software advances. Given the importance of dynamic imaging under physiologic weight for detection of foot and ankle conditions, especially subtle ones, research done by Gunio and colleagues on suspected Lisfranc joint injuries and instability focused on using an MRI-compatible, joint-specific foot stressor device engineered to replicate weight-bearing conditions, finding that the device was able to consistently generate stress-induced changes in the joint during the process of the MRI when comparing morphologically known normal and abnormal ligaments. Also, the certain degree of ligament injury and accompanying joint instability in Lisfranc joint injuries was revealed by the stress-induced alterations in the midfoot. Moreover, compared with chronic injuries, acute-to-subacute injuries showed more inducible alterations under stress (P = .047).[45] Compared with other weight-bearing imaging modalities, soft tissue pathologies can be remarkably accentuated and hence more adequately outlined by radiologists using weight-bearing MRI. The idea of adding weight-bearing component has been mentioned by several researchers but perhaps due to technical limitations and barriers this has not been widely developed and investigated by orthopedic providers and researchers.[12] This implies the need for future research on the applications of weight-bearing along with computer-assisted measurement and decision-making models to foot and ankle MRI that will potentially expand our understanding of ligamentous and other soft tissue diseases.

CONCLUSION AND FUTURE DIRECTIONS

Further research conducted with the aim of developing advanced imaging techniques and modalities will tremendously improve the accuracy, indications, standard values, and detection of foot and ankle pathologies along with their associated imaging characterizations. On weight-bearing, it seems that the imaging condition with the advent of AI tools is allowing us to observe more insightful dimensions that allow orthopedists and radiologists to more accurately, efficiently, safely, and economically deliver targeted care to their patients. In addition, automation will curb the measurement variability and boost its reliability as standardization will become inevitable.

Our review highlights advantageous emerging developments in foot and ankle imaging, concluding that there are wide and promising applications of AI and computer-assisted measurements and decision-making, that could substantially improve orthopedic health care for patients. Moreover, as the use of the contralateral uninjured side for comparison is provided by today's bilateral radiographs and WBCT, calibration, and standardization of the measurements and comparisons using the uninjured side of the same patient as the control, can lead to a more specific and reliable method of diagnosis and can be even useful for postoperative assessment of the quality of treatment. Last, to improve the accuracy and reliability of AI-based methods, developing larger data sets screened and annotated by highly skilled clinicians is of great necessity and important and should be considered by health care settings.

CLINICS CARE POINTS

- When obtaining weight-bearing dynamic images, make sure that the patient is in a standard and balanced position, particularly if obtaining bilateral images.

- Incorporating AI into practice will need knowledge on how the AI models were developed and on what database, thus, before deciding to use any AI-based decision-support tool, ask about the size of the database, validity, and reliability of the database and its developers, and ask for explainable AI protocols that show how the model makes the decision and is not based on a "black box."

- Portable ultrasound devices can detect ligament injuries, but the current devices have limitation in the viewing field and might not cover the gaps between to two ends of the tendons, that is, Achilles tendon, and this might need further assessment and might increase the chance of missing the injury under the probe.

CONTRIBUTION OF EACH AUTHOR

S. Ghandour: Literature search and acquisition, literature screening, drafting the manuscript, editing, and finalizing the manuscript. S.A. Esfahani: Study design, drafting, and editing the manuscript, finalizing the manuscript. J.Y. Kwon: Study design, editing the manuscript, finalizing the manuscript.

DECLARATION OF COMPETING INTEREST

None.

ACKNOWLEDGMENTS

The authors would like to thank Ms Ghalia Al-Alwani, for helping in literature review, obtaining the literature, and proof-reading the manuscript. Also, they would like to thank Dr Noor Nassour for her guidance during the literature acquisition process.

REFERENCES

1. Scatliff JH, Morris PJ. From Roentgen to magnetic resonance imaging: the history of medical imaging. N C Med J 2014;75(2):111–3.

2. Malhotra K., Welck M., Cullen N., et al., The effects of weight bearing on the distal tibiofibular syndesmosis: A study comparing weight bearing-CT with conventional CT, *Foot Ankle Surg*, 25 (4), 2019, 511–516.

3. Mohaideen K, Negi A, Verma DK, et al. Current understanding on artificial intelligence and machine learning in orthopedics - A scoping review. J Orthop 2022;34:201–6.

4. Lintz F., Beaudet P., Richardi G., et al., Weight-bearing CT in foot and ankle pathology, *Orthop Traumatol Surg Res*, 107 (1S), 2021, 102772.

5. Liew C. The future of radiology augmented with Artificial Intelligence: A strategy for success. Eur J Radiol 2018;102:152–0.

0. Lauder J, Harris J, Layton B, et al. A fully automatic system to assess foot collapse on lateral weight-bearing foot radiographs: A pilot study. Comput Methods Progr Biomed 2022;213:106507.

7. Carrara C., Caravaggi P., Belvedere C., et al., Radiographic angular measurements of the foot and ankle in weight-bearing: A literature review, *Foot Ankle Surg*, 26 (5), 2020, 509–517.

8. Wagner P, Lescure N, Siddiqui N, et al. Validity and Reliability of a New Radiological Method to Estimate Medial Column Internal Rotation, *Hallux Valgus Using Foot Weight-Bearing X-Ray*. Foot Ankle Spec 2021. https://doi.org/10.1177/19386400211029162. 19386400211029162.

9. Amin A., Janney C., Sheu C., et al., Weight-Bearing Radiographic Analysis of the Tibiofibular Syndesmosis, *Foot Ankle Spec*, 12 (3), 2019, 211–217.

10. Shelton T.J., Singh S., Robinson E.B., et al., The Influence of Percentage Weight-Bearing on Foot Radiographs, *Foot Ankle Spec*, 12 (4), 2019, 363–369.

11. Miller CP, Ghorbanhoseini M, Ehrlichman LK, et al. High Variability of Observed Weight Bearing During Standing Foot and Ankle Radiographs. Foot Ankle Int 2017;38(6):690–3.

12. Bruno F, Arrigoni F, Palumbo P, et al. Weight-bearing MR Imaging of Knee, Ankle and Foot. Semin Muscoskel Radiol 2019;23(6):594–602.

13. Nitris L, Varfolomeeva A, BLinov D, et al. Artificial Intelligence-Based Solution for x-Ray Longitudinal Flatfoot Determination and Scaling. Imag Med 2019;11:6.

14. Pei Y., Yang W., Shangqing W., et al., Automated measurement of hip-knee-ankle angle on the unilateral lower limb X-rays using deep learning, *Phys Eng Sci Med*, 44 (1), 2021, 53–62.

15. Koo J., Hwang S., Han S.H., et al., Deep learning-based tool affects reproducibility of pes planus radiographic assessment, *Sci Rep*, 12 (1), 2022, 12891.

16. Kitamura G., Chung C.Y., Moore B.E., Ankle Fracture Detection Utilizing a Convolutional Neural Network Ensemble Implemented with a Small Sample, De Novo Training, and Multiview Incorporation, *J Digit Imag*, 32 (4), 2019, 672–677.

17. Ashkani-Esfahani S, Yazidi RM, Bhimani R, et al. Detection of ankle fractures using deep learning algorithms. Foot Ankle Surg 2022;S1268-7731(22) 00102-00103..

18. Day J., de Cesar Netto C., Richter M., et al., Evaluation of a weightbearing CT artificial intelligence-based automatic measurement for the M1-M2 intermetatarsal angle in Hallux Valgus, *Foot Ankle Int*, 42 (11), 2021, 1502–1509.

19. Ashkani-Esfahani S., Mojahed-Yazidi R., Bhimani R., et al., Deep Learning Algorithms Improve the Detection of Subtle Lisfranc Malalignments on Weightbearing Radiographs, *Foot Ankle Int*, 43 (8), 2022, 1118–1126.

20. Conti MS, Scott JE. Weight-bearing CT Scans in Foot and Ankle Surgery. J Am Acad Orthop Surg 2020;28(14):e595–603.

21. Lawlor M.C., Kluczynski M.A., Marzo J.M., et al., Weight-Bearing Cone-Beam CT Scan Assessment of Stability of Supination External Rotation Ankle Fractures in a Cadaver Model, *Foot Ankle Int*, 39 (7), 2018, 850–857.

22. Willey M.C., Compton J.T., Marsh, J.L., et al., Weight-Bearing CT Scan After Tibial Pilon Fracture Demonstrates Significant Early Joint-Space Narrowing, *J Bone Joint Surg*, 102 (9), 2020, 796–803.

23. Krähenbühl N., Bailey T.L., Presson A.P., et al., Torque application helps to diagnose incomplete syndesmotic injuries using weight-bearing computed tomography images, *Skeletal Radiol*, 48 (9), 2019, 1367–1376.

24. Patel S., Malhotra K., Cullen N.P., et al., Defining reference values for the normal tibiofibular syndesmosis in adults using weight-bearing CT, *Bone & Joint J*, 101-B (3), 2019, 348–352.

25. Hagemeijer N.C., Chang S.H., Abdelaziz M.E., et al., Range of Normal and Abnormal Syndesmotic Measurements Using Weightbearing CT, *Foot Ankle Int*, 40 (12), 2019, 1430–1437.

26. Elghazy M.A., Hagemeijer N.C., Guss D., et al., Screw versus suture button in treatment of syndesmosis instability: Comparison using weightbearing CT scan, *Foot Ankle Surg*, 27 (3), 2021, 285–290.

27. Bhimani R., Ashkani-Esfahani S., Lubberts B., et al., Utility of Volumetric Measurement via Weight-Bearing Computed Tomography Scan to Diagnose Syndesmotic Instability, *Foot Ankle Int*, 41 (7), 2020, 859–865.

28. Bhimani R., Ashkani-Esfahani S., Lubberts B., et al., Utility of WBCT to Diagnose Syndesmotic Instability in Patients with Weber B Lateral Malleolar Fractures, *J Am Acad Orthop Surg*, 30 (3), 2022, e423–e433.

29. Guss D., Lucchese O., Ashkani-Esfahani S., et al., Automated Volume Measurement of the Syndesmosis Using 3D Weightbearing CT, *Foot & Ankle Orthopaedics*, 7, 2022, 1, 2473011421S00031.

30. Borjali A., Chen A.F., Muratoglu O.K., et al., Detecting total hip replacement prosthesis design on plain radiographs using deep convolutional neural network. *J Orthop Res*, 38(7), 2020, 1465-1471.

31. Sripanich Y., Weinberg M.W., Krähenbühl N., et al., Reliability of measurements assessing the Lisfranc joint using weightbearing computed tomography imaging, *Arch Orthop Trauma Surg*, 141 (5), 2021, 775–781.

32. Bhimani R., Sornsakrin O.P., Ashkani-Esfahani S., et al., Using area and volume measurement via weightbearing CT to detect Lisfranc instability, *J Orthop Res*, 39 (11), 2021, 2497–2505.

33. Sangoi D., Ranjit S., Bernasconi A., et al., 2D Manual vs 3D automated assessment of alignment in normal and Charcot-Marie-Tooth Cavovarus feet using weightbearing CT, *Foot Ankle Int*, 43 (7), 2022, 973–982.

34. Bernasconi A., Cooper L., Lyle S., et al., Pes cavovarus in Charcot-Marie-Tooth compared to the idiopathic cavovarus foot: A preliminary weightbearing CT analysis, *Foot Ankle Surg*, 27 (2), 2021, 186–195.

35. De Cesar Netto C., Shakoor D., Roberts L., et al., Hindfoot alignment of adult acquired flatfoot deformity: A comparison of clinical assessment and weightbearing cone beam CT examinations, *Foot Ankle Surg*, 25 (6), 2019, 790–797.

36. De Carvalho K.A.M., Walt J.S., Ehret A., et al., Comparison between Weightbearing-CT semiautomatic and manual measurements in Hallux Valgus, *Foot Ankle Surg*, 28 (4), 2022, 518–525.

37. Van den Wyngaert T., Elvas F., De Schepper S., et al., SPECT/CT: Standing on the Shoulders of Giants, It Is Time to Reach for the Sky, *J Nuclear Med*, 61 (9), 2020, 1284–1291.

38. Claassen L., Yao D., Ettinger S., et al., Relevance of SPECT-CT in complex cases of foot and ankle surgery: a comparison with MRI, *Foot Ankle Spec*, 13 (6), 2020, 451–462.

39. Alagic Z., Bujila R., Enocson A., et al., Ultra-low-dose CT for extremities in an acute setting: initial experience with 203 subjects, *Skeletal Radiol*, 49 (4), 2020, 531–539.

40. Falkowski A.L., Jacobson J.A., Freehill M.T., et al., Hand-Held Portable Versus Conventional Cart-Based Ultrasound in Musculoskeletal Imaging, *Orthopaedic J Sports Med*, 8, 2020, 2, 2325967119901017.

41. Beard N.M. and Gousse R,P,, Current Ultrasound Application in the Foot and Ankle, *Orthop Clin N Am*, 49 (1), 2018, 109–121.

42. Saengsin J., Lubberts B., Sornsakrin P., et al., Dynamic Portable Ultrasound Cut-off Values for Diagnosing Medial Ankle Instability in Supination External Rotation Ankle Injury: A Cadaveric Study, *Foot & Ankle Orthopaedics*, 7, 2022, 1, 2473011421S00427.

43. Saengsin J., HAgemeijer N., Bhimani R., et al., Using Portable Ultrasound to Measure the Effect of Lateral Ankle Ligament Injury on Syndesmotic Stability: A Cadaveric Study, *Foot & Ankle Orthopaedics*, 5, 2020, 4, 2473011420S00423.

44. Saengsin J., Bhimani R., Sato G., et al., Use of portable ultrasonography for the diagnosis of lateral ankle instability, *J Orthop Res*, 40 (10), 2022, 2421–2429.

45. Gunio DA Vulcano E, Benitez CL,. Dynamic MR imaging analysis of instability in the injured Lisfranc joint with an MRI-compatible foot stressor device. Eur J Radiol 2020;131:109263.

MRI of Pediatric Foot and Ankle Conditions

Bruno Cerretti Carneiro, MD[a,b], Alípio G. Ormond Filho, MD[a],
Júlio Brandão Guimarães, MD, PhD[a,c],*

KEYWORDS

- MRI • Pediatric • Foot • Ankle

KEY POINTS

- Skeletal maturation is a dynamic process, and although it is somewhat predictable, it also has several variable particularities that can be easily misinterpreted as diseases on imaging, especially on MRI fluid-sensitive sequences.

- On MRI, cartilage shows high signal intensity on fluid-sensitive sequences, so its bright appearance may draw the reader's attention erroneously to fractures, apophysitis and other mechanical overload situations, besides tumors, osteonecrosis, and inflammatory pathologic conditions, among other conditions.

- Normal primary ossification centers of the foot and ankle in children can have heterogeneous marrow signal intensity, with multiple foci of high signal intensity on fluid-sensitive sequences, known as a starry sky appearance, especially in tarsal bones. It was hypothesized that this might represent small islands of residual red marrow, areas of increased vascularity, or normal developmental stress caused by regular weight-bearing and weight gain. This pattern rarely persists in adults and usually disappears by the age of 15 years.

- The foot apophysis has single or multiple secondary ossification centers (SOCs) that may show multiple/fragmented aspects, high signal intensity on T2 fat-saturated weighted imaging/short tau inversion recovery, a sclerotic appearance (either on radiographs or other imaging examinations) and irregular margins that are consistent with normal development changes and should not be mistaken for disease. In the calcaneus and medial malleolus apophyses, these characteristics might be even more prominent. Extension of the edema outside of the SOCs to the bone marrow, and soft tissues of course, when associated with an appropriate clinical picture, favors the presence of pathologic conditions, such as mechanical overload, osteochondrosis, or fractures.

[a] Department of Musculoskeletal Radiology, Fleury Medicina e Saúde, São Paulo, SP, Brazil;
[b] Department of Diagnostic Imaging, United Health Group Brazil, São Paulo, SP, Brazil;
[c] Department of Diagnostic Imaging, Federal University of São Paulo, São Paulo, SP, Brazil
* Corresponding author. Fleury Medicina e Saúde Higienópolis, R. Mato Grosso, 306 - Higienópolis, São Paulo 01239-040.
E-mail address: julio.guimaraes@grupofleury.com.br

Foot Ankle Clin N Am 28 (2023) 681–695
https://doi.org/10.1016/j.fcl.2023.04.007
foot.theclinics.com

INTRODUCTION

Increasing participation and intensity of training in organized sports among the pediatric population, associated with the higher availability, lower costs, and lack of ionizing radiation, has increased the demand for MRI in children and adolescents. On MRI, cartilage shows high signal intensity on fluid-sensitive sequences—T2 fat-saturated weighted imaging (T2FS) and short tau inversion recovery (STIR)—so its bright appearance may draw the reader's attention erroneously to fractures, apophysitis and other mechanical overload situations, besides tumors, osteonecrosis, and inflammatory pathologic conditions, among other conditions. The foot and ankle have several bones with abundant radiolucent and high signal intensity growth cartilages that gradually ossify and may create undulating or irregular margins, making the interpretation of the images even more problematic. Moreover, the immature skeleton has red marrow and hypervascularized areas in metaphyseal equivalents that also have a bright appearance on T2FS/STIR. The MR imaging appearance of the pediatric foot and ankle reflects the dynamic process of skeletal growth and maturation.[1–3]

In this article, the authors will review MRI aspects of medullar conversion, endochondral and intramembranous ossification, physis, apophysis and periosteum characteristics and anatomic variations, as well as traumatic and atraumatic disease presentations, highlighting how to differentiate them on imaging examinations, especially MRI.

BONE FORMATION

Bone formation occurs by intramembranous and endochondral ossification. Endochondral ossification is the dominant process in the skeleton and occurs in the extremities, as well as in several other parts of the body. It uses a preexisting cartilage model that is gradually replaced by bone.[4] Longitudinal (in long bones) and centrifugal (in tarsal bones) growth occurs by endochondral ossification, whereas an increase in diameter occurs by intramembranous deposition from the surrounding periosteum in long bones.[5]

The primary ossification center is located in the center of the bone and forms the future diaphysis and tarsal bones, whereas the secondary ossification centers (SOCs) are located at the ends of the bone and form the epiphysis and apophysis.[2]

Cartilaginous precursors develop in utero and form blueprints for both primary and SOCs about the ankle and foot.[1] Some ossification centers are partially ossified before birth, such as the primary ossification centers of the talus and calcaneus. However, other ossification centers are not ossified, and they are called nonossified precursors at this stage. Nonossified precursors are radiolucent on radiographs; however, they are well visualized on MRI, and how they are constituted by cartilage shows high signal intensity on T2/STIR images.[6]

Preossification centers develop within cartilaginous precursors and bring about SOCs. They represent local biochemical alterations in the hyaline cartilage matrix, which allow osteoblastic activity. They are visible on MRI, mostly in the medial malleolus, calcaneal apophysis, and navicular cartilaginous precursors. Later, they convert into ossification centers and disappear on MRI.[1] The age of the radiographic appearance and fusion of the primary and SOCs are shown in **Fig. 1**.

RED TO YELLOW MARROW CONVERSION

Early in development, the ossification centers are rich in red marrow, which has low T1 and intermediate/high signal intensity on T2/STIR, and enhancement after gadolinium

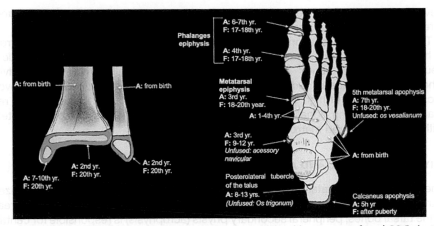

Fig. 1. The important primary and SOCs of the foot and ankle. Some unfused SOCs in the mature skeleton are accessory ossicles. A, age of radiographic appearance; F, age of radiographic fusion.

injection on MRI. Afterward, it will show fat marrow signal intensity, similar to adults, that is, high T1 and low T2/STIR signal intensity, without enhancement in postcontrast sequences. Bone marrow in newborns is composed mostly of hematopoietic marrow. Its conversion to fat marrow starts shortly after birth[7] or even before birth in the toes.[8] Conversion of the tarsal and metatarsal bones also initiates very early and is complete in 7-year-old children in the talus and calcaneus, for example.[9] However, even after this age, on MRI, normal primary ossification centers can have heterogeneous marrow signal intensity, with multiple foci of high signal intensity on fluid-sensitive sequences, known as a starry sky appearance (**Fig. 2**). It was hypothesized that this might represent small islands of residual red marrow, areas of increased vascularity, or normal

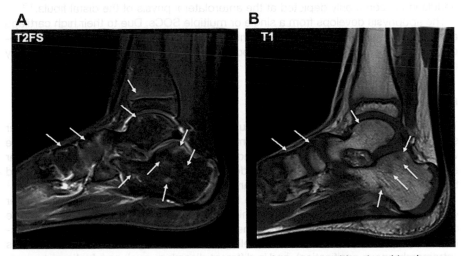

Fig. 2. Diffuse starry sky—normal bone marrow signal in a 7-year-old male ankle, characterized by focal areas of hypersignal intensity on T2FS (*A*) and low signal intensity on T1 (*B*) in the bone marrow of the talus, calcaneus, tibia, and tarsal bones (*arrows*).

developmental stress caused by regular weight-bearing and weight gain.[7] This pattern rarely persists in adults[1] and normally disappears by the age of 15 years.[7]

The most common locations for high signal intensity on T2/STIR of the bone marrow in healthy children are the talar dome, head and posterior tubercle, posterior calcaneus, and navicular bone.[7] These bones are developmentally similar to the pelvis, where similar islands of red marrow have been previously described.[10] Moreover, most of these foci of high signal are endosteal, which is similar to the residual red marrow seen in long bones, thus supporting that these findings can be consistent with the remaining red marrow.[7]

PHYSIS, ACROPHYSIS, AND APOPHYSIS

The tibial, fibula, metatarsal, and phalangeal primary physes are highly organized cartilaginous structures responsible for linear growth of the ankle and foot, whereas in the tarsal bones, peripheral secondary physis (acrophysis) is responsible for centrifugal growth. The physis is organized into 3 layers from the epiphysis to the metaphysis: the germinal, proliferative, and hypertrophic zones. The hypertrophic zone can be further subdivided into zones of maturation and degeneration and the zone of provisional calcification. In the adjacent metaphyseal side is the primary spongiosa, a highly vascularized structure in which osteoclasts and osteoblasts replace the calcified cartilage matrix to produce new bone. The cartilage layers of the physis, the zone of provisional calcification, and the primary spongiosa produce a characteristic trilaminar appearance on T2FS MRI.[1–3]

In toddlers, the physis has a regular, flat, and wide aspect. During weight-bearing and gait, it develops irregular, wavy, and thinner characteristics, with more conspicuous 3 layers on MRI; however, it always maintains a uniform physiologic thickness. Later, in adolescence, it will finally narrow and close. Usually, the physis fuses from the center to the periphery. However, the distal tibial physis has a more undulating pattern with a focal anteromedial upward deviation called Kump's bump or Poland's hump.[11] This represents the site of initial physiologic physeal closure, which is completed in girls from 12 to 15 years and boys from 15 to 18 years. A similar physeal undulation is commonly depicted at the anterolateral physis of the distal fibula.[1,3]

The apophysis develops from a single or multiple SOCs. Due to their high cartilage and red marrow content, they can show high signal intensity on MRI fluid-sensitive sequences. Similar to the epiphysis, the apophysis will also develop a physiologic wavy appearance.

PERIOSTEUM

The periosteum covers most bone structures, with the exception of their intra-articular surfaces and the carpal, tarsal, and sesamoid bones. In children, it is a loose structure with a well-defined outer fibrous layer and an inner cambial layer that is highly cellular and exhibits osteoblastic potential. Underneath its layers, there is the cortex, and together, they show a characteristic trilaminar aspect on MRI.

The inner layer is at its thickest in the fetus, and it becomes progressively thinner with age. In the adult, it becomes so thin that its inner and outer layers cannot be distinguished from themselves or from the cortex. The periosteum is a dynamic structure that plays a major role in bone modeling and remodeling under normal conditions (intramembranous ossification), and in different disorders, such as infections, tumors, hematomas, and systemic diseases, the osteogenic potential of the periosteum is stimulated, and new bone is produced.[5,12]

The perichondrium lies at the junction of the physis and the periosteum, surrounding the main physeal cartilage. The perichondrium is tightly fixed to the underlying physis, preventing its separation and acting as a barrier to the spread of subperiosteal hematomas, abscesses, and tumors to the epiphysis.[13]

ANATOMIC VARIANTS

There are several anatomic variations of the foot and ankle related to different bone morphologies, accessory ossification centers, nonfusion of ossification centers, sesamoid bones, and accessory muscles, among others, that go beyond the scope of this review. Thus, we will highlight just some examples that can cause some confusion during daily routine.

The foot apophysis has single or multiple SOCs that may show multiple/fragmented aspects, high signal intensity on T2FS/STIR, a sclerotic appearance (either on radiographs or other imaging examinations) and irregular margins that are consistent with normal development changes and should not be mistaken for disease. In the calcaneus and medial malleolus apophyses, these characteristics might be even more prominent (**Figs. 3** and **4**). Extension of the edema outside of the SOCs to the bone marrow (see **Fig. 3**), and soft tissues (see **Fig. 4**), of course, when associated with an appropriate clinical picture, favors the presence of pathologic conditions, such as mechanical overload, osteochondrosis or fractures.

Other SOCs may also suffer from mechanical overload or osteochondrosis, such as the navicular and fifth metatarsal tuberosities (see **Fig. 4**; **Fig. 5**) and the lateral tubercle of the posterior process of the talus (**Fig. 6**). The cleft epiphysis of the proximal phalanx of the hallux is an anatomic variant that might be misdiagnosed as a fracture.

Focal periphyseal edema (FOPE) zones are areas of periphyseal edema seen near the time of physeal closure that are thought to be a physiologic phenomenon related to changes in the distribution of forces around the physis as it closes, most often around the knee but they have also been described in other sites. They have also been reported to be a cause of nontraumatic pain; however, other conditions must first be excluded before attributing symptoms to FOPE.[14,15] It manifests with focal bone marrow edema centered at an open but narrow physis that extends into the metaphysis and sometimes involves the epiphysis. Periphyseal edema greater than 3 cm and/or a nonuniform physeal width should raise a suspicion about other pathologic processes.[1,2]

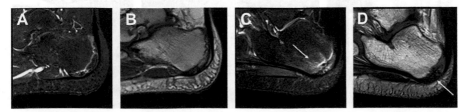

Fig. 3. Normal apophysis versus apophysitis (Sever)—normal calcaneous apophysis in a 13-year-old boy (*A, B*), with a fragmented aspect that is normal during developmental ossification identified on T2WFS (*A*) and T1 (*B*) MR images. Another apophysis in a 10-year-old boy with hindfoot pain (*C, D*), showing mild sclerosis accompanied by bone marrow edema (*arrows*) that extends to the adjacent calcaneus tuberosity, on T2WFS (*C*) and T1 (*D*) MR images signs that support the diagnosis of apophysitis in this clinical scenario.

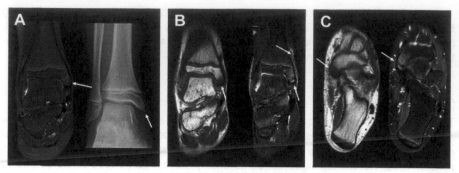

Fig. 4. SOCs: normal x overload. (*A*) Normal aspect of the secondary ossifying center of the medial malleolus in a coronal T2WFS MR image and frontal digital radiography of an 8-year-old boy (*arrows*). (*B*) A 7-year-old girl with medial ankle pain presenting with bone marrow (*lower arrows*) and overlying soft tissue edema that extends to the subcutaneous planes (*upper arrow*), suggestive of mechanical apophysitis. (*C*) MR images of a 9-year-old girl's foot depicting bone marrow edema at the SOC and at the navicular bone (*arrow*) (apophysitis).

PHYSEAL OR PERIPHYSEAL INJURIES
Traumatic or Microtraumatic

Growth plates are weaker than ankle ligaments and are vulnerable to shear and rotational forces. Therefore, injury mechanisms that may result in ankle sprains in adults can manifest as physeal or avulsion fractures in children, although ligament injuries in children are more common than previously thought.[16–18]

The incidence of ankle sprains has been estimated at 2.1 per 1000 person-years in the United States, and the peak incidence of ankle sprain occurs between 15 and 19 years of age. Half of all ankle sprains occur during sports activity, with lateral ankle sprain and syndesmotic sprain being the most common ankle and foot injuries in collegiate football players, occurring in 31% and 15% of players, respectively.[19] The

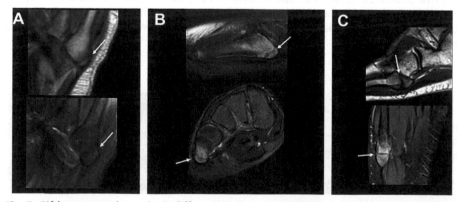

Fig. 5. Fifth metatarsal apophysis differential diagnoses. (*A*) MRI showing normal apophysis of the fifth metatarsal in a 12-year-old boy, lying laterally and longitudinally oriented (*arrows*). (*B*) MRI of the foot of a 13-year-old female gymnast with recurrent lateral pain, showing signs of apophysitis with bone marrow edema on the apophysis and adjacent proximal metaphysis of the fifth metatarsal (*arrows*). (*C*) MRI showing the transverse fracture line in a 6-year-old boy after a sports injury (*arrows*).

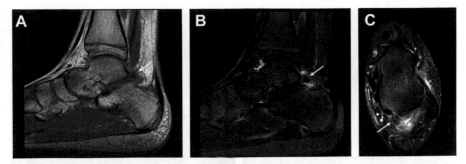

Fig. 6. Posterior impingement of the ankle. T1W (*A*) and T2W fat saturation (*B, C*) MR images of a 13-year-old boy depicting bone marrow edema on a nonfused SOC of the lateral tuberosity of the posterior process of the talus, with small articular effusion, reactional synovitis and Kager fat pad edema (*arrows*).

lateral ankle ligaments are most commonly injured, and they comprise the anterior talofibular ligament (ATFL), posterior talofibular ligament (PTFL), and calcaneofibular ligament (CFL).

Growth plate injury usually occurs near physeal maturity, that is, approximately between 12 and 15 year old. Of all physeal injuries, fractures of the distal tibial physis have among the highest rates of complications. Salter-Harris is the most common anatomic classification system for fractures involving unfused growth plates. It also has valuable prognostic significance. Complications are uncommon with types I and II. However, fractures that cross the physis into the epiphysis (Salter Harris III and IV types) may damage the germinative layer and thus are at a higher risk of causing physeal bars, growth arrest, angular deformities, articular incongruity, and precocious osteoarthritis.[16–18] On MRI, it is possible to visualize nondisplaced radiographically occult Salter-Harris I fractures, with physeal thickening, irregularities, and higher signal intensity on T2/STIR images. Comparison with other physis may be helpful in differentiating normal physis with high signal intensity from fracture. Of course, other types of Salter-Harris fractures that extend to the bone are also well defined on MRI. Other imaging findings might be associated with Salter-Harris acute fractures, such as osteochondral lesions (OCLs), periosteum displacement, subperiosteal hematoma, and periosteal entrapment, within the physis (**Fig. 7**). Avulsion of the superior extensor retinaculum of the ankle and subperiosteal hematoma of the distal fibula in children, although well described on ultrasound,[20] is not an uncommon finding on MRI after ankle sprain. A single traumatic event can cause one or multiple focal physeal widening, with a cartilaginous high signal extending from the physis into the adjacent metaphysis, showing a tongue-like morphology that is greater in its longitudinal dimension than in its width. These findings may be associated with growth disturbances and growth recovery lines.[21]

Chronic physeal stress injuries may affect the feet of young athletes, although more classically described in the wrist (gymnast wrist) and in the shoulder (little leaguer shoulder). It seems as a focal T2 hyperintense widening of the physis on MR, usually associated with bone marrow edema.[22]

Fatigue fractures or stress reactions are not uncommon in the pediatric athletic population and can be found in virtually any bone; however, the most common locations are the second and third metatarsals (**Fig. 8**), calcaneus (see **Fig. 8**) and distal tibia.[23,24] In stress reactions, there is a periosteal reaction and subcortical bone

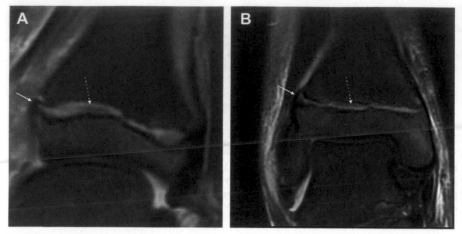

Fig. 7. Salter-Harris I fracture and periosteal entrapment. Sagittal (*A*) and coronal (*B*) T2FS MRI of the ankle of a 10-year-old boy after an ankle sprain. Note the enlargement and loss of the trilaminar pattern of the distal physis of the tibia, compatible with Salter-Harris type I fracture (*dotted arrow*). There is also periosteal interposition on the anterolateral epiphyseal plate (*arrow*).

marrow edema. In stress fractures, a fracture line is visible, usually incomplete and perpendicular to the bony trabeculae or sometimes longitudinal in the cortex of the long bones. Subchondral stress fractures are rare in children but are frequently observed in the elderly (insufficiency fractures).[23,24]

Inflammatory or Infectious

Foot and ankle pathologic conditions are common in juvenile idiopathic arthritis (JIA) and include joint disease, tenosynovitis, muscle atrophy, enthesitis, digital deformities, and biomechanical abnormalities. In a previous study surveying foot problems

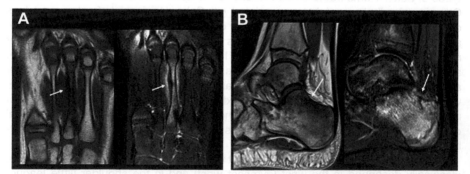

Fig. 8. Stress fractures. (*A*) MRI of the forefoot of a 6-year-old girl with intensive ballet practice and recurrent forefoot pain, without trauma history, showing bone marrow edema, periosteal reaction and a small transverse fracture line on the third metatarsal (*arrow*), compatible with a stress fracture. (*B*) MRI of the ankle of a 14-year-old boy with hindfoot pain related to soccer practice, showing a line of incomplete fracture involving cortical and medullary bone on the dorsal surface of the calcaneus, perpendicular to the trabecular bone, suggestive of a stress fracture.

in children with JIA, 63% reported some degree of foot-related impairment, and 60% reported foot-related participation restriction.[25]

Joint disease in JIA may include joint swelling, tenderness, pain, warmth, and stiffness. These symptoms typically occur because of synovitis (**Fig. 9**). Tenosynovitis (see **Fig. 9**) in JIA commonly affects the tibialis posterior and peroneal tendons, and muscle atrophy—plantar-flexor muscle atrophy may be observed in children with JIA.[26] Enthesitis is common at the Achilles tendon, and the medial tubercle of the calcaneus is typically seen in male patients with the enthesitis-related subtype of JIA.[27]

Chronic nonbacterial osteomyelitis (CNO), also known as chronic recurrent multifocal osteomyelitis (CRMO) (**Fig. 10**), is a noninfectious, autoinflammatory, and rare disorder that occurs primarily in children and adolescents (peak of incidence between 7 and 12 years) and is characterized by episodic skeletal pain with a protracted course.[28] Although consistent epidemiologic data are lacking, recent studies suggest that CNO is more common than previously thought[29] and may be one of the most prevalent autoinflammatory diseases.[30]

The most common sites of disease are the metaphyses or metaphyseal equivalents, especially in the lower extremities. The tibia has been reported as the most common bone involved. Typical lesions occur adjacent to the physis, are lytic and geographic on radiographs with bone marrow edema on MRI in the early stages and might be associated with periosteal reaction. They also may show a mirror-like appearance involving the epiphysis. Chronic lesions become sclerotic, with low signal intensity in all MRI sequences.[31]

Whole-body MRI (WBMRI) is a useful diagnostic approach. If the child has a good general condition, mild or absent fever, white blood cell count and inflammatory markers are normal or mildly changed, with most patients being healthy between recurrent episodes, and WBMRI shows multifocal typical lesions throughout the skeleton, both symptomatic and asymptomatic, a diagnosis of CRMO can be considered (see **Fig. 10**).[32] Abscess formation, fistulas, and/or sequestra must be excluded. However, traditionally, CNO is a diagnosis of exclusion, and biopsy can be required to exclude tumors or pyogenic osteomyelitis, showing sterile osteitis, especially in doubtful cases.[33]

However, in pyogenic osteomyelitis, symptoms are usually acute and more dramatic, and most of the cases are unifocal. MRI findings (**Fig. 11**) are present early in disease onset, unlike radiographs, in which at least 1 or 2 weeks are required to see bone destruction or periosteal reaction. MRI early findings are metaphyseal

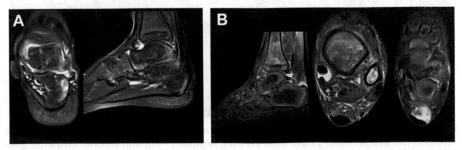

Fig. 9. Juvenile idiopathic arthritis. Ankle MR images of a 3-year-old girl (*A*) and an 8-year-old boy (*B*) with ankle pain, showing tibiotalar and subtalar joint effusion, marked tenosynovitis and retrocalcaneal bursitis (*arrows*). The findings and clinical correlation were compatible with oligoarticular juvenile idiopathic arthritis.

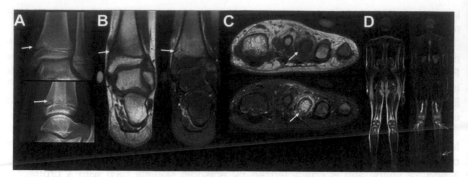

Fig. 10. Chronic nonbacterial osteomyelitis. A 13-year-old girl with fever, pain, and swelling of the left ankle for 10 days. Radiographs (A) showing discrete hypodense foci and bone irregularities on the medial side of the distal tibial metaphysis (*arrows*), with bone marrow edema on T1 and T2FS MRI images (*arrows*) (B). Biopsy and bacterial culture did not isolate any pathogens. After 1 year, bilateral midfoot pain presented with similar MRI findings on the metatarsals (*arrows*) (C). Due to the clinical hypothesis, the patient was submitted to WBMRI (D) that showed other bone alteration sites, some of them asymptomatic, which contributed to the diagnosis of chronic nonbacterial osteomyelitis.

heterogeneous bone marrow edema of ill-defined limits adjacent to the growth plates, with characteristic very low signal intensity on T1 (related to substitution of the bone marrow), associated with periosteal reaction and soft tissue edema. In the subacute phase, Brodie's intraosseous abscess with the penumbra sign is classically present (see **Fig. 11**), either associated or not associated with fistulae, soft tissue, or subperiosteal abscess. Sequestrum, involucrum, and cloaca are classic chronic osteomyelitis findings that can be assessed by radiographs, CT scans, or MRI.[34]

Fixed Flatfoot Deformity

There are a few causes of fixed flatfoot deformities in children, such as congenital vertical talus and the most common tarsal coalitions, especially calcaneonavicular and talocalcaneal, which are usually easily diagnosed on radiographs. However, in difficult

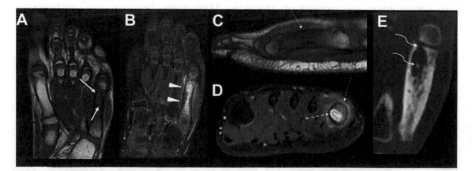

Fig. 11. Bacterial osteomyelitis. A 7-year-old girl presenting with pain and swelling of the forefoot. MR images (axial T1 (A), axial T2FS (B), sagittal T1 (C), and coronal T1FS after gadolinium injection (D)) showing bone marrow edema (*arrowheads*) and intraosseous abscess with the penumbra sign (*arrows*) on the distal metaphysis of the fifth metatarsal, with a solid corticoperiosteal reaction (*dotted arrows*) and enhancement (*dashed arrows*). CT scan (E) showing a bony sequestrum and extension to the distal physis (*curved arrows*).

or atypical cases, cross-sectional studies can be helpful[35] such as in extra-articular posteromedial talocalcaneal coalition[36] (**Fig. 12**) or the accessory anterolateral talar facet.[37]

Moreover, there are also other types of tarsal coalitions, such as widespread coalition, and between the third metatarsal and the lateral cuneiform joint (see **Fig. 12**).[38]

Osteochondritis Dissecans of the Talar Dome

OCL is an umbrella term for focal injury of the articular cartilage and underlying bone, and it does not imply cause or age of injury (either acute or chronic).[39] However, OCL in clinical practice is used as a synonym for traumatic osteochondral fracture. However, osteochondritis dissecans (OCD) is a chronic and idiopathic type of OCL with a risk for instability and disruption of adjacent articular cartilage that may result in premature osteoarthritis.[40] The cause is unclear; there are probably multiple contributing factors, such as genetic, vascular, or (micro)traumatic, leading to deficiency in subchondral bone formation and subsequent chondral lesions, which may result in an unstable subchondral fragment. OCD is frequently related to repetitive athletic stress (**Fig. 13**); therefore, microtraumatic stress is the favored cause. OCD can be further subdivided into juvenile (children and young adolescents who have open growth plates) or adult (older adolescents and young adults after the growth plates have closed) forms. The adult form of OCD is an incompletely healed juvenile OCD.[39]

Bone Tumors of the Foot

A comprehensive review of bone tumors is not the aim of this review; however, a few bone tumors might be confused with stress reaction/fracture, inflammatory or infectious diseases, such as osteoid osteoma (OO), chondroblastoma, and Ewing sarcoma (ES), although uncommon in the foot and ankle.

Osteoid Osteoma

Some OO cases, when in atypical locations, such as the foot, may present unusual clinical and imaging findings that can lead to misdiagnosis. Medullary OO is the most common type that occurs in tarsal bones and is usually accompanied by less

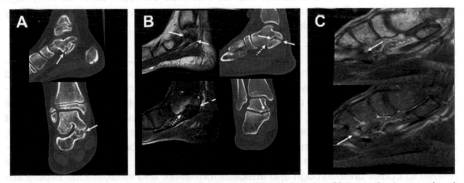

Fig. 12. Tarsal coalition. (A) Ankle CT of a 9-year-old girl showing fibrocartilaginous talocalcaneal coalition at the middle subtalar joint, with irregularity of the apposed bone surfaces and subcortical cysts. (B) Ankle MRI and CT of an 18-year-old boy after an ankle sprain showing fibrocartilaginous extra-articular posteromedial coalition (*arrow*). Note the middle (*dotted arrow*) and posterior (*dashed arrows*) subtalar joints with the usual bone and chondral morphology. The areas of marrow edema have a contusional etiology. (C) Foot MRI of a 12-year-old boy showing partial plantar fibrocartilaginous coalition between the lateral cuneiform and the base of the third metatarsal, also with mechanical overload edema.

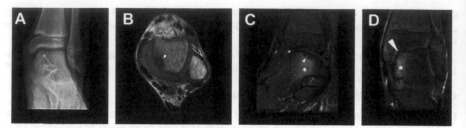

Fig. 13. Osteochondritis dissecans. An 8-year-old boy with deep ankle pain for 2 years, which worsened after physical activities. (A) CR mortise shows mild irregularity of the bone plate at the medial segment of the talar dome (*arrow* in A). (B–D): MRI showing osteochondritis dissecans at the posterior medial shoulder of the talus, with mild impaction of the subchondral bone plate (*arrowheads*), and adjacent bone marrow edema (*asterisk*).

cortical thickening than typical OO and it may induce bone expansion. Because the bones of the hands and feet are small and close to each other, it may be difficult to locate the cause of inflammation, which may spread to adjacent bones, joints, and soft tissues. Additionally, there may be prominent soft tissue swelling, resembling infection, or inflammatory arthritis. When OO is located in the distal phalanx, it may also cause nail deformities, which are also confounding factors. In addition, the clinical presentation may be unusual, with atypical pain or even the absence of pain.[41,42]

CHONDROBLASTOMA

Chondroblastoma is a benign cartilage tumor developing in the epiphysis or apophysis of skeletally immature individuals that, in the majority of cases, presents with a periosteal reaction and edema/inflammation in the adjacent cortex, marrow, and soft tissue that can lead to misdiagnosis of stress reaction/fracture, osteomyelitis, or arthritis. On imaging, it is usually a geographic lytic lesion with sclerotic margins, heterogeneous high signal intensity on T2FS/STIR and intermediate signal intensity on T1WI. Only one-third to a half of the cases present the characteristic chondroid matrix on MRI (at least in some part of the lesion), that is, lobulated contours with markedly high signal intensity on fluid-sensitive sequences, associated with low signal intensity foci, related to chondroid calcifications.[43,44]

Ewing Sarcoma

ES is a highly aggressive bone and soft-tissue tumor that usually affects children and young adults. ES in bone may mimic osteomyelitis clinically and radiologically. On imaging examinations, both ES and osteomyelitis may present as aggressive permeative lesions, periosteal reactions, and soft tissue masses. ES, however, usually does not destroy the cortex, and the periosteal reaction might be more aggressive (spiculated) and shows avidly solid enhancement after gadolinium injection, whereas in osteomyelitis, the periosteal reaction tends to be linear and thicker, soft tissue masses are related to cortex breakthrough and abscess formation, and intraosseous Brodie abscess may be present in the subacute phase. In addition, signs of chronic osteomyelitis, such as sequestrum, involucrum, and cloaca, typically do not cause diagnostic doubts.[45,46]

Dysplasia Epiphysealis Hemimelica

Dysplasia epiphysealis hemimelica (DEH) is a rare disease that usually affects boys (3 M:1F) aged younger than 8 years and is also known as Trevor Fairbank disease or *tarsomégalie*. It is characterized by epiphyseal overgrowth and osteocartilaginous epiphyseal lesions caused by idiopathic benign cell proliferation. DEH may manifest as a painless deformity, limited range of motion, impingement, mechanical pain, and/or localized growth disturbances. It tends to affect the epiphyses or apophysis of the same side of one lower extremity. On imaging, there is abnormal hypertrophy of the epiphyseal cartilage and subsequent excessive ossification, which results in lobulated ossified masses, asymmetric epiphyseal enlargement, irregular ossification centers within one side (ie, medial vs lateral) of an affected epiphysis, or any combination of these features. MRI provides a better understanding of epiphyseal cartilage overgrowth that is not yet ossified on radiographs, presenting high signal intensity on fluid-sensitive sequences.[47]

SUMMARY

Skeletal maturation is a dynamic process, and although it is somewhat predictable, it also has several variable particularities that can be easily misinterpreted as diseases on imaging, especially on MRI fluid-sensitive sequences. Therefore, knowledge of the physiologic patterns of development in children and adolescents and disease presentations are crucial for making the correct diagnoses and providing proper treatment to the pediatric population.

CLINICS CARE POINTS

- Increasing participation and intensity of training in organized sports among the pediatric population has increased the demand for MRI in children and adolescents. Therefore, MRI aspects of physeal fractures or overload, apophysitis, stress reactions and fractures, periosteal avulsions, subperiosteal hematomas and ligament injury, among other mechanical and traumatic pathologic conditions must be well known by orthopedists and radiologists.

- Knowledge of the physiologic patterns of development in children and adolescents and disease presentations are crucial for making the correct diagnoses and providing proper treatment to the pediatric population.

- Autoinflammatory disorders, infectious diseases, and bone tumors that show bone marrow and soft tissue edema on MRI, although not frequent in the foot and ankle, might be confused with stress reaction/fracture. Imaging associated with clinical history play a pivot role differentiating then.

DISCLOSURE

The authors have nothing to disclose.

REFERENCES

1. Walter WR, Goldman LH, Rosenberg ZS. Pitfalls in MRI of the Developing Pediatric Ankle. Radiographics 2021;41(1):210–23.
2. Augusto ACL, Goes PCK, Flores DV, et al. Imaging Review of Normal and Abnormal Skeletal Maturation. Radiographics 2022;42(3):861–79.
3. Ma GM, Ecklund K. MR Imaging of the Pediatric Foot and Ankle: What Does Normal Look Like? Magn Reson Imaging Clin N Am 2017;25(1):27–43.
4. Mackie EJ, Ahmed YA, Tatarczuch L, et al. Endochondral ossification: how cartilage is converted into bone in the developing skeleton. Int J Biochem Cell Biol 2008;40(1):46–62.

5. Dwek JR. The periosteum: what is it, where is it, and what mimics it in its absence? Skeletal Radiol 2010;39(4):319–23.

6. Nguyen JC, Markhardt BK, Merrow AC, et al. Imaging of Pediatric Growth Plate Disturbances. Radiographics 2017;37(6):1791–812.

7. Shabshin N, Schweitzer ME, Morrison WB, et al. High-signal T2 changes of the bone marrow of the foot and ankle in children: red marrow or traumatic changes? Pediatr Radiol 2006;36(7):670–6.

8. EMERY JL, FOLLETT GF. Regression of bone-marrow haemopoiesis from the terminal digits in the foetus and infant. Br J Haematol 1964;10:485–9.

9. Taccone A, Oddone M, Dell'Acqua AD, et al. MRI "road-map" of normal age-related bone marrow. II. Thorax, pelvis and extremities. Pediatr Radiol 1995;25(8):596–606.

10. Schweitzer ME, Levine C, Mitchell DG, et al. Bull's-eyes and halos: useful MR discriminators of osseous metastases. Radiology 1993;188(1):249–52.

11. Love SM, Ganey T, Ogden JA. Postnatal epiphyseal development: the distal tibia and fibula. J Pediatr Orthop 1990;10(3):298–305.

12. Bisseret D, Kaci R, Lafage-Proust MH, et al. Periosteum: characteristic imaging findings with emphasis on radiologic-pathologic comparisons. Skeletal Radiol 2015;44(3):321–38.

13. Laor T, Jaramillo D. It's time to recognize the perichondrium. Pediatr Radiol 2020;50(2):153–60.

14. Beckmann N, Spence S. Unusual Presentations of Focal Periphyseal Edema Zones: A Report of Bilateral Symmetric Presentation and Partial Physeal Closure. Case Rep Radiol 2015;2015:465018.

15. Zbojniewicz AM, Laor T. Focal Periphyseal Edema (FOPE) zone on MRI of the adolescent knee: a potentially painful manifestation of physiologic physeal fusion? AJR Am J Roentgenol 2011;197(4):998–1004.

16. Su AW, Larson AN. Pediatric Ankle Fractures: Concepts and Treatment Principles. Foot Ankle Clin 2015;20(4):705–19.

17. Chaturvedi A, Mann L, Cain U, et al. Acute Fractures and Dislocations of the Ankle and Foot in Children. Radiographics 2020;40(3):754–74.

18. Rougereau G, Noailles T, Khoury GE, et al. Is lateral ankle sprain of the child and adolescent a myth or a reality? A systematic review of the literature. Foot Ankle Surg 2022;28(3):294–9.

19. Shawen SB, Dworak T, Anderson RB. Return to Play Following Ankle Sprain and Lateral Ligament Reconstruction. Clin Sports Med 2016;35(4):697–709.

20. Ding J, Moraux A, Nectoux É, et al. Traumatic avulsion of the superior extensor retinaculum of the ankle as a cause of subperiosteal haematoma of the distal fibula in children. A retrospective study of 7 cases. Skeletal Radiol 2016;45(11):1481–5.

21. Laor T, Hartman AL, Jaramillo D. Local physeal widening on MR imaging: an incidental finding suggesting prior metaphyseal insult. Pediatr Radiol 1997;27(8):654–62.

22. O'Dell MC, Jaramillo D, Bancroft L, et al. Imaging of Sports-related Injuries of the Lower Extremity in Pediatric Patients. Radiographics 2016;36(6):1807–27.

23. Mandell JC, Khurana B, Smith SE. Stress fractures of the foot and ankle, part 2: site-specific etiology, imaging, and treatment, and differential diagnosis. Skeletal Radiol 2017;46(9):1165–86.

24. Welck MJ, Hayes T, Pastides P, et al. Stress fractures of the foot and ankle. Injury 2017;48(8):1722–6.

25. Hendry G, Gardner-Medwin J, Watt GF, et al. A survey of foot problems in juvenile idiopathic arthritis. Muscoskel Care 2008;6(4):221–32.

26. Javadi S, Kan JH, Orth RC, et al. Wrist and ankle MRI of patients with juvenile idiopathic arthritis: identification of unsuspected multicompartmental tenosynovitis and arthritis. AJR Am J Roentgenol 2014;202(2):413–7.
27. Ravelli A, Martini A. Juvenile idiopathic arthritis. Lancet 2007;369(9563):767–78.
28. Zhao Y, Ferguson PJ. Chronic Nonbacterial Osteomyelitis and Chronic Recurrent Multifocal Osteomyelitis in Children. Pediatr Clin North Am 2018;65(4):783–800.
29. Bader-Meunier B, Van Nieuwenhove E, Breton S, et al. Bone involvement in monogenic autoinflammatory syndromes. Rheumatology 2018;57(4):606–18.
30. Schnabel A, Range U, Hahn G, et al. Unexpectedly high incidences of chronic non-bacterial as compared to bacterial osteomyelitis in children. Rheumatol Int 2016;36(12):1737–45.
31. Khanna G, Sato TS, Ferguson P. Imaging of chronic recurrent multifocal osteomyelitis. Radiographics 2009;29(4):1159–77.
32. von Kalle T, Heim N, Hospach T, et al. Typical patterns of bone involvement in whole-body MRI of patients with chronic recurrent multifocal osteomyelitis (CRMO). Röfo 2013;185(7):655–61.
33. Falip C, Alison M, Boutry N, et al. Chronic recurrent multifocal osteomyelitis (CRMO): a longitudinal case series review. Pediatr Radiol 2013;43(3):355–75.
34. Jaramillo D, Dormans JP, Delgado J, et al. Hematogenous Osteomyelitis in Infants and Children: Imaging of a Changing Disease. Radiology 2017;283(3):629–43.
35. Lin YC, Kwon JY, Ghorbanhoseini M, et al. The Hindfoot Arch: What Role Does the Imager Play? Radiol Clin North Am 2016;54(5):951–68.
36. Phyo N, Pressney I, Khoo M, et al. The radiological diagnosis of extra-articular posteromedial talocalcaneal coalition. Skeletal Radiol 2020;49(9):1413–22.
37. Aydıngöz Ü, Topcuoğlu OM, Görmez A, et al. Accessory Anterolateral Talar Facet in Populations With and Without Symptoms: Prevalence and Relevant Associated Ankle MRI Findings. AJR Am J Roentgenol 2016;207(4):846–51.
38. Stevens BW, Kolodziej P. Non-osseous tarsal coalition of the lateral cuneiform-third metatarsal joint. Foot Ankle Int 2008;29(8):867–70.
39. Gorbachova T, Melenevsky Y, Cohen M, et al. Osteochondral Lesions of the Knee: Differentiating the Most Common Entities at MRI. Radiographics 2018;38(5):1478–95.
40. Edmonds EW, Polousky J. A review of knowledge in osteochondritis dissecans: 123 years of minimal evolution from König to the ROCK study group. Clin Orthop Relat Res 2013;471(4):1118–26.
41. Carneiro BC, Da Cruz IAN, Ormond Filho AG, et al. Osteoid osteoma: the great mimicker. Insights Imaging 2021;12(1):32.
42. Andalib A, Sajadie-Khajouei S. Osteoid osteoma of distal phalanx: A rare disorder and review of literature. J Res Med Sci 2013;18(3):264–6.
43. Gao S, Zhou R, Xu Q, et al. Edema Surrounding Benign Tumors and Tumor-Like Lesions. BioMed Res Int 2019;2019:8206913.
44. Blancas C, Llauger J, Palmer J, et al. [Imaging findings in chondroblastoma]. Radiologia 2008;50(5):416–23.
45. Murphey MD, Senchak LT, Mambalam PK, et al. From the radiologic pathology archives: ewing sarcoma family of tumors: radiologic-pathologic correlation. Radiographics 2013;33(3):803–31.
46. Kasalak Ö, Overbosch J, Adams HJ, et al. Diagnostic value of MRI signs in differentiating Ewing sarcoma from osteomyelitis. Acta Radiol 2019;60(2):204–12.
47. Degnan AJ, Ho-Fung VM. More Than Epiphyseal Osteochondromas: Updated Understanding of Imaging Findings in Dysplasia Epiphysealis Hemimelica (Trevor Disease). AJR Am J Roentgenol 2018;211(4):910–9.

High-resolution Ultrasound of the Foot and Ankle

Marcelo Bordalo, MD, PhD[a],*,
Marcos Felippe de Paula Correa, MD[b], Eduardo Yamashiro, MD[a]

KEYWORDS

- Foot • Ankle • Ultrasound • Musculotendinous • Ligament • Strains • Tears
- Injuries

KEY POINTS

- Ultrasound (US) evaluation of foot and ankle injuries provides high spatial resolution and is a valuable tool in this assessment.
- US is an excellent option to MRI for soft tissue assessment of the foot and ankle.
- US of tendinous injuries allows visualization of the tendon itself, the synovial sheath, the paratenon and the presence of increased blood flow (inflammation) and calcifications.
- US can aid clinical examination on the diagnosis of a ligament disruption.
- US is an excellent imaging method to assess the small nerves of the foot.

INTRODUCTION

The use of ultrasound (US) in diagnosis and procedural guidance has increased significantly in recent years and involves multiple medical specialties. US is a very useful alternative for imaging the foot and the ankle. Compared to MRI, it is mainly indicated in soft tissue assessment and has a lower cost, is widely available, allows portability, has the possibility of dynamic evaluation, is easy to compare contralaterally, allows high spatial resolution assessment, and is directly correlated with the painful area. We will review the main clinical indications and pathologic conditions diagnosed by US.

TECHNICAL CONSIDERATIONS

US is an imaging method that utilizes high-frequency sound waves to produce images. The image formation depends on the tissue characteristics and, consequently, on the balance between US reflection and absorption by the tissue. The images are acquired in real time and dynamically.

[a] Radiology Department, Aspetar Orthopedic and Sports Medicine Hospital, Al Waab Street, Zone 54, PO Box 29222, Doha, Qatar; [b] Radiology Department, Hospital Sirio Libanes, Rua Dona Adma Jafet, 115, Sao Paulo 01308-050, Brazil
* Corresponding author.
E-mail address: marcelo.bordalo@aspetar.com

Foot Ankle Clin N Am 28 (2023) 697–708
https://doi.org/10.1016/j.fcl.2023.04.008
1083-7515/23/© 2023 Elsevier Inc. All rights reserved.

foot.theclinics.com

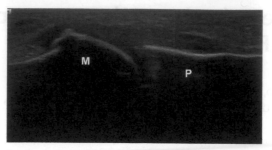

Fig. 1. *Acoustic shadowing of bone.* US longitudinal image of the metatarsal head (M) and proximal phalanx (P) shows hyperechoic cortex and posterior acoustic shadowing.

The echogenicity of a tissue is its ability to reflect or absorb US waves. It can be characterized as hyperechoic (white—US wave reflection is greater than absorption), hypoechoic (gray—US wave reflection is similar to absorption) and anechoic (black—US wave absorption is greater than reflection).[1]

US does not penetrate osseous tissue; bone appears with a bright hyperechoic rim, and posteriorly, it is black, which represents acoustic shadowing (**Fig. 1**). Fluid appears anechoic or hypoechoic (**Fig. 2**). Fat is hypoechoic, and muscles are hypoechoic with a striated structure (**Fig. 3**). Ligaments and tendons have a characteristic striated hyperechoic structure with interspersed hypoechoic lines[2,3] (**Fig. 4**).

Foot and ankle structures are usually superficial, and US evaluation requires high-frequency probes (higher than 7 MHz), usually 10 to 15 MHz, which have better resolution and less penetration.

CLINICAL INDICATIONS

US evaluation of the foot and ankle is indicated in the following acute and chronic conditions[4]:

1. Musculotendinous injuries
2. Ligament sprains
3. Peripheral nerve evaluation
4. Metatarsalgia

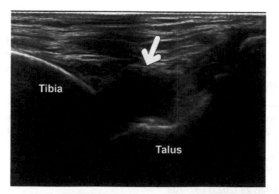

Fig. 2. *Fluid appearance.* US longitudinal image of the tibiotalar joint. Anterior tibiotalar articular recess (*arrow*) with significant amount of fluid, which appears anechoic.

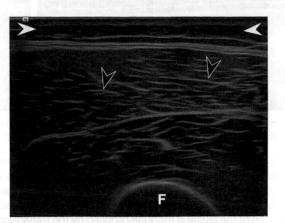

Fig. 3. *US appearance of fat and muscle.* US transverse image of the thigh shows hypoechoic aspect of subcutaneous fat (*white arrowhead*) and striated appearance of muscle structures (black *arrowhead*). Note the hyperchoic rim and posterior acoustic shadowing caused by the femur (F).

5. Evaluation of synovitis, joint fluid, and loose bodies
6. Plantar fascia injuries
7. Guiding interventional procedures (injections, aspirations)

MUSCULOTENDINOUS INJURIES

Tendinitis is defined as inflammation of the tendon, and the US appearance is tendon hypoechogenicity with possible increased vascular flow on Doppler.[5] Tendinosis is a chronic tendon condition with collagenous degeneration, and its US features are tendon hypoechogenicity with diameter increase, with or without flow on Doppler (**Fig. 5**). Calcific tendinopathy is easily diagnosed on US (**Fig. 6**). Inflammation of the tendon's synovial sheath is called tenosynovitis and it shows characteristic thickening of the synovial sheath (**Fig. 7**). The inflammation of the paratenon surrounding a tendon that does not have a synovial sheath (for example, the Achilles tendon) is called paratenonitis (**Fig. 8**). Tendon disruption (or tear) can be partial or full thickness (**Figs. 9** and **10**). A partial tear can be intrasubstance or superficial (see **Fig. 10**). A longitudinal split tear is common on peroneal tendons. Tendon avulsion occurs at the bony attachment.

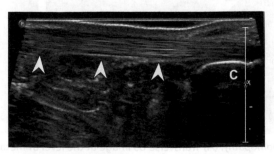

Fig. 4. *Normal tendon.* US longitudinal image of the distal Achilles tendon. Normal hyperechoic striated aspect of a tendon (*arrowheads*).

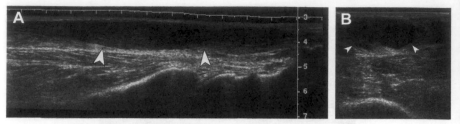

Fig. 5. *Tendinosis of the Achilles.* Longitudinal (*A*) and transverse (*B*) US images of the Achilles tendon show diffuse thickening and hypoechogenicity (*arrowheads*).

US elastography is a recently introduced method that allows for evaluation of the mechanical properties of the tissue. It is based on the principle that stress applied to a tissue causes changes within it that depend on its elastic properties.[6] The most common method applied to musculoskeletal US is strain elastography or compression elastography. In this method, compression of the tissue is manually applied by the transducer. The tissue stiffness is calculated through differences in tissue displacement after the compression is applied. Elasticity information is provided in a qualitative or semiquantitative manner. It is widely used for evaluation of the Achilles tendon, and it has been demonstrated that elastography shows increased stiffness in abnormal tendons compared with asymptomatic tendons which are softer.[7] However, elastography alterations in asymptomatic and sonographically normal tendons are not completely understood.

LIGAMENT TEARS

The diagnosis of ligament injuries is based on clinical findings. US can aid in the evaluation of a ligamentous tear, appearing as a thickened and hypoechoic structure (**Fig. 11**) in comparison with the normal asymptomatic contralateral side. A complete tear is represented by a complete loss of the continuity of the ligamentous substance (**Fig. 12**). Hyperechoic foci at the ligamentous insertion can represent a bony avulsion (**Fig. 13**).

PLANTAR FASCIA

US examination of the plantar fascia is performed with the patient in a prone position and the foot hanging freely over the examination table. The US aspect of the normal

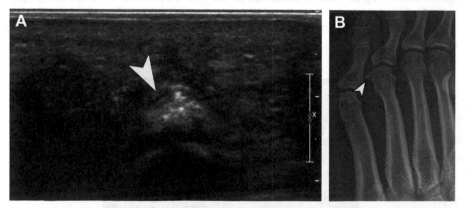

Fig. 6. *Calcific tendinopathy.* (*A*) Transverse US image at the level of metatarsal heads shows calcification (*arrowhead*) within the distal aspect of the dorsal interosseous tendon (*arrowhead*), which is confirmed by radiographic image (*B*) of the foot.

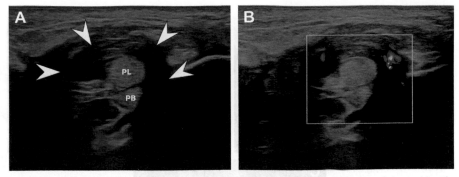

Fig. 7. *Tendinopathy on US.* (A) US transverse images of the lateral aspect of the ankle. Significant thickening and hypoechogenicity of the common tendon peroneal tendon sheath (*arrowheads*), surrounding the peroneus longus (PL) and Brevis (PB) tendons. (B) Transverse US image at the same point with Doppler shows increased blood flow at the tendon sheath, indicating acute inflammation.

plantar fascia is a fibrillar hyperechoic linear structure, usually with up to 4 mm thickness[8] (**Fig. 14**). Plantar fasciitis is a frequent cause of heel pain and it appears as a thickened and hypoechoic plantar fascia (**Fig. 15**).

PERIPHERAL NERVES IN THE FOOT AND ANKLE

Visualization of nerves at the foot and ankle may be difficult on MRI, as they have a similar appearance to adjacent vessels. On US, the usage of high-frequency probes

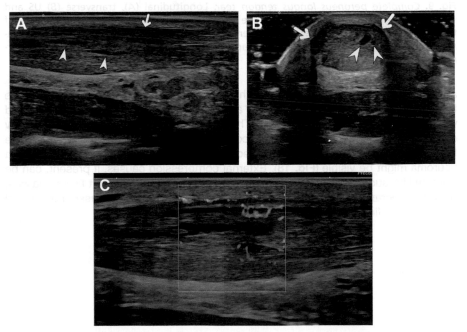

Fig. 8. *Achilles tendinopathy, partial tear and paratenonitis.* US longitudinal (A) and transverse (B) images of the Achilles tendon. Thickening and heterogenicity of the Achilles tendon with partial intrasubstance tears (*arrowheads*) and thickening of the paratenon (*arrows*), indicating paratenonitis. On power Doppler assessment (C), increased tendon and paratendon blood flow is depicted.

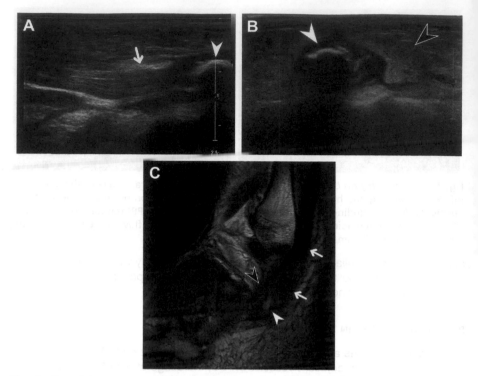

Fig. 9. *Complete peroneus longus tendon tear.* Longitudinal (*A*), transverse (*B*) US and sagittal T1-weightes MR (*C*) images of the lateral aspect of the ankle. Complete tear of the distal aspect of the peroneus longus tendon (*white arrows*) with an accessory *os peroneum* bone retracted proximally (*arrowheads*). Note the peroneus brevis tendon (*black arrowheads*) adjacent to the *os peroneum.*

allows high spatial resolution, making the nerves easier to identify and differentiate from adjacent vasculature. They appear as hypoechoic linear structures interspersed with hyperechoic linear lines (**Fig. 16**). The vessels are anechoic, and the blood flow can be seen on color Doppler US.[9] In compression neuropathies, the nerve can be focally or diffusely thickened and hypoechoic (**Fig. 17**). In traumatic nerve lesions, a neuroma might be visible (**Fig. 18**). External compression causes, if present, can be seen on US, such as muscle hernias, accessory muscles, cysts, soft tissue masses, bone protuberances, and scar tissue. However, in the majority of cases, no external cause is identified.[10]

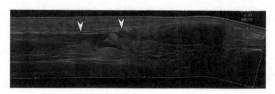

Fig. 10. *Complete Achilles tendon tear.* Longitudinal panoramic US image of the posterior aspect of the ankle shows a complete rupture of the middle third of the Achilles tendon with a gap between the tendon stumps (*arrowheads*). Note the tendinopathy (thickening and hypoechogenicity) of the distal aspect of the Achilles.

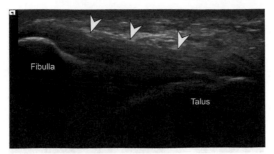

Fig. 11. *Partial tear of the anterior talofibular ligament.* Transverse US image of the anterolateral aspect of the ankle showing ATFL thickening, hypoechogenicity and loss of fibrillar pattern (*arrowheads*), corresponding to a partial tear.

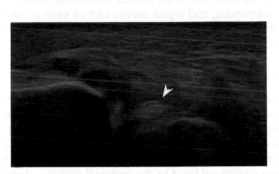

Fig. 12. *Complete tear of the anterior talofibular ligament.* Transverse US image of the anterolateral aspect of the ankle. Complete tear of the ATFL, with distal retraction of ligament fibers (*arrowhead*).

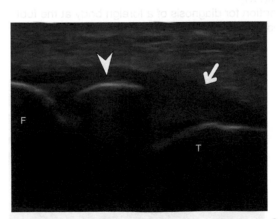

Fig. 13. *Anterior talofibular ligament avulsion.* Transverse US image of the anterolateral aspect of the ankle shows avulsed ATFL, with a bone fragment (*arrowhead*) detached to distal fibula and connected to the distal ATFL (*arrow*).

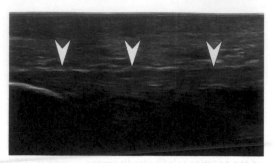

Fig. 14. *Normal plantar fascia.* Longitudinal US image of the plantar fascia (*arrowheads*) shows a fibrillar linear structure arising from the calcaneal tuberosity.

Superficial and deep peroneal, tibial, medial, and lateral plantar, medial and inferior calcaneal, sural, saphenous, and digital nerves can be seen on high-resolution US.[11]

Morton neuroma is also visualized by dorsal probe placement with web space compression[9] (**Fig. 19**).

METATARSALGIA

Pain in the metatarsal region is a common problem and is caused by many different structures. High-resolution US can diagnose most causes, including adventitial and intermetatarsal bursitis, Morton's neuroma, metatarsophalangeal synovitis, plantar plate injury, tendon disorders, venous thrombosis, and soft tissue masses.

The plantar plate is visualized in the longitudinal plane by a thin hyperechoic band extending from the metatarsal head to the proximal phalanx, deep to the flexor tendons.[12] US evaluation of plantar plate tears is comparable to MRI in terms of sensitivity and appears as focal or complete discontinuity, thickening and loss of normal hyperechoic homogeneous aspects[13] (**Fig. 20**). They typically occur at the distal insertion onto the proximal phalanx. This is frequently associated with metatarsophalangeal joint effusion and tendinosis of the dorsal interosseous tendons.[14]

Metatarsal stress fractures can also be seen on US, with periosteal thickening and hemorrhage[14] (**Fig. 21**).

US is also an option for diagnosis of a foreign body at the foot. Not all of them are radio-opaque and may be clearly seen on US (**Fig. 22**).

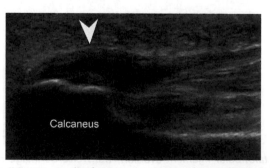

Fig. 15. *Plantar fasciitis.* Longitudinal US image of the plantar fascia (*arrowhead*) depicts thickening and hypoechogenic proximal plantar fascia, corresponding to plantar fasciitis.

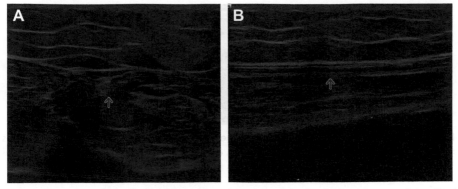

Fig. 16. *Normal peripheral nerve.* Transverse (*A*) and longitudinal (*B*) US image of the distal leg with normal morphology of the superficial peroneal nerve (*arrow*).

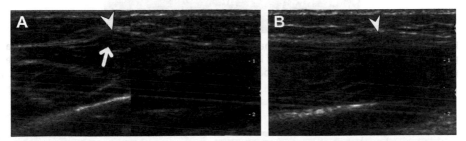

Fig. 17. *Compressive neuropathy.* Longitudinal US image (*A*) of the distal leg shows a small anterior tibial muscle herniation (*arrowhead*) and compression of the superficial peroneal neuropathy (*arrowheads*). (*B*) US image of the superficial peroneal neuropathy shows focal thickening and hypoeecgicity

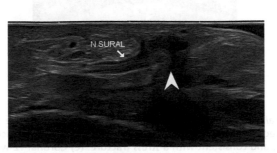

Fig. 18. *Traumatic US image.* US longitudinal image of the foot shows a complete sural nerve transection with a small stump neuroma (*arrowheads*).

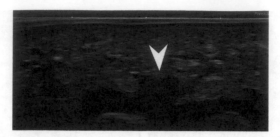

Fig. 19. *Morton neuroma.* US transverse image at the level of distal intermetatarsal spaces shows a neuroma at the plantar aspect of foot, at the space between second and third metatarsals (*arrowheads*).

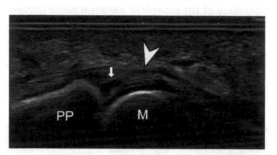

Fig. 20. *Plantar plate injury.* Longitudinal US image of the metatarsophalangeal joint with a partial intrasubstance tear at the distal insertion of the plantar plate (*arrow*). Note that the proximal plate has normal striated appearance.

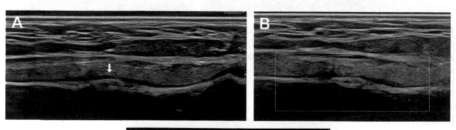

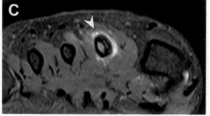

Fig. 21. *Metatarsal stress fracture.* (*A*) Longitudinal US image of the second metatarsal shows cortical irregularities and periosteal thickening (*arrow*) with increased blood flow on US Doppler (*B*) and consistent with a stress fracture. (*C*) Coronal T2-weighted MR image of the forefoot confirms diagnosis, showing increased bone marrow and periosteal edema (*arrowhead*).

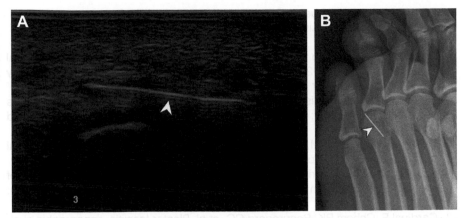

Fig. 22. *Foreign body.* (*A*) Longitudinal US image of the plantar aspect of the forefoot. There is a linear soft tissue foreign body (*arrowhead*) adjacent to the metatarsophalangeal joint. (*B*) Foot x-ray was done to confirm the presence of the foreign body (needle).

SUMMARY

High-resolution US is an excellent imaging modality for the evaluation of tendons, ligaments, and nerves in the ankle and is a useful alternative to MRI. The major advantages of US are wide availability, lower cost, and the possibility of dynamic evaluation and contralateral side comparison.

CLINICS CARE POINTS

- Is high-resoltion ultrasound indicated for peripheral neuropathy of the foot? Yes, based on our experience and in the literature, US evaluation of peripheral nerves in the foot can provide images with higher spatial resolution, compared to MRI.
- Can US detect metatarsal stress fractures: US is an useful alternative tool to x-ray and MRI for detection of metatarsal stress fractures > It might show periosteal thickening and hemorrhage at the fracture site.
- Is US indicated for evaluation of foreign bodies? Based on our experience, US is an option for detection of foreign bodies not visible on plain radiographs.
- What are the advantages and disadvantages of high-resoltion US of the foot compared to MRI? US is more available, has a lower cost and the possibility of dynamic evaluation and comparison with contralateral side. It is less useful for detection of associated injuries in the bone and cartilage and is user-dependant.

DISCLOSURE

The authors have nothing to disclose.

REFERENCES

1. Ihnatsenka B, Boezaart AP. Ultrasound: Basic understanding and learning the language. Int J Shoulder Surg 2010;4(3):55–62.
2. Fessell DP, van Holsbeeck M. Ultrasound of the Foot and Ankle. Semin Musculoskelet Radiol 1998;2(3):271–82.

3. Fessell DP, Vanderschueren GM, Jacobson JA, et al. US of the ankle: technique, anatomy, and diagnosis of pathologic conditions. Radiographics 1998;18(2): 325–40.
4. Sconfienza LM, Albano D, Allen G, et al. Clinical indications for musculoskeletal ultrasound updated in 2017 by European Society of Musculoskeletal Radiology (ESSR) consensus. Eur Radiol 2018;28(12):5338–51.
5. Hall MM, Allen GM, Allison S, et al. Recommended musculoskeletal and sports ultrasound terminology: a Delphi-based consensus statement. Br J Sports Med 2022;56(6):310–9.
6. Drakonaki EE, Allen GM, Wilson DJ. Ultrasound elastography for musculoskeletal applications. Br J Radiol 2012;85(1019):1435–45.
7. Sconfienza LM, Silvestri E, Cimmino MA. Sonoelastography in the evaluation of painful Achilles tendon in amateur athletes. Clin Exp Rheumatol 2010;28(3): 373–8.
8. Cardinal E, Chhem RK, Beauregard CG, et al. Plantar fasciitis: sonographic evaluation. Radiology 1996;201(1):257–9.
9. De Maeseneer M, Madani H, Lenchik L, et al. Normal Anatomy and Compression Areas of Nerves of the Foot and Ankle: US and MR Imaging with Anatomic Correlation. Radiographics 2015;35(5):1469–82.
10. Donovan A, Rosenberg ZS, Cavalcanti CF. MR imaging of entrapment neuropathies of the lower extremity. Part 2. The knee, leg, ankle, and foot. Radiographics 2010;30(4):1001–19.
11. Delfaut EM, Demondion X, Bieganski A, et al. Imaging of foot and ankle nerve entrapment syndromes: from well-demonstrated to unfamiliar sites. Radiographics 2003;23(3):613–23.
12. Gregg J, Marks P. Metatarsalgia: an ultrasound perspective. Australas Radiol 2007;51(6):493–9.
13. Carlson RM, Dux K, Stuck RM. Ultrasound imaging for diagnosis of plantar plate ruptures of the lesser metatarsophalangeal joints: a retrospective case series. J Foot Ankle Surg 2013;52(6):786–8.
14. Gregg JM, Schneider T, Marks P. MR imaging and ultrasound of metatarsalgia– the lesser metatarsals. Radiol Clin North Am 2008;46(6):1061–78, vi-vii.

Moving?

Make sure your subscription moves with you!

To notify us of your new address, find your **Clinics Account Number** (located on your mailing label above your name), and contact customer service at:

Email: journalscustomerservice-usa@elsevier.com

800-654-2452 (subscribers in the U.S. & Canada)
314-447-8871 (subscribers outside of the U.S. & Canada)

Fax number: 314-447-8029

Elsevier Health Sciences Division
Subscription Customer Service
3251 Riverport Lane
Maryland Heights, MO 63043

*To ensure uninterrupted delivery of your subscription, please notify us at least 4 weeks in advance of move.